Calcific Aortic Valve Disease

Calcific Aortic Valve Disease

Edited by **Samuel Ostroff**

hayle
medical

New York

Published by Hayle Medical,
30 West, 37th Street, Suite 612,
New York, NY 10018, USA
www.haylemedical.com

Calcific Aortic Valve Disease
Edited by Samuel Ostroff

International Standard Book Number: 978-1-63241-072-6 (Hardback)

Printed in the United States of America.

Contents

Preface

Calcific aortic valve disease (CAVD) has become the most widespread cardiac valve disease in the economically advanced nations. Population ageing is one of the major reasons for this increasing rate. There is no definite treatment which may slow down the disease progression; valve replacement is the only adequate treatment. This book encompasses the understandable fundamental biology of cardiac valve and procedures of CAVD. It also discusses genetics, proteomics and metabolism of CAVD, depicts novel methods in valve tissue engineering and regenerative medicines. This book will facilitate people to know about CAVD and other aspects concerning valve biology. It also emphasizes on the prospective chances of curbing the disease from rising in future.

This book is a result of research of several months to collate the most relevant data in the field.

When I was approached with the idea of this book and the proposal to edit it, I was overwhelmed. It gave me an opportunity to reach out to all those who share a common interest with me in this field. I had 3 main parameters for editing this text:

1. Accuracy – The data and information provided in this book should be up-to-date and valuable to the readers.

2. Structure – The data must be presented in a structured format for easy understanding and better grasping of the readers.

3. Universal Approach – This book not only targets students but also experts and innovators in the field, thus my aim was to present topics which are of use to all.

Thus, it took me a couple of months to finish the editing of this book.

I would like to make a special mention of my publisher who considered me worthy of this opportunity and also supported me throughout the editing process. I would also like to thank the editing team at the back-end who extended their help whenever required.

Editor

Biology and Function of Normal Aortic Valve

Anatomy and Function of Normal Aortic Valvular Complex

Ioan Tilea, Horatiu Suciu, Brindusa Tilea,
Cristina Maria Tatar, Mihaela Ispas and
Razvan Constantin Serban

Additional information is available at the end of the chapter

1. Introduction

Recently, the interest in the anatomy of the normal aortic valve complex has augmented, mostly because of the increasing use of conservative surgical techniques for repairing or re-placing cardiac valves. The knowledge of the anatomy also has important implications in the manufacture of prostheses that must conform to this anatomical configuration.

1.1. Historical perspective

The earliest documented interest in the anatomy of the aortic valvular complex stems from the Renaissance, with the description and drawings by Leonardo da Vinci. [1]

Leonardo da Vinci had an almost perfect understanding of the physiology of the human heart. But he had no inkling of the circulation of the blood, and the existence of one-way valves was incompatible with the ancient belief that the heart simply churned blood in and out of the ventricles, thus generating heat and 'vital spirit'. Unable to reconcile what he had observed with what he believed to be true, Leonardo reached an impasse. He became trap-ped in describing the motion of the blood through the valves in even more detail. And there, it seems, his anatomical work came to an end. [2]

The next anatomist to study the aortic valve was Andreas Vesalius. Then, for almost 400 years the study of the human heart was very sporadic and limited.

The 19th century brought in the era of anatomic dissection and the knowledge on the aortic valve grew wider. Henle was the first to introduce the term "arterial root". During the first half of the 20th century the rise in autopsy rates in Europe and North America facilitated the study of cardiac anatomy. [3]

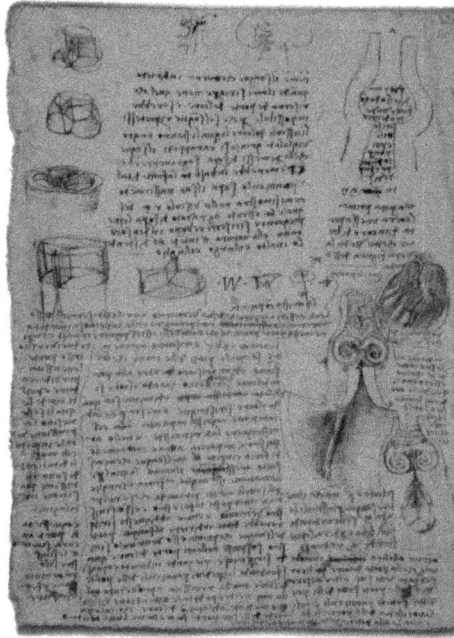

Figure 1. Leonardo da Vinci - The aortic valve, from the Royal Collection © Her Majesty Queen Elizabeth II - http:// www.royalcollection.org.uk/collection/919082/the-aortic-valve

Nowadays the need to understand the anatomy of the aortic valve is crucial, therefore the books and articles devoted to this topic are numerous.

1.2. Definitions

There is still no consensus on the best way to describe the anatomy of the aortic root [4].

The term "aortic root" refers to the aortic valve from its position at the left ventricular outlet to its junction with the ascending portion of the aorta. [5] It is the direct continuation of the left ventricular outflow tract.

Aorto-ventricular junction refers to the junction between the left ventricular structures and the aortic valvular sinuses, this representing the anatomic junction, or the semilunar lines of attachment of the arterial valvular leaflets, this locus representing the haemodynamic ventriculo-arterial junction [4].

Annulus is conventionally described as the virtual ring, formed by joining the basal attachment points of the leaflets within the left ventricle.

Nodule of Arantius is the small fibrous mound that forms at the center of each leaflet when the closing edge meets the free edge.

Between the free and closing edges, to each side of the nodule are two crescent-shaped areas known as the lunulae, which represent the sites of cusp apposition during valve closure. [6]

1.3. Embryology

The development of the aortic valve complex is extremely complicated and not yet fully understood.

The heart begins as a single tube that separates into two tubes and begins to twist rightward onto itself, called "d" looping.

Cells from the primary cardiac crescent, formed bilaterally within the embryonic disc, migrate into the cervical region of the developing embryo to form the primary heart tube. With further growth, cells from a second cardiogenic area, located posterior to the dorsal wall of the developing pericardial cavity, migrate into the cardiac region. The cells from this secondary heart field populate the outflow tract and the aortic arches. [7]

The heart tube is composed of an outer layer of myocardium and an inner lining of endocardial cells, separated by an extensive extracellular matrix referred to as the cardiac jelly. After rightward looping of the heart, the cardiac jelly overlying the future atrioventricular canal and outflow tract expands into swellings known as cardiac cushions. [8]

Subsequent to looping, the outflow tract possesses a characteristic dog-leg bend which divides the outflow tract into proximal and distal portions.

The cushions contained within the myocardial wall go through significant changes. In addition to the cushions that have fused to separate the proximal outflow tract into prospective aortic and pulmonary components, two further intercalated cushions have grown in the opposite quadrants of the common outflow tract. Formation of cavities in the fused distal parts of the proximal cushions, along with similar cavitation in the intercalated cushions, now produces the primordiums of the arterial valvular leaflets and sinuses. These structures, therefore, are formed in the most distal part of the proximal outflow tract, immediately upstream relative to the developing sinotubular junction. The cavitation of the cushions leaves the central luminal part of each cushion to form the arterial valvular leaflets, with the peripheral part arterialising to form the wall of the supporting valvular sinuses. The rightward and inferior of the intercalated cushions forms one sinus of the aortic valve, while the opposite leftward and superior intercalated cushion forms the non-adjacent sinus of the pulmonary valve. The adjacent sinuses and valvular leaflets, in contrast, are excavated from the fused distal parts of the proximal cushions, with each of the two fused cushions forming one sinus and leaflet of the aortic valve, together with the adjacent sinus and leaflet of the pulmonary valve. [7]

The definitive fetal cardiac structure is developed by 8 weeks.

2. Histological structure

Function of normal heart valves is based on their properties of ensuring unidirectional blood flow without regurgitation. They open and close 40 million times a year and 3 billion times over a lifetime. This property depends on the mobility, pliability, and structural integrity of their leaflets. The competency of the aortic valvular complex depends on the stretching and molding of its 3 cusps to fill the orifice during the closed phase of the cardiac cycle. [9]

2.1. Dynamic relations between the aortic valvular complex and its histological structure

The substantial changes in size and shape of the valve cusps and leaflets that occur during the cardiac cycle are facilitated by a highly complex internal microarchitecture. The layered structure of the aortic valve is formed by: a dense collagenous layer close to the outflow surface, which provides the primary strength component, a central core of loose connective tissue, and an elastin layer below the inflow surface. The essential functional components of the heart valves comprises the valvular endothelial cells (VECs), the valvular interstitial cells (VICs), and extracellular matrix (ECM), including collagen, elastin and glycosaminoglycans. [9]

The major component of valve cusps is collagen, 43% to 55% (predominantly type I but also some type III) [10] and 11% elastin. The quantity, quality, and architecture of the valvular ECM, particularly collagen, elastin, and glycosaminoglycans, are the major determinants of not only the cyclical functional mechanics over the second-to-second periodicity of the cardiac cycle, but also the lifetime durability of a valve. The cells of the heart valves through complex cell-ECM interactions, transduce forces into molecular changes that mediate normal valve function and pathobiology. Through such mechanisms, healthy heart valves are able to maintain homeostasis, adapt to an altered stress state, and repair injury via connective tissue remodeling mediated by the synthesis, repair, and remodeling of the several ECM components. [9]

The most abundant cell type in the aortic valve are VICs. They are distributed throughout all of its layers, are crucial for valvular function [11] and synthesize the ECM. VICs mediate matrix remodeling and continuously repair functional damage to collagen and the other ECM components. As a response to injury VICs may translate from one phenotypic state to another during valvular homeostasis. The 5 distinct VIC phenotypes include embryonic progenitor endothelial/mesenchymal cells (eVICs), quiescent VICs (qVICs), activated VICs (aVICs), postdevelopmental/adult progenitor VICs (pVICs), and osteoblastic VICs (ob-VICs). [12] Adult heart valve VICs have characteristics of resting fibroblasts, are quiescent, without synthetic or destructive activity for extracellular matrix. They are activated by abrupt changes in the mechanical stress during intrauterine maturation. Once activated VICs can differentiate into a variety of other cell types, including myofibroblasts and osteoblasts. [11]

The blood-contacting surfaces of the aortic valve are lined by endothelial cells. VECs resemble to endothelial cells but evidence is increasing that VECs are phenotypically different from vascular endothelial cells elsewhere in the circulation, which is consistent with the increasing recognition of more widespread endothelial heterogeneity across circulatory sites,

[13] and the possibility that VECs may interact with VICs to maintain the integrity of valve tissues. [14] Evidence indicates that different transcriptional profiles are expressed by VECs on the opposite faces of a normal adult pig aortic valve and these may contribute to localization of early pathological aortic valve calcification [15]. Abnormal hemodynamic forces can cause tissue remodeling and inflammation which may lead to aortic valve diseases. [11]

2.2. Normal aortic valve development

An understanding of valve architecture and cellular changes that occur in cardiac valves during fetal development, maturation, and aging would provide mechanistic insights into the pathogenesis of congenital and acquired valve abnormalities and aid assessment of therapeutic strategies for valve disease. A study which performed quantitative histological assessment of 91 human semilunar valves obtained from second and third trimester fetus, neonates, children and normal adults found very interesting results. [16]

Valves must accommodate to substantial hemodynamic changes throughout lifetime. Large populations of VICs undergo phenotypic modulation to become activated myofibroblasts and return to quiescent fibroblasts during adaptive remodeling in response to changing environmental conditions. [17-19] VICs and VECs functions likely influence ECM synthesis and remodeling. Fetal valves possess a dynamic/adaptive structure and contain cells with an activated/immature phenotype. During postnatal life, activated cells gradually become quiescent, whereas collagen matures through increased fiber thickness and alignment. Fetal second-trimester semilunar (aortic and pulmonary) valves lack distinguishable layers, are composed primarily of proteoglycans, have no detectable elastin, small amounts of disorganized collagen, and are histologically identical. [20] Fetal valves structure differs, even late in gestation, from that of adult valves, which have a trilayered architecture with a highly specialized and functionally adapted ECM. The study demonstrated that fetal valves have much higher cellular densities than adult valves, associated with an increased cell proliferation-to-apoptosis ratio. VICs density was highest in the second trimester and decreased progressively throughout gestation and postnatally. Fetal VICs proliferation indices were likewise greater than those of adult valves. Valvular cell turnover is high during fetal development and continues at a low rate postnatally. [16]

They also demonstrated physiological activation of endothelial cells that consistently expressed high levels of SMemb, MMP-1, MMP-13, ICAM-1, and VCAM-1 in fetal and children's valves in contrast to adult valves. Valvular cells that are activated in utero undergo phenotypic changes at birth and gradually become quiescent, whereas collagen matures through increased fiber thickness and alignment. This suggests a progressive adaptation to the prevailing hemodynamic environment. [16]

3. Structure and anatomy of the aortic root

The aortic valve is the cardiac centerpiece and forms the bridge between the left ventricle and the ascending aorta. Its components are the sinuses of Valsalva, the fibrous interleaflet triangles, and the valvular leaflets themselves. [1]

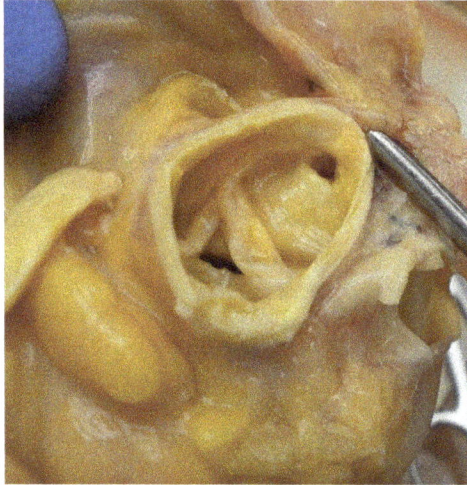

Figure 2. View of a dissected heart (the atrial chambers and the arterial trunks are removed). The heart is photographed from above. [4]

3.1. The "Annulus" controversy

When defined literally "annulus" refers to a little ring. The aortic root contains at least 3 circular rings and 1 crown-like ring. [21] The valvular leaflets are attached throughout the length of the root. Therefore, seen in 3 dimensions, the leaflets take the form of a 3-pronged coronet, with the hinges from the supporting ventricular structures forming the crown-like ring (Figure 1). The base of the crown is a virtual ring, commonly known as "annulus". This plane represents the inlet from the left ventricular outflow tract into the aortic root and is the diameter that is typically analysed by the echocardiographer when providing measurements of the diameter of the annulus.

The controversy arises from the fact that on one hand there are multiple rings described and on the other hand, the term "annulus" appears to describe a circle, a fibrous ring on which the leaflets are inserted, but such a structure does not exist in the anatomy of the aortic valve. No consensus has been found yet.

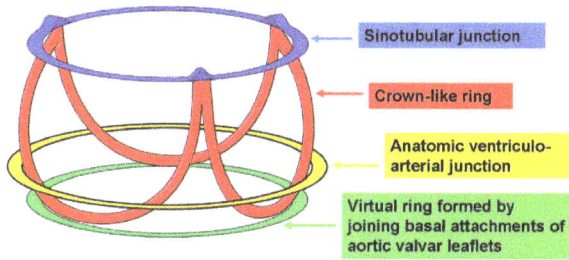

Figure 3. The "rings" of the aortic root [1]

3.2. Anatomic versus hemodynamic ventriculo-arterial junction

As we have shown in figure 3, there is a marked discrepancy between the circular anatomic junction and the semilunar hemodynamic junction. [22] The hemodynamic junction separates the root into those compartments exposed to aortic as opposed to left ventricular pressures. By virtue of the semilunar attachments of the leaflets, portions of the fibrous aortic root are exposed to ventricular pressures, these being the superior portions of the interleaflet triangles, whereas portions of the left ventricle are exposed to aortic pressures, these being the most basal portions within the sinus of Valsalva. [1]

3.3. Aortic sinuses, location of the coronary arteries and sinotubular junction

The spaces between the luminal surface of the three bulges on the aortic root and their respective valvular leaflets are known as the aortic sinuses of Valsalva. [5] The sinuses are named according to the arteries arising from within them (right, left, and noncoronary). The right sinus structures have the greatest dimensions followed by the non coronary sinus, and finally the left coronary sinus. [23]

Distance between the ostium and Valsalva's sinus		Sex	
		Male	Female
Left commissure	left coronary	9.7	9.3
	right coronary	11.2	10.7
Right commissure	left coronary	10.9	10.8
	right coronary	11.3	9.9
Bottom of the Valsalva's sinus	left coronary	13.4	13.0
	right coronary	15.0	13.8

Table 1. Mean values of the distances of the ostium and its relation to the corresponding Valsalva's sinus (in mm) in both sexes (adapted from [24])

In the majority of cases, the orifices of the coronary arteries arise within the 2 anterior sinuses of Valsalva, usually positioned just below the sinotubular junction, but are rarely cen-
trally located. It is not unusual, however, for the arteries to be positioned superior relative to
the sinotubular junction. Accessory coronary arterial orifices are found in the majority of the
anterior aortic sinuses. [25]

Several studies emphasize on the importance of large variations of coronary ostia origins.
Also, there are significant differences between in vivo and ex vivo measurements regarding
the right coronary ostium. [26,27]

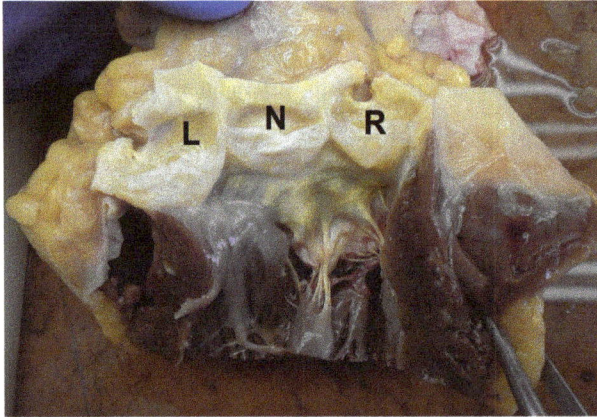

Figure 4. Left (L) and right (R) aortic sinuses that give origin to the main coronary arteries and the non-coronary (N) sinus. [5]

The superior border of the sinuses is the sinotubular junction (also known as the supra-aort-
ic ridge). On the outside, the sinotubular junction is where the tubular portion of the aorta
joins onto the sinusal portion. Inside, there is usually a slightly raised ridge of thickened
aortic wall. But the sinotubular junction is not perfectly circular. It takes on the contour of
the three sinuses, giving it a mildly trefoil or scalloped outline. [5]

A comparison between the circumferences measured at the level of the sinotubular junction
and at the level of the aortic root base shows that the circumference of the sinotubular junction is 95% of the circumference measured at the aortic root base. [23]

3.4. Aortic valvular leaflets

The normal aortic valve has three leaflets. Each of the three leaflets has a free margin and a margin where it is attached in semilunar fashion to the aortic root. The maximal height of each leaflet is considerably less than that of its sinus on account of its scoop-shaped free margin. When
the valve opens, the leaflets fall back into their sinuses without the potential of occluding any
coronary orifice. The semilunar hingelines of adjacent leaflets meet at the level of the sinotubu-

lar junction, forming the commissures. The body of the leaflets are pliable and thin in the young, although its thickness is not uniform. With age, the leaflets become thicker and stiffer.

Each leaflet has a somewhat crimped surface facing the aorta and a smoother surface facing the ventricle. The leaflet is slightly thicker towards its free margin. On its ventricular surface is the zone of apposition, known as the lunulae, occupying the full width along the free margin and spanning approximately one-third of the depth of the leaflet. This is where the leaflet meets the adjacent leaflets during valvular closure. At the midportion of the lunulae, the ventricular surface is thickened to form the nodule of Arantius that extends along 60% of the inferior margin of the lunulae. When the valve is in closed position, the inferior margin of the lunulaes meet together, separating blood in the left ventricular cavity from blood in the aorta. Fenestrations in the lunulaes are common, especially in the elderly, but the valve remains competent because they are above the closure line. [5]

The leaflets have a core of fibrous tissue, with endothelial linings on their arterial and ventricular aspects. Their origin from the supporting left ventricular structures, where the ventricular components give rise to the fibroelastic walls of the aortic valvular sinuses, marks the anatomic ventriculo-arterial junction. Significantly, in those areas where the leaflets arise from the ventricular myocardium, their basal attachments are well below the level of the anatomic ventriculo-arterial junction. [1]

Leaflet	Measure	Sex	
		Male	Female
Left coronary	Leaflet height	15.2	14.9
	Lunulae width	4.6	4.3
	Lunulae length	30.7	29.3
	External intercommissural distance	25.4	23.5
	Internal Intercommissural distance	20.0	18.5
Right coronary	Leaflet height	15.2	14.5
	Lunulae width	4.4	4.2
	Lunulae length	30.4	27.9
	External intercommissural distance	24.5	23.8
	Internal Intercommissural distance	19.2	18.7
Noncoronary	Leaflet height	15.0	14.6
	Lunulae width	4.3	4.2
	Lunulae length	30.3	28.2
	External intercommissural distance	24.4	22.1
	Internal Intercommissural distance	20.1	19.1

Table 2. Mean values of the height of the leaflets and size of the lunulae (width and length) and internal intercommissural distances in mm in both sexes (adapted from [24])

Variations exist among individuals in the dimensions of the root, but in the same individual, there can be marked variations in all aspects of the dimensions of the individual leaflets, including the height, width, surface area and volume of each of the supporting sinuses of Valsalva. [28, 29, 30] A study of 200 normal hearts revealed that the average width, measured between the peripheral zones of attachment along the sinus ridge, for the right, the noncoronary, and the left coronary leaflets was 25.9, 25.5, and 25.0 mm, respectively. [28]

3.5. Interleaflet fibrous triangles

As a result of the semilunar attachment of the aortic valvular leaflets, there are 3 triangular extensions of the left ventricular outflow tract that reach to the level of the sinotubular junction. [31] These triangles, however, are formed not of ventricular myocardium but of the thinned fibrous walls of the aorta between the expanded sinuses of Valsalva. Their most apical regions represent areas of potential communication with the pericardial space or, in the case of the triangle between the right and left coronary aortic leaflets, with the plane of tissue interposed between the aorta and anteriorly located sleeve-like subpulmonary infundibulum. [1]

The triangles are thinner and less collagenous than the hingelines or the sinusal walls. These areas are potential sites of aneurysmal formation. [32]

3.6. The relationships of the aortic root

The aortic root is positioned to the right and posterior relative to the subpulmonary infundibulum. The leaflets of the aortic valve are attached only in part to the muscular walls of the left ventricle, since so as to fit the orifices of both aortic and mitral valves within the circular profile of the left ventricle, there is no muscle between them in the ventricular roof. The aortic root, furthermore, is wedged between the orifices of the two atrioventricular valves. The root is related to all four cardiac chambers. [4]

The plane of the aortic valve tilts inferiorly at an angle to the pulmonary valve. The nadirs of the aortic sinuses lie in a plane at an angle of 30º from the horizontal. [32] Thus, the arterial surface of the closed leaflets of the aortic valve is directed not only upwards but also rightward at an angle of at least 45º to the median plane. [33]

3.6.1. Relationship between the left ventricular outflow tract and the aortic root

The left ventricular outflow tract is composed of a muscular component and a more extensive fibrous component. The orientation of the outflow tract is known to change with aging. In individuals aged under 20 years, the angle varies between 135 and 180 degrees and the left ventricular outflow tract represents a more direct and straight extension into the aortic root. In hearts from individuals aged over 60 years, the angle varies between 90 and 120 degrees and the left ventricular outflow tract may not extend in straight fashion into the aortic root but rather in a rightward "dog leg". [1]

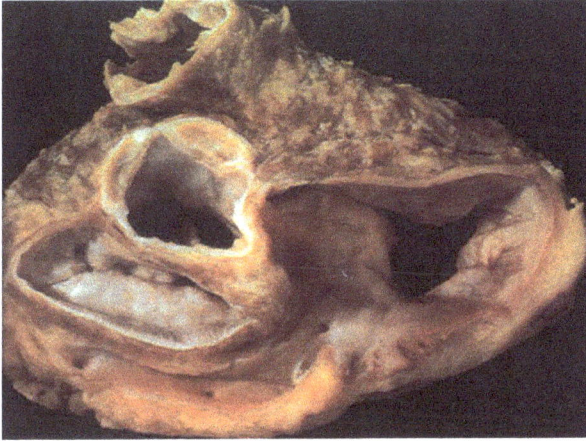

Figure 5. A dissected atrioventricular junction viewed from above showing how the aortic valve wedges itself between the mitral and tricuspid valves (reproduced from http://www.rjmatthewsmd.com)

3.6.2. Interleaflet triangles and their relationship to the mitral valve and membranous septum

Guarding the left ventricular outflow tract, the aortic root also has an intimate relationship with the ventricular septum and the mitral valve. In attitudinal orientation, it is apparent that the aortic root leans rightward slightly, over the ventricular septum, to overly the right ventricle. In the elderly, the relationship between septal crest and aortic root changes to give a sigmoid-shaped ventricular septum. [4]

Relative to the aorta, the mitral valve is located posterior and to the left, the tricuspid valve is located inferiorly and to the right.

The ends of the area of fibrous continuity are thickened to form the left and right fibrous trigones. The interleaflet triangle between the noncoronary and left coronary leaflet is part of the area of fibrous continuity because the aortic-mitral curtain seen from within the left ventricular outflow tract represents the equivalent of the anterior mitral valvular annulus. The interleaflet triangle located between the right coronary and noncoronary aortic leaflets is confluent with the membranous septum. Together, the membranous septum and the right fibrous trigone form the central fibrous body of the heart. This is the area within the heart where the membranous septum, the atrioventricular valves and the aortic valve join in fibrous continuity. [1]

3.6.3. Relationship between the aortic valve and the conduction system

The atrioventricular node, located in the wall of the right atrium at the apex of the triangle of Koch, is relatively distant from the root. As the conduction axis, penetrates to the left, through the central fibrous body, however, it is positioned at the base of the interleaflet triangle between the non- and right coronary aortic sinuses. Having penetrated through the fibrous plane providing atrioventricular insulation, the bundle then branches on the crest of the muscular ventricular septum, the left bundle branch fanning out on the smooth left ventricular side, while the cord-like right bundle branch penetrates back through the muscular septum, emerging on the septal surface in the environment of the medial papillary muscle (figure 6). [4]

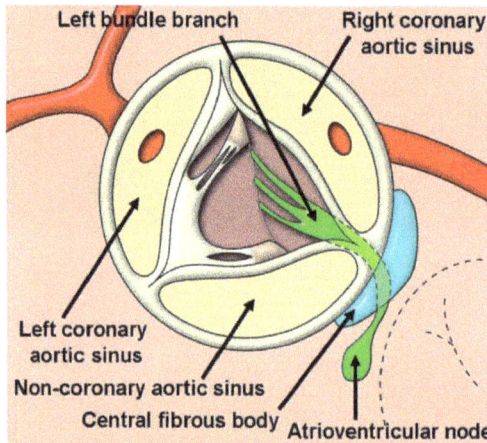

Figure 6. Aortic sinuses, coronary arteries and the the location of the atrioventricular conduction axis, as seen by looking down through the aortic root (schematic from [4])

4. Microscopic anatomy

The aortic valve is composed of different structures, each one with its own histological profile. The histology of the aortic root is characterized by a gradual shift from the primarily elastic aorta to the muscular ventricle. [31]

The annulus is a dense collagenous meshwork, in which elastic and collagenous fibrils and also neuronal structures are present. At the commissure level originate the collagen fibres of the intermediate layer, which are orientated in a radial fashion. Here, they do not only infiltrate the intima layer of the aortic root, but they also radiate into the media layer where they are anchored. The endothelial cells are separated by the basal layer from the elastic fibres and collagenous fibrils. The endothelial cells show microvilli at their surface, which increase the overall surface area for an increased exchange of substances.

The interleaflet triangles are different in their microscopic structure. The triangle between the left-coronary and non-coronary sinus forms part of the aortic–mitral valvular curtain, is histologically fibrous and equivalent to the mitral valve leaflet structure. The triangle between the non-coronary and the right-coronary aortic sinus is incorporated within the membranous part of the septum and is also made of fibrous tissue. In contrast, the triangle between the right-coronary and left-coronary sinus in the area of the subpulmonary infundibulum is supported by muscular tissue and only fibrous at its apex.

The sinuses are arranged with very different components, but the largest part of all the three sinuses is composed in a similar manner to the three layers of the aortic wall: tunica intima, tunica media and tunica externa (adventitia). The inner layer of the intima is composed of endothelial cells arranged in the direction of the vessel. The subendothelial connective tissue is arranged in the same manner as the endothelial cells. This layer is divided from the intima by the membrana elastica interna. The media is composed of circular arranged structures: smooth muscle cells, elastic fibres, collagen fibres type II and III and proteoglycans. The adventitia is the external layer. It is separated from the intima by the membrana elastica externa. Similar to the intima, the elements of the adventitia are arranged in a longitudinal fashion and composed of collagen fibres of type I. The sinotubular junction shows the same principal arrangement of tissue elements compared with the sinuses and the ascending aorta, but the diameter of the wall is thicker. [34]

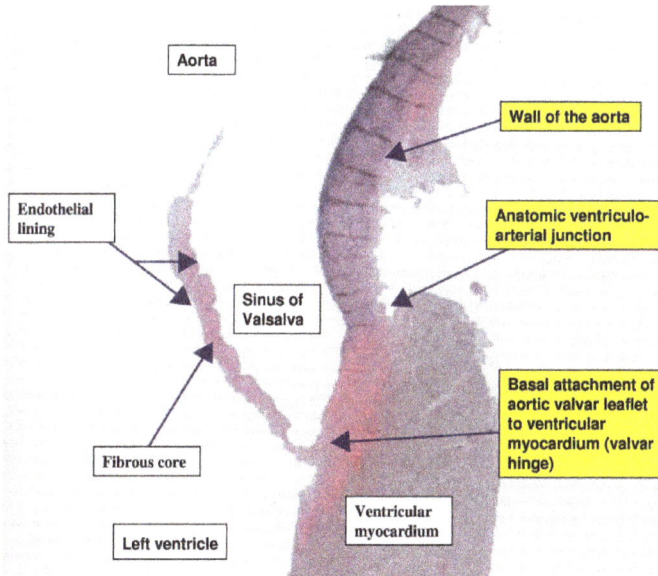

Figure 7. Histology of the aortic valvular complex [1]

The aortic valve leaflet is a three-layered structure (lamina ventricularis, lamina spongiosa and lamina fibrosa) composed of differing amounts of collagen, elastin, and glycosamino-glycans, that form a well-defined honeycomb or spongelike structure, suggesting that elastin forms a matrix that surrounds and links the collagen fiber bundles. [35] The leaflets are covered by a continuous layer of endothelial cells with a smooth surface on the ventricular side and numerous ridges on the arterial side. The arrangement of the endothelial cells is across, not in line with the direction of flow. [36]

5. Surgical anatomy

A thorough knowledge of the anatomy of the aortic valve and its relations to the surrounding cardiac structures is a prerequisite for the successful completion of the repair or replacement performed by the surgeon.

Surgical descriptions of the aortic root are not always similar with the anatomical descriptions, leading to a series of confusional data. Also the in vivo measurement of the valve components don't always correspond to the ex vivo measurements, in part due to the movement of the heart and its structures during the cardiac cycle.

By sequentially following the line of attachment of each leaflet, the relationship of the aortic valve to its surrounding structures can be clearly understood. Beginning posteriorly, the commissure between the noncoronary and left coronary leaflets is positioned along the area of aorto-mitral valvular continuity. The fibrous subaortic curtain is beneath this commissure. To the right of this commissure, the noncoronary leaflet is attached above the posterior diverticulum of the left ventricular outflow tract. Here the valve is related to the right atrial wall. As the attachment of the noncoronary leaflet ascends from its nadir toward the commissure between the noncoronary and right coronary leaflets, the line of attachment is directly above the portion of the atrial septum containing the atrioventricular node. The commissure between the noncoronary and right coronary leaflets is located directly above the penetrating atrioventricular bundle and the membranous ventricular septum. The attachment of the right coronary leaflet then descends across the central fibrous body before ascending to the commissure between the right and left coronary leaflets. Immediately beneath this commissure, the wall of the aorta forms the uppermost part of the subaortic outflow. An incision through this area passes into the space between the facing surfaces of the aorta and pulmonary trunk. As the facing left and right leaflets descend from this commissure, they are attached to the outlet muscular component of the left ventricle. Only a small part of this area in the normal heart is a true outlet septum, since both pulmonary and aortic valves are supported on their own sleeves of myocardium. Thus, although the outlet components of the right and left ventricle face each other, an incision below the aortic valve enters low into the infundibulum of the right ventricle. As the lateral part of the left coronary leaflet descends from the facing commissure to the base of the sinus, it becomes the only part of the aortic valve that is not intimately related to another cardiac chamber. [37]

6. Ecocardiographic anatomy

The ability to record high-quality echocardiographic images and obtain accurate Doppler flow recordings are essential determinants of the overall value of the echocardiographic examination. As such, echocardiography is highly operator dependent. It is difficult to overemphasize the critical role of the person who performs the imaging. To obtain a comprehensive and accurate echocardiogram, the echocardiographer must understand the anatomy and physiology of the aortic valve and have a thorough knowledge of the ultrasound equipment to optimize the quality of the recording. [38]

6.1. Transthoracic Echocardiography (TTE)

Anatomic evaluation of the aortic valve is based on a combination of short- and long-axis images to identify the number of leaflets, and to describe leaflet mobility, thickness, and calcification.

Two-dimensional imaging of the normal aortic valve in the parasternal long axis view demonstrates two leaflets (right and noncoronary), while the parasternal short axis demonstrates a symmetrical structure with three uniformly thin leaflets that open equally, forming a circular orifice during most of systole. During diastole, the normal leaflets form a three pointed star with a slight thickening or prominence at the central closing point formed by the aortic leaflet nodules, known as the nodules of Arantius. The three aortic valve leaflets may also be visualized in a subcostal view.

The aortic valve leaflets appear thin and delicate and may be difficult to visualize. In the long-axis view, the leaflets open rapidly in systole and appear as linear parallel lines close to the walls of the aorta. With the onset of diastole, they come together and are recorded as a faint linear density within the plane of the aortic annulus. Because the velocity of valve motion during opening and closing is high relative to the frame rate of most echocardiographic systems, the normal aortic valve is usually visualized either fully opened or closed but rarely in any intermediate position. In the basal short-axis view, the three aortic leaflets can be visualized within the annulus during diastole. The three lines of coaptation can be recorded, normally forming a Y (sometimes referred to as an inverted Mercedes-Benz sign). With the onset of systole, the leaflets open out of the imaging plane, providing a view of the aortic annulus. The short-axis perspective is most helpful to determine the number of leaflets and whether fusion of one or more commissures is present. In patients who are difficult to image, normal leaflets are so delicate that they are hard to visualize, generally an indication that they are morphologically normal. [38]

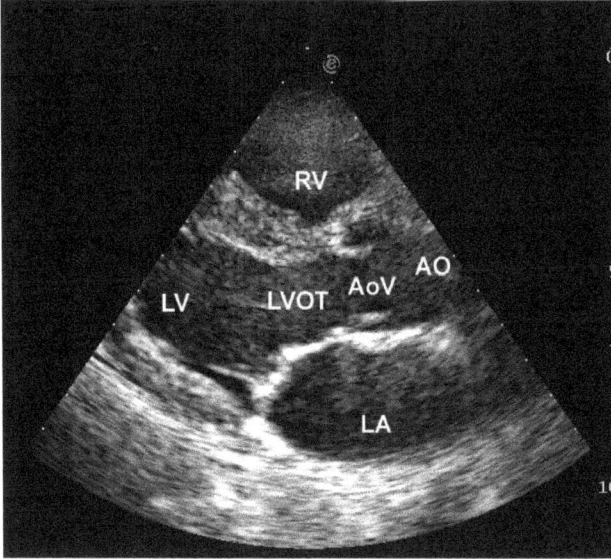

Figure 8. Transthoracic echocardiogram, parasternal long axis view. Aortic valve is open (author's collection).

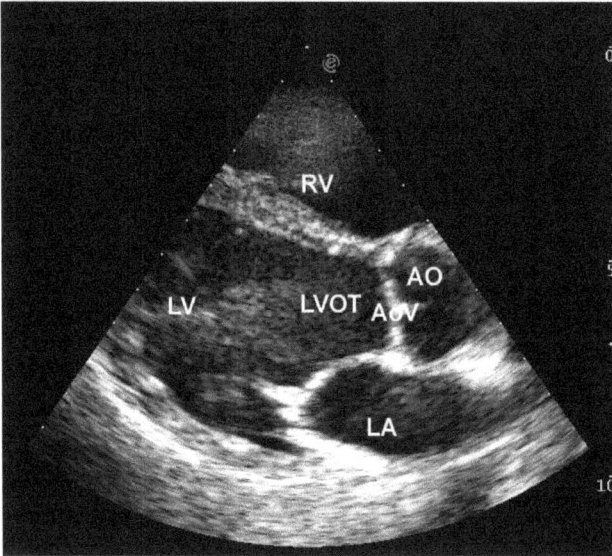

Figure 9. Transthoracic echocardiogram, parasternal long axis view. Aortic valve is closed (author's collection).

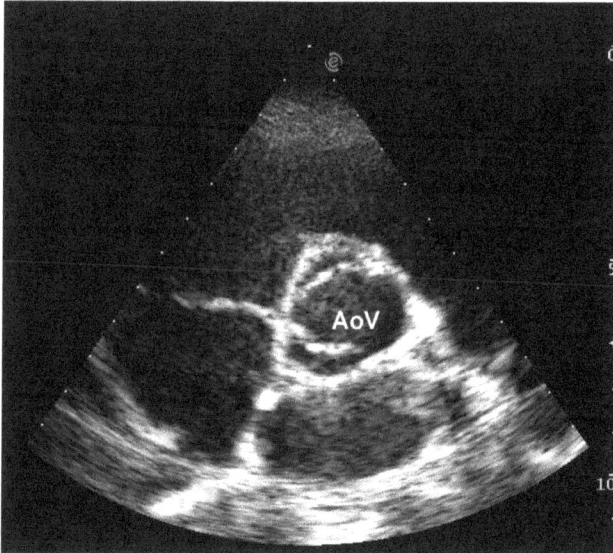

Figure 10. Transthoracic echocardiogram, suprasternal view. Aortic valve is open (author's collection).

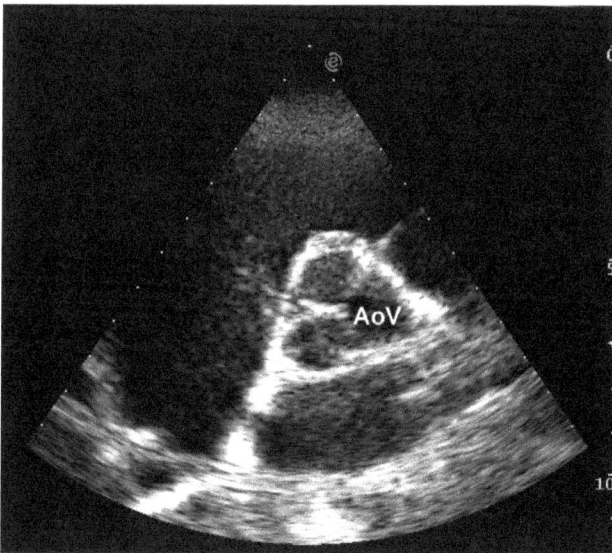

Figure 11. Transthoracic echocardiogram, suprasternal view. Aortic valve is closed (author's collection).

6.2. Transesophageal Echocardiography (TEE)

Transthoracic imaging usually is adequate, although TEE may be helpful when image quality is suboptimal.

To characterize the aortic valve using TEE, the valve should be imaged in short-axis view (the aortic valve can generally be visualized in a plane between 30 to 60º from the transverse 0º) and long-axis view (typically at 120 to 160° from transverse 0º).

The short-axis view is the only view that provides a simultaneous image of all three leaflets. The leaflet adjacent to the atrial septum is the noncoronary leaflet, the most anterior is the right coronary leaflet, and the other is the left coronary leaflet. The probe is withdrawn or anteflexed slightly to move the imaging plane superiorly through the sinuses of Valsalva to bring the right and left coronary ostia and then the sinotubular junction into view. The probe is then advanced to move the imaging plane through and then proximal to the AV annulus to produce a short axis view of the left ventricular outflow tract. The mid esophageal short-axis view at the level of the leaflets is used to measure the length of the free edges of the leaflets and the area of the aortic valve orifice by planimetry.

In the long axis view, the left ventricular outflow tract appears toward the left of the display and the proximal ascending aorta toward the right. The leaflet that appears anteriorly or toward the bottom of the display is always the right coronary, but the leaflet that appears posteriorly in this cross-section may be the left or the noncoronary, depending on the exact location of the imaging plane as it passes through the valve. The mid esophageal long-axis view is the best cross-section for assessing the size of the aortic root by measuring the diameters of the annulus, sinuses of Valsalva, sinotubular junction and proximal ascending aorta, adjusting the probe to maximize the internal diameter of these structures. The diameter of the annulus is measured during systole at the points of attachment of the aortic valve leaflets to the annulus and is normally between 1.8 and 2.5 cm.

The deep transgastric view is obtained by advancing the probe deep into the stomach and positioning the probe adjacent to the left ventricular apex. The exact position of the probe and transducer is more difficult to determine and control deep in the stomach, but some trial and error flexing, turning, advancing, withdrawing, and rotating of the probe develops this view in most patients. In the deep transgastric long-axis view, the aortic valve is located in the far field at the bottom of the display with the left ventricular outflow tract directed away from the transducer. Detailed assessment of valve anatomy is difficult in this view because the left ventricular outflow tract and aortic valve are so far from the transducer, but Doppler quantification of flow velocities through these structures is usually possible. [39]

The TEE examination is also performed intraoperative to refine and confirm preoperative diagnosis, to assess the etiology and severity of aortic valve disease, to measure the annulus and to prepare the surgeon for other alternatives.

6.3. Three-Dimensional Echocardiography (3DE)

3DE represents a major innovation in cardiovascular ultrasound. Advancements in computer and transducer technologies permit real-time 3DE acquisition and presentation of cardiac structures from any spatial point of view.

A complete 3D TTE exam requires multiple acquisitions from the parasternal, apical, subcostal, and suprasternal transducer positions. Because the volume-rendered 3D data set can be cropped to display a variety of intracardiac structures by choosing different cut planes as an alternative to "view" (referred to heart's orientation to the body axis), "anatomic planes" (referred to the heart itself) can be used to describe image orientation. [40]

For the visualization of the aortic valve the 3DE TTE protocol is the parasternal long-axis view with and without color (narrow angle and zoomed acquisitions) and the 3DE TEE protocol is the 60º mid-esophageal, short-axis view with and without color (zoomed or full-volume acquisition) and the 120º mid-esophageal, long-axis view with and without color (zoomed or full-volume acquisition).

The common approaches for imaging the aortic valve by 3D TTE are from the parasternal and apical views. Three-dimensional data sets including the aortic root can be cropped and rotated for a dynamic 3D rendering of the aortic valve, which can be visualized from both the aortic and ventricular perspectives, as well as sliced in any desired longitudinal or oblique plane.

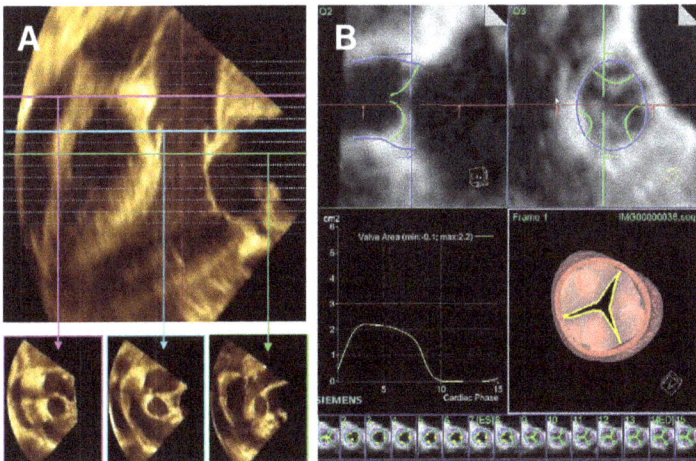

Figure 12. Three-dimensional TEE data set cropped to demonstrate the aorta in long axis (A, top). Using this image, in face views of the sinotubular junction (A, bottom left), sinus of Valsalva (A, bottom middle), and aortic annulus (A, bottom right) can be obtained for assessment. Dynamic, automatic tracking of the aortic valve leaflets (B, top left) and annulus (B, top right) can be performed, providing aortic valve area throughout the cardiac cycle (B, middle left and bottom strip). A model derived from the automated tracking is also produced (middle right). [41]

Real-Time 3D can be realized by obtaining a TEE 2D image of the aortic valve at either the 60º midesophageal, short-axis view or the 120º midesophageal, long-axis view. After the 2D image is optimized, narrow-angled acquisitions can be used to optimize the 3D image and to examine aortic valve and root anatomy. After acquisition, the aortic valve should be oriented with the right coronary cusp located inferiorly, regardless of whether the aortic or the left ventricular outflow tract perspective is presented.

Color Doppler 3D TEE imaging should also be performed to detect the initial appearance of flow at the onset of systole. [41]

7. Functional anatomy

The aortic root is a complex structure that requires analysis part by part but always remembering that all the parts contribute to form one functional unit, a three-dimensional structure adjoining distally to the aorta and proximally to the ventricle.

The aortic valve, like the pulmonary valve, has no tensor apparatus (i.e., chordae tendineae or papillary muscles). The commissures form tall, peaked spaces between the attachments of adjacent leaflets and attain the level of the aortic sinotubular junction, the ridge that separates the sinus and tubular portions of the ascending aorta. The functional aortic valve orifice can be at the sinotubular junction or proximal to it. [42]

The three half moon-shaped leaflets form pocket-like tissue flaps that are avascular. Just below the free edge of each leaflet is a ridgelike closing edge. At the center of each leaflet, the closing edge meets the free edge and forms the nodule of Arantius. Between the free and closing edges, to each side of the nodule are two crescent-shaped areas known as the lunulae, which represent the sites of leaflet apposition during valve closure. Lunular fenestrations, near the commissures are common and increase in size and incidence with age. [43] However, owing to their position distal to the closing edge, they rarely produce valvular incompetence. [42] When viewed from above, the linear distance along the closing edge of a leaflet is much greater than the straight-line distance between its two commissures. This extra length of leaflet tissue is necessary for nonstenotic opening and nonregurgitant closure of the valve. [6] Normally, the diameter of the aortic annulus at the hinge points of the aortic valve is about equal to the diameter of the ascending aorta at the sinotubular junction. [44] When the valve opens, the leaflets fall back into their sinuses without the potential of occluding any coronary orifice. The semilunar hingelines of adjacent leaflets meet at the level of the sinotubular junction, forming the commissures. The body of the leaflets are pliable and thin in the young, although its thickness is not uniform.

The commissure between the right and posterior aortic leaflets overlies the membranous septum and contacts the commissure between the anterior and septal leaflets of the tricuspid valve. The commissure between the right and left aortic leaflets contacts its corresponding pulmonary commissure and overlies the infundibular septum. The intervalvular fibrosa, at the commissure between the left and posterior aortic cusps, fuses the aortic valve to the anterior mitral leaflet. [6, 42]

A study of 100 formalin-fixed hearts from adult patients with normally functioning aortic valves found that the luminal area of the aorta at the sinotubular junction increased with age and with heart weight, where increased heart weight was attributed to systemic hypertension. [45] Volume-wise, the sinuses are largest when the valve closes, serving as reservoirs during ventricular diastole and allow filling of the coronary arteries.

When left ventricular pressure exceeds that in the aortic root, the valvular leaflets are pushed apart and fall back into their respective sinuses, allowing unimpeded ejection of blood. The orifices of the coronary arteries are commonly found close to the level of the sinotubular junction. [25]

8. Conclusion

In the new era of cardiac surgery, now more then ever, the need to further study the aortic valve complex anatomy and function is greater.

A thorough knowledge of the anatomy of the aortic valve and its relationships is essential to understanding aortic valve pathology and many congenital cardiac malformations. Also it is crucial for the diagnosis and treatment (both surgical and conservatory) of aortic valve pathology.

Accurate understanding of the anatomy of interest is of cardinal importance for the development of devices and treatment protocols. We emphasize the importance of considering anatomic variations in the development of treatments, an understanding of the intraindividual and interindividual variations that may exist can lead to refinements in current designs of valvular prostheses.

Although the aortic valve is the most intensely studied cardiac valve, there is still no consensus on how to describe its components and a universal terminology is yet to be found. The multidisciplinary approach will continue to be crucial in working through these challenges.

Author details

Ioan Tilea[1], Horatiu Suciu[3], Brindusa Tilea[2], Cristina Maria Tatar[1], Mihaela Ispas[3] and Razvan Constantin Serban[3]

1 Internal Medicine Clinic, Division of Cardiology, University of Medicine and Pharmacy Tirgu Mures, Romania

2 Infectious Disease Clinic, University of Medicine and Pharmacy Tirgu Mures, Romania

3 Cardiology Clinic, Emergency Clinical County Hospital Tirgu Mures, Romania

References

[1] Piazza N, de Jaegere P, Schultz C, Becker AE, Serruys PW, Anderson RH. Anatomy of the aortic valvular complex and its implications for transcatheter implantation of the aortic valve. Circ Cardiovasc Interv. 2008; 1:74–81. DOI: 10.1161/CIRCINTERVENTIONS.108. 780858

[2] Clayton M, Nature 484, 19 April 2012, 314–316, doi:10.1038/484314a

[3] Hurst WJ, King SB, Walter PF, Freisinger GC, Edward JE. Atherosclerotic coronary heart disease: angina pectoris, myocardial infarction, and other manifestations of myocardial ischemia. In: Hurst's the Heart. 6th ed. New York: McGraw-Hill; 1986:882–1008.

[4] Anderson RH. The surgical anatomy of the aortic root, in: Multimedia Manual of Cardiothoracic Surgery, doi:10.1510/ mmcts. 2006.002527

[5] Siew YH, Structure and anatomy of the aortic root, European Journal of Echocardiography (2009) 10, i3–i10 doi:10.1093/ejechocard/jen243

[6] Edwards WD., Anatomy of the Cardiovascular System: Clinical Medicine. Vol 6. Philadelphia: Harper & Row; 1984:1–24.

[7] Anderson RH, Webb S, Brown NA, Lamers W, Moorman A. Development of the heart: (3) Formation of the ventricular outflow tracts, arterial valves, and intrapericardial arterial trunks, September 2003;89:1110–18.

[8] Anderson RH, Webb S, Brown NA, Lamers W, Moorman A. Development of the heart (1): septation of the atriums and ventricles. Heart. 2003; 89: 949–958.

[9] Schoen FJ. Evolving Concepts of Cardiac Valve Dynamics: The Continuum of Development, Functional Structure, Pathobiology, and Tissue Engineering. Circulation 2008;118:1864-1880.

[10] Bashey RI, Bashey HM, Jimenez SA. Characterization of pepsinsolubilized bovine heart-valve collagen. Biochem J. 1978;173:203–208.

[11] Rajamannan NM, Evans FJ, Aikawa E, Grande-Alen KJ, Demer LL, Heistad DD at al. Calcific aortic valve disease: not simply a degenerative process. Review and Agenda for Research From the National Heart and Lung and Blood Institute Aortic Stenosis Working Group. Circulation. 2011;124:1783-1791.

[12] Liu AC, Joag VR, Gotlieb AI. The emerging role of valve interstitial cell phenotypes in regulating heart valve pathobiology. Am J Pathol. 2007; 171:1407–1418.

[13] Aird WC. Phenotype heterogeneity of the endothelium, I: Structure, function, and mechanisms. II. Representative vascular beds. Circ Res. 2007;100:158 –173, 174–190.

[14] Butcher JT, Nerem RM. Valvular endothelial cells regulate the phenotype of interstitial cells in co-culture: effects of steady shear stress. Tissue Eng. 2006;12:905–915.

[15] Simmons CA, Grant GR, Manduchi E, Davies PF. Spatial heterogeneity of endothelial phenotypes correlates with side-specific vulnerability to calcification in normal porcine aortic valves. Circ Res. 2005;96:792-799.

[16] Aikawa E, Whittaker P, Farber M, Mendelson K, Padera RF, Aikawa M at al. Human semilunar cardiac valve remodeling by activated cells from fetus to adult: implications for postnatal adaptation, pathology, and tissue engineering. Circulation. 2006;113:1344-1352

[17] Rabkin-Aikawa E, Aikawa M, Farber M, Kratz JR, Garcia-Cardena G, Kouchoukos NT, Mitchell MB, Jonas RA, Schoen FJ. Clinical pulmonary autograft valves: pathologic evidence of adaptive remodeling in the aortic site. J Thorac Cardiovasc Surg. 2004;128:552–561.

[18] Rabkin-Aikawa E, Farber M, Aikawa M, Schoen FJ. Dynamic and reversible changes of interstitial cell phenotype during remodeling of cardiac valves. J Heart Valve Dis. 2004;13:841–847.

[19] Rabkin E, Hoerstrup SP, Aikawa M, Schoen FJ. Evolution of cell phenotype and extracellular matrix in tissue-engineered heart valves during in-vitro maturation and in-vivo remodeling. J Heart Valve Dis. 2002;11:308–314.

[20] Maron BJ, Hutchins GM. The development of the semilunar valves in the human heart. Am J Pathol. 1974;74:331–344.

[21] Anderson RH. Clinical anatomy of the aortic root. Heart. 2000;84:670–673

[22] Davies MJ. Pathology of Cardiac Valves. London: Butterworths & Co; 1980. p1–61.

[23] Berdajs D, Lajos P, Turina M. The anatomy of the aortic root. Cardiovasc Surg 2002. 10(4):320–327

[24] Jatene MB, Monteiro R, Guimarães MH, Veronezi SC, Koike MK, Jatene FB et al. Aortic valve assessment. Anatomical study of 100 healthy human hearts. Arq. Bras. Cardiol. 1999; 73(1):81-86.

[25] Muriago M, Sheppard MN, Ho SY, Anderson RH. Location of the coronary arterial orifices in the normal heart. Clin Anat. 1997;10: 297–302.

[26] Cavalcanti JS, de Melo NC, de Vasconcelos RS. Morphometric and topographic study of coronary ostia. Arq Bras Cardiol 81(4).2003; 359–362, 355-358

[27] Knight J, Kurtcuoglu V, Muffly K, Marshall W Jr, Stolzmann P, Desbiolles L et al, Ex vivo and in vivo coronary ostial locations in humans, Surgical and Radiologic Anatomy October 2009, Volume 31, Issue 8, pp 597-604

[28] Vollebergh FE, Becker AE. Minor congenital variations of cusp size in tricuspid aortic valves: possible link with isolated aortic stenosis. Br Heart J. 1977; 39:1006 –1011.

[29] Silver MA, Roberts WC. Detailed anatomy of the normally functioning aortic valve in hearts of normal and increased weight. Am J Cardiol. 1985; 55:454–461.

[30] [30]. Roberts WC. The structure of the aortic valve in clinically isolated aortic steno-
      sis: an autopsy study of 162 patients over 15 years of age. Circulation. 1970; 42:91–97.

[31] Sutton JP III, Ho SY, Anderson RH. The forgotten interleaflet triangles: a review of
      the surgical anatomy of the aortic valve. Ann Thorac Surg. 1995; 59:419–427.

[32] McAlpine WA. Heart and Coronary Arteries. Berlin: Springer-Verlag. 1975. p9–26.

[33] Walmsley R. Anatomy of left ventricular outflow tract. Br Heart J. 1979; 41:263–7.

[34] Misfeld M, Sievers H-H. Heart valve macro and micro structure. Phil. Trans. R. Soc.
      B. 2007; 362:1421–1436. doi:10.1098/rstb.2007.2125

[35] Scott M, Vesely I. Aortic valve cusp microstructure: the role of elastin. Ann Thorac
      Surg. Aug 1995; 60(2 Suppl):S391-4

[36] Deck J.D. Endothelial cell orientation on aortic valve leaflets. Cardiovasc. Res. 1986;
      20: 760–767.

[37] Mill MR, Wilcox BR, Anderson RH. Surgical Anatomy of the Heart. Cohn LH, Ed-
      munds LH Jr, eds. Cardiac Surgery in the Adult. New York: McGraw-Hill,
      2003:31-52.

[38] Feigenbaum H, Armstrong WF and Ryan T. Feigenbaum's Echocardiography, 6th
      edn. (2004). Lippincott Williams & Wilkins, Philadelphia, USA. ISBN 0-7817-3198-4

[39] Shanewise JS, Cheung AT, Aronson S, Stewart WJ, Weiss RL, Mark JB et al. ASE/SCA
      guidelines for performing a comprehensive intraoperative multiplane transesopha-
      geal echocardiography examination: recommendations of the American Society of
      Echocardiography Council for Intraoperative Echocardiography and the Society of
      Cardiovascular Anesthesiologists Task Force for Certification in Perioperative Trans-
      esophageal Echocardiography. J Am Soc Echocardiogr 1999; 12:884.

[40] Muraru D, Cardillo M, Livi U, Badano LP. 3-dimensional transesophageal echocar-
      diographic assessment of papillary muscle rupture complicating acute myocardial
      infarction. J Am Coll Cardiol. 2010; 56:e45.

[41] Lang RM, Badano LP, Tsang W, Adams DH, Agricola E, Buck T, et al, EAE/ASE Rec-
      ommendations for Image Acquisition and Display Using Three-Dimensional Echo-
      cardiography, J Am Soc Echocardiogr 2012; 25:3-46.

[42] Edwards WD. Applied anatomy of the heart. In: Giuliani ER, Fuster V, Gersh BJ, et
      al, eds. Cardiology Fundamentals and Practice. Vol 1. 2nd ed. St Louis: Mosby-Year
      Book; 1991: 47–112.

[43] Malouf JF, Edwards WD, Tajik AJ, Seward JB. Functional anatomy of the heart. In:
      Fuster V, Alexander RW, O'Rourke RA, et al, eds. The heart. 11th ed. New York, NY:
      McGraw-Hill, 2004; 75–83.

[44] Stewart W. Intraoperative echocardiography. In: Topol EJ, ed. Textbook of Cardio-
      vascular Medicine. Philadelphia: Lippincott-Raven; 1998:1497–1525.

[45] Sliver MA, Roberts WC. Detailed anatomy of the normally functioning aortic valve in hearts of normal and increased weight. Am J Cardiol. 1985; 55:454–61.

Chapter 2

Extracellular Matrix Organization, Structure, and Function

Dena Wiltz, C. Alexander Arevalos, Liezl R. Balaoing,
Alicia A. Blancas, Matthew C. Sapp, Xing Zhang and
K. Jane Grande-Allen

Additional information is available at the end of the chapter

1. Introduction

Heart valves are thin, complex, layered connective tissues that direct blood flow in one direction through the heart. There are four valves in the heart, located at the entrance to and exit from the ventricular chambers. The normal function of the heart valves is essential to cardiovascular and cardiopulmonary physiology. The opening and closing of valve leaflets at precise times during the cardiac cycles contributes to the generation of sufficiently high pressure to eject blood from the ventricles, and also prevents blood from flowing backwards into the heart instead of forward towards the systemic circulation and the lungs.

The ability of heart valves to open and close repeatedly, as well as the maintenance of the phenotypes of valvular cells, is made possible by their tissue microstructure, specifically the composition and orientation of extracellular matrix (ECM). The ECM within heart valves is primarily comprised of collagen, elastic fibers, and proteoglycans and glycosaminoglycans, although other ECM components are present as well. Taken together, the ECM performs several roles in heart valves. First, the ECM plays a biomechanical role: it is responsible for the unique mechanical behavior of the valve tissue and thus the overall valve function. Second, the valvular cells are bound to and surrounded by the ECM that is located within the immediate vicinity of the cell; this ECM is specifically known as the pericellular matrix (PCM). The PCM influences cell function by serving as a source of ligands for cell surface receptors, which transfers mechanical strains (experienced by the leaflet tissues) to the cells and initiates intracellular signaling pathways. Third, the various types of ECM have different innate mechanical behaviors, for example with collagen being stiffer than elastic fibers, and a growing body of research has demonstrated that the phenotype and function of cells, including valve cells, are influenced by the stiffness of the substrate to which they are adhered [1]. These two latter functions of the ECM are considered to be mechanobiological as opposed to merely biomechanical since they affect cell behavior. Fourth, ECM has binding sites for growth factors and other soluble molecules found in the extracellular space, and thus the ECM serves as a reservoir for numerous bioactive factors than can affect cell behavior if they are released (such as when the ECM is degraded) or if a cell migrates close to this ECM reservoir.

Overall, the heart valve field is beginning to appreciate that there are numerous interactions between the ECM, valve cells, and valve mechanics. Given the complicated relationships that are being demonstrated, it is not surprising that alterations to the normal arrangement or composition of ECM, which frequently occur in valve disease, significantly and detrimentally impact valve function in a rather vicious cycle. For this reason, there has been an increasing effort to characterize the ECM within normal heart valves not only to elucidate valve biomechanics and mechanobiology, but also to obtain a solid basis for comparison with diseased valves.

This chapter will provide an overview of the ECM within heart valves, focusing on the aortic valve. After detailing the layered structure of the valve leaflets, each type of ECM component will be described and discussed in relation to its role in valve function and, in some instances, valve dysfunction.

2. The aortic valve leaflets are layered structures

Aortic valve leaflets consist of three main layers: the fibrosa, spongiosa, and ventricularis. Each layer has a distinct composition that aids in the normal mechanical and biochemical behavior of the valve. In diseased states, however, the composition of the layered structures can be altered compared to healthy tissues.

The fibrosa layer, close to the outflow surface, is mainly composed of collagen fibers with a small amount of elastic fibers, which are the major stress-bearing components and provide strength to maintain coaptation during diastole [2]. The circumferential alignment and orientation of collagen fibers contribute to the biological stress-strain relationship for aortic valve leaflets (Figure 1). This bilinear stress-strain curve represents the high extension with a low load and high elastic modulus with a high load applied [3]. Moreover, the particular architecture of collagen fibers contributes to the anisotropic mechanical behavior of the fibrosa layer. It has been found that the fibrosa is 4-6 times stiffer in the circumferential direction than in the radial direction [4].

The middle spongiosa layer of the leaflet predominantly consists of glycosaminoglycans and proteoglycans, particularly hyaluronan, which form a foam-like structure and bind a large amount of water. The spongiosa layer absorbs energy during compression, and facilitates the arrangement of collagen fibrils in the fibrosa and elastin in the ventricularis during the cardiac cycles [5].

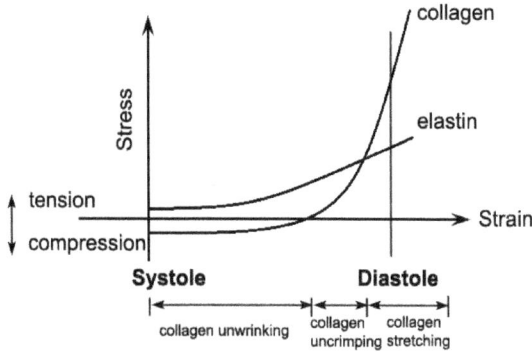

Figure 1. Schematic drawing of stress-strain relationships for collagen and elastin fibers during valve motion, reproduced with permission [3]

The ventricularis layer, close to the inflow surface, is rich in elastin with a moderate amount of collagen, which extends in diastole and recoils during systole [6]. The recoil of elastin restores the crimp of collagen fibrils and decreases the surface area of the stretched tissue from the closing phase [5]. The thickness of the three layers varies from the base to the free edge of the cusp [7].

It is worth noting that elastic fibers were found to span the whole leaflet, and connect or anchor three discrete layers together [6,8]. In addition, elastin provides intrafibrillar connections between collagen bundles in the fibrosa layer, whereas it forms a three-dimensional interconnected network in the spongiosa layer [8]. During unloading, the intrafiber elastin, which has high extensibility, helps the collagen fibers return to their wavy and crimped state [6]. These interconnected structures of elastic fibers anchor the discrete layers together, and prevent delamination, which therefore improves the continuity of material behavior of the whole leaflet. Table 1 summarizes the key ECM components in the layers and their major functions.

Location	Main Component(s)	Major Function(s)
Fibrosa	Collagen	Stress bearing
Spongiosa	Glycosaminoglycans and proteoglycans	Conferring flexibility, dampening vibrations from closing, and resisting delamination
Ventricularis	Elastin	Restoration of the wavy and crimped state of collagen fibers

Table 1. The key ECM components in each layer of the leaflet and their major functions

The structures of the leaflets described above provide the following critical functions [6,9–11]: 1) anisotropic mechanical behavior withstanding circumferential stress and extending radially; 2) bilinear biological stress-strain behavior allowing the leaflet to extend before bearing load in the closed phase; 3) elastic recoil to fully open the valve and restore the layer structures for the next cycle. The particular shape of the leaflets and their unique macro- and micro-structures cause the anisotropic mechanical behavior along the circumferential and radial directions of the leaflets [9–11].

During the closed phase (diastole), the leaflets experience the maximum load. Collagen bundles in the fibrosa layer are the major stress-bearing component withstanding approximately 80 mm Hg pressure while the valve is closed and bulging back towards the ventricle [3]. Collagen fibrils are assembled into parallel collagen fiber bundles oriented along the circumferential direction in the leaflet, which are able to withstand such high tensile forces. However, collagen fibers cannot be compressed, making the alignment of collagen (waviness and crimping) important for decreasing the area of the stretched fibrosa layer. Although the collagen fibrils have limited extensibility (approximately 1-2% yield strain), the waviness and crimping allows the fibrosa to withstand roughly 40% strain under loading. Straightening of wavy fibers provides approximately 17% strain, whereas the crimping allows additional approximately 23% strain [6]. In addition, the strains of the cusps in the closed phase are anisotropic, i.e., the strains differ in the radial and circumferential directions [11].

During valve opening, cusps become relaxed through recoil of the elongated, taut elastin. This restores the wavy and crimped state of collagen fibers while decreasing the surface area of the cusps. The GAG-rich spongiosa layer facilitates the rearrangements of the collagen and elastic fibers during the cardiac cycle, dampens vibration from closing, and resists delamination between layers [6,8].

It is evident that normal aortic valve function is maintained, in part, by not only the composition but also the arrangement and orientation of ECM components, particularly collagen, elastin, and GAGs, in the leaflets. Furthermore, it is important to note that alteration of the composition [12] and mechanics [13] of ECM in the aortic valve leaflets was found in diseased conditions. In calcific aortic valve disease (CAVD), collagen bundles and elastin fibers in the fibrosa layer were disrupted and disorganized [14]; meanwhile, there was increased proteoglycan deposition [12]. Matrix metalloproteinases (MMPs) [14,15] and the potent elastase cathepsin S [16], which are produced by macrophages, contribute to this ECM remodeling. Moreover, ECM proteins related to bone, i.e., osteocalcin and osteonectin, were present in the calcified fibrosa layer [17]. These proteins promote mineralization, and their presence suggests the osteoblastic differentiation of valve interstitial cells (VICs).

In addition, excessive myofibroblast differentiation from VICs, leading to ECM accumulation and fibrosis, was influenced by remodeling of ECM in the fibrosa and facilitated by elastin degradation [18]. Furthermore, myofibroblast differentiation from VICs and calcification in vitro have been shown to be dependent on ECM composition [19].

Taken together, the macroscopic layered structure and the microscopic structure in each layer of the leaflets impart pronounced anisotropic mechanical behavior that allows the valve to open and close during a great number of cardiac cycles throughout life. These structures are tailored to fulfill the normal functions and maintain the homeostasis of the leaflets in a healthy condition. However, abnormal alteration of composition and mechanics of ECM in these structures may lead to calcific heart valve disease.

3. Collagen comprises a significant portion of the aortic valve leaflet fibrosa

Collagen is an essential component of the aortic valve's layered structure and is vital for maintaining the tissue's mechanical integrity. Mainly responsible for tensile strength, collagen is a strong load-bearing protein created and regulated by VICs. Although present throughout the entire valve, collagen is largely located in the fibrosa where it reduces high tensile stresses. In addition to its central role in valve mechanics, collagen acts as a regulator of VIC phenotype and calcification. Insight into the structure of collagen reveals its unique mechanical properties that support aortic valve function.

Fibrillar collagens are high strength fibers that comprise nearly all of the valve's collagen content. Fibrillar collagens are groups of 3 coiled polypeptide chains that assemble together in tightly packed parallel arrangements. These coils are approximately 300 nm long and join together in a staggered banding pattern with a periodicity of 67 nm [20]. The aortic valve is mainly composed of fibrillar collagen types I, III, and V. Each of these collagens is constructed from different types of alpha chains that govern the overall function of the collagen molecule. Together, these three collagen types work to provide the aortic valve with unique mechanical properties suited for maintaining unidirectional blood flow.

Synthesis of fibrillar collagen is an essential mechanism for maintaining the valve's mechanical integrity. This complex process originates within VICs and is completed in the valve ECM. Production of collagen begins with the intracellular creation of polypeptide alpha chains. There exist ten distinct polypeptide chains that consist of approximately 300 consecutive Gly-X-Y amino acid sequences flanked by small terminal domains. The secondary structure of collagen is created by folding alpha chains into a right-handed alpha helix with the peptide bonds localized at the backbone of the helix and the amino acid side chains facing outward. With slightly less than three residues per turn and a pitch of approximately 8.6 nm, glycine residues are positioned in such a way that the side chains of these residues allow for the formation of the helix. The single hydrogen side chains of these glycine residues allows for the formation of a triple helix structure [21].

The tertiary structure of collagen involves the formation of a left-handed triple helix constructed in the C to N direction. These triple helices exist as both homotrimers and heterotrimers of alpha chains. Collagen type III is a homotrimer of $\alpha1(III)$ while collagen type I is a heterotrimer of $\alpha1(I)$ and $\alpha2(I)$. Additionally, collagen type V is a heterotrimer of $\alpha1(V)$ and $\alpha2(V)$. Known as procollagen, the tertiary structure molecule is approximately 1.5 nm wide and longer than 300 nm. For creation of the final supramolecular structure, the procollagen molecule is transported into the ECM for crosslinking and fibril formation. After modification in the extracellular space, procollagen is converted into tropocollagen, which undergoes fibrillogenesis where the triple helices are packed together into bundles. Crosslinking of the fibrils ensures the stability of the complex [21].

The arrangement of collagen fiber bundles is crucial to the proper functioning of the aortic valve. Collagen fibers are organized into multilayer structures linked by thin membranes containing variably aligned collagen. Ranging from 10 to 50 μm in size, these membranes are believed to be much more extensible than the collagen fiber bundles they connect. These multilayer structures can easily slide past one another during valve movement, providing the combination of flexibility and tensile strength necessary for the required mechanics during valve opening and closing [22].

Collagen constitutes approximately 90% of the protein content of the valve insoluble matrix [23]. The vast majority of the valve's content is composed of collagens type I, III, and V. Together, these fibrillar collagens account for 60% of the valve's dry weight [24]. There is approximately 74% collagen type I, 24% collagen type III, and 2% collagen type V distributed throughout the valve [25–27]. Whereas collagen type I mainly exists in the fibrosa, collagen type III is expressed ubiquitously throughout all three layers [25].

Collagen fibers mainly function to reduce stress on the leaflets during systole and diastole. While elastin controls initial valve opening and closing, collagen fibers reduce peak stresses in the leaflet matrix by an estimated 60%. These fibers have an important role in stabilizing leaflet motion [28]. Throughout leaflet movement, collagen fibers adjust position to resist tensile forces. As transvalvular pressure increases, the ventricularis expands in the circumferential direction, causing collagen fibers to become highly aligned. This is believed to increase the cuspal stiffness of the valve during diastole and prevent overextension of the valve [29].

The heterogeneous distribution of collagen throughout the aortic valve provides high strength in areas of greater stress while also allowing the valve to achieve a large degree of flexibility. Within the fibrosa, the primary tensile load-bearing layer, collagen fibers are highly aligned in the circumferential direction, resulting in tissue anisotropy. The arrangement of these fibers corresponds to the direction of highest tensile stress. In contrast, the ventricularis endures smaller tensile forces involved with initial opening and closing of the valve [30]. In addition to circumferentially oriented collagen, the largest and strongest collagen fiber bundles are localized in the areas of greatest tensile stress along the lower part of the commissure and coapting regions [22]. This unique arrangement and positioning of collagen reduces high tensile loads on the valve while allowing flexibility to open and close.

Comparisons between the fibrosa and ventricularis indicate that the fibrosa has a greater elastic modulus in the circumferential direction but a similar elastic modulus in the radial direction. These mechanical differences are largely the result of the number of aligned collagen fibers in each direction. With fewer collagen fibers, the ventricularis is approximately half as stiff as the fibrosa in the circumferential direction. In the radial direction, however, each layer contains approximately the same amount of collagen fibers and has similar elastic moduli [31]. Taken together, the multilayer valve structure causes aortic valves to be less stiff and more extensible radially than circumferentially [32].

Collagen achieves high strength and extensibility with the aid of additional mechanisms that contribute to the valve's mechanical properties. These include collagen cross-links, collagen crimp, and layer corrugations. Collagen cross-links function to increase the strength of aligned collagen. In the circumferential direction, the number of collagen cross-links per collagen molecule directly corresponds to the elastic modulus. However, this relationship does not apply to the radial direction, possibly due to the presence of elastin [31]. When there is no mechanical stress on the leaflet, the fibrosa exists as a number of folds in the radial direction known as corrugations. Large extensibility is achieved through these collagen corrugations in combination with collagen crimp. When stress is applied to the leaflet, initial extension is accomplished by straightening of the collagen crimp. Further stress causes the corrugations to unfold in the radial direction [30]. Together, collagen crimp and corrugations allow the fibrosa to extend further in the radial direction when compared to the circumferential direction.

Throughout the lifetime of the aortic valve, collagen synthesis and degradation are responsible for maintaining adequate valve strength and extensibility. Constant turnover of collagen allows the valve to adapt to regional changes in tensile strength. *In vitro* studies show that VICs respond to cyclic mechanical loading as a way to balance collagen synthesis and degradation. Cyclic stretch of valve leaflets stimulates VIC collagen type III production. In particular, the amount and duration of the stretching can have an effect on the amount of collagen produced [27]. Additionally, VICs in culture express collagen type I and collagen type III mRNA for new matrix synthesis [33]. New collagen production is localized to specific regions of the valve depending on the collagen type that is produced. Collagen type I synthesis occurs in the fibrosa around, but not within, areas of mature collagen. Collagen type III synthesis, however, mainly occurs outside of the fibrosa [34]. Collagen degradation is also an important function of VICs and acts as an essential control to collagen production. Studies have shown that VICs seeded into collagen scaffolds express MMPs that degrade the scaffold in a heterogeneous manner [33]. Thus, VICs continuously regulate the mechanical properties of the surrounding ECM through collagen synthesis and degradation.

Aside from its mechanical functions, collagen has been shown to regulate VIC phenotype and calcification potential. *In vitro* studies were unable to induce calcification in VICs cultured on collagen proteins in standard media. It is believed that collagen actively inhibits VIC calcification [19]. Other studies have shown that scaffold collagen content also affects VIC proliferation. Specifically, one study reported that VICs adhered and spread on collagen surfaces but were not able to proliferate [35]. Another study showed that VIC proliferation decreased on scaffolds containing higher collagen content [36]. An *in vitro* study indicated that matrix stiffness regulates VIC differentiation to myofibrogenic or osteogenic phenotypes in calcific conditions [37].

4. Elastic fibers comprise a significant portion of the ventricularis layer of the aortic valve leaflets

Elastic fibers are macromolecular assemblies of several different molecules. The majority of the elastic fiber consists of elastin, an insoluble protein generated by lysyl oxidase crosslinking of soluble tropoelastin monomers (approximately 70 kDa). The elastin tends to be located in the inner core of the elastic fiber and is surrounded by a fine mesh of microfibrils.

These microfibrils are predominantly fibrillin-1, but to a lesser extent Fibrillin-2. Microfibril associated glycoproteins (MAGPs), fibulins, and other proteins are also present in the microfibrillar sheath [38]. At the light microscope level, one can observe the fine elastic fibers by histological staining with Voerhoff's stain or related methods, but when tissue sections are viewed with transmission electron microscopy, there is a clear distinction between the electron-dense elastin core and the microfibrillar sheath [39].

The unique mechanical behavior of the elastic fiber is conferred primarily by the mechanical function of elastin and fibrillin. Crosslinked elastin is remarkable for its ability to undergo high amounts of deformation when subjected to small amounts of load, as well as to recoil back to its original dimensions, when the load is removed, with very little loss of energy. Fibrillin-1, the most widely studied of the microfibrillar components, is also highly extensible. Fibrillin and the other microfibrillar components also coordinate, in a complicated manner still under investigation [38], to aid in the cross-linking of tropoelastin and assemble the final elastic fiber. Interestingly, fibrillin is not always associated with elastic fibers. Fibrillin can often be found by itself, in which it may independently function as a mechanical, load-bearing but highly extensible scaffold [40]. Numerous domains in fibrillin exist for binding integrins, heparan sulfate proteoglycans, and growth factors, which point to substantial roles for alone fibrillin and mature elastic fibers in mediating cell signaling and adhesion [41].

In semilunar heart valves, elastin is found primarily within the ventricularis layer on the inflow side of the leaflet, but is also abundant in the middle spongiosa layer. A thin, frequently imperceptible layer of elastic fibers, the aterialis, is found atop the collagen-rich fibrosa layer. These elastic fibers merge with the intima of the adjacent arterial well, but the overall function of the arterialis has not been well characterized [42].

In the ventricularis, elastic fibers are present in dense and continuous sheets across the whole of the leaflet. These fiber sheets are the most significant contributor to the mechanical properties of the ventricularis [6,30], which can be demonstrated when all ECM components but elastin are removed when using NaOH digestion. After this treatment, the digested ventricularis matches the mechanical behavior of the undigested ventricularis radially, indicating a strong presence of elastin in the radial direction [30]. The elastic fibers within the ventricularis undergo considerable, continual stretch from the initial stage of closure, when blood flow vortices are starting to push the leaflets towards the valve orifice, to the final coapted position of the leaflets. The extension of these elastic fibers accommodates the unfolding of the fibrosa layer, which is normally corrugated in the unloaded position. During this unfolding process, the elastic fibers are bearing the loading of the entire leaflet [43]. Even at high strains, when the collagen in the fibrosa is considered to dominate mechanical properties, the elastin in the ventricularis still plays a significant role. This effect was shown when separated ventricularis was preloaded to mimic its intact configuration; the separated ventricularis was shown to bear load before the separated fibrosa [44]. It has been speculated that this response acts as a safety mechanism to prevent radial overextension of the aortic valve leaflet. Then, when the pressure across the valve is reduced, the elastic fiber sheet in the ventricularis recoils and retracts the leaflets back toward the annular attachment to the arterial wall, a process that involves the re-folding of the corrugations in of the fibrosa. This action restores the original shape and orientation of collagen quickly and consistently to prepare for the next cycle of valve closing. Although the elastic sheet in the ventricularis has fibers that are also oriented circumferentially as well as radially, elastin does not appear to play an important role in the mechanical behavior of the leaflet in the circumferential direction. Valve leaflets exposed to cyclic circumferential stretch and cultured under flow for 48 hours maintained a constant concentration of elastic, suggesting that elastogenesis was not activated during the duration of stretch [45]. However, it is speculated that connections between the elastic fiber and collagen networks facilitate the radial extensibility of the ventricularis layer and the overall leaflet [43]. There are also some elastic fibers in the fibrosa, which surround and connect the collagen fibers, thus preserving collagen crimp and the characteristic corrugated nature of the fibrosa [6,46,47].

The elastic fiber structure in the spongiosa has been characterized much less than in the ventricularis, partly due to the difficulty in isolating its structure from the rest of the leaflet [30]. This elastic structure, however, has been observed during microdissection separating the leaflet [30,48], with scanning electron microscopy (SEM) [6,46], micro-computed tomography (micro-CT) [6], immunohistochemistry (IHC) [25], and autofluorescence imaging [49,50], which all have shown a fine elastic fiber network emanating from the ventricularis and connecting to the fibrosa. We have recently reported that the thickness of this elastic fiber network in the spongiosa is significantly thicker in the hinge and coaptation region than in the belly region of the aortic valve leaflet [8]. We also found two distinct patterns of spongiosa elastic fibers within the leaflet: (i) a rectilinear pattern in the hinge and coaptation region; and (ii) a radially oriented stripe pattern in the belly. Overall, it is believed that the elastic fibers in the spongiosa contribute to valve function in three ways. First, they connect the elastic fibers in the ventricularis to collagen in the fibrosa, which allows coupling of the mechanics of the two layers and matrix components, while using elastic recoil to exert preload on the fibrosa. Second, they distribute stress between collagen and elastic fibers, particularly at low strains. Third, they passively allow relative movement and shear between the outer layers [5,6,48].

Given the presence of a thick, rectilinearly-arranged structure of elastic fibers in the spongiosa of the hinge and coaptation regions, it is speculated that this elastin structure plays a role in leaflet flexure [5,30]. Flexure of the leaflet towards the outflow direction compresses the fibrosa and applies tension to the ventricularis. Rather than undergoing compression, however, the fibrosa may attempt to buckle separately from the leaflet, thereby exaggerating its corrugated configuration. The leaflet would subsequently bend at the troughs of this corrugation, where the second moment of inertia would be locally reduced, albeit temporarily. Buckling would only occur with shearing between the fibrosa and ventricularis, which is allowed by both the compliant elastic fibers in the spongiosa connecting the two outer layers as well as by GAGs in the spongiosa lubricating the outer layer movement [5,30,51,52]. Recoil from the elastic fibers in the spongiosa would then return the fibrosa to its original configuration so it could undergo the next cycle of loading [5,30]. At the hinge, where bending occurs in the opposite direction, it is speculated that the elastic fiber-rich ventricularis compresses readily without buckling, most likely due to the tensile preload already exerted on the ventricularis, but that leaflet deflection may be limited by the stiff fibrosa, which would not allow the leaflet to bend [4,53]. Limited flexure at the hinge would allow the leaflet to absorb pressure from reverse blood flow in diastole, but prevents distention of the leaflet. Thus, our finding of a thicker spongiosa and elastic fiber structure in flexural regions provides evidence of a significant role for elastin in flexure [8]. In addition, the thick network of elastic fibers that we have observed in the spongiosa of the coaptation region may play a role in dampening vibrations that result from valve closing [5].

5. The middle layer, the spongiosa, is comprised mainly of glycosaminoglycans and proteoglycans

Glycosaminoglycans and proteoglycans (GAGs and PGs, respectively) comprise a significant part of the aortic valve leaflets. PGs and GAGs are mainly found in the spongiosa layer of the valve, located between the ventricularis and fibrosa, where they play a vital role in maintaining normal valve function. Previous work has shown that GAGs and PGs serve to not only provide mechanical support to the tissue but also aid in the normal biological functions of the valve [54]. Therefore, it is crucial to fully understand the function of GAGs and PGs in both the normal and possible diseased states of tissues.

GAGs are composed of long and unbranched chains of repeating disaccharides, which consist of a hexosamine and either, depending on the GAG type, uronic acid or galactose. There exist the following families of GAGs with each group being defined by its composition: hyaluronan (HA), heparin, heparan sulfate (HS), chondroitin sulfate (CS), dermatan sulfate (DS), and keratan sulfate (KS) (Table 2) [55–58].

GAGs are primarily formed in the lumen of the Golgi apparatus. The formation process occurs, except in the case of HA, with glycosyltransferases alternatively adding a uronic acid or galactose with a hexosamine to a protein core. The attachment to the protein core varies based on the GAG type. Heparin, HS, CS, and DS are attached to a serine residue, connected to the protein core, via xylose. KS can attach to the protein core either by an asparagine residue at the N-terminus or linked to serine or threonine at the O-terminus. HA does not attach to a protein core. It is synthesized by the addition of sugars to the non-reducing termini of the forming polysaccharide by HA synthase, without a protein backbone. In all cases, modifications can be made to the resulting polysaccharides. Two noteworthy changes include sulfation of the chains and epimerization of the uronic acid. These changes do not occur, however, with HA. Sulfation and epimerization modifications can give a more distinct characteristic to the GAG chains. The epimerization of the uronic acid of CS leads to the production of DS. Epimerization also occurs on heparin and HS. Sulfation can occur in CS, DS, heparin, HS, and KS. N-sulfation takes place in heparin and HS; whereas, O-sulfation can take place in heparin, HS, CS, and DS. In addition to epimerization and sulfation, phosphorylation of the xylose linkage—occurring among CS, DS, heparin, and HS to their respective protein cores—can take place [54,58,59]. Through gel electrophoresis, it has been found that

HA comprises approximately half of the total GAG content in aortic valves [60]. It is important to note that all GAGs, with the exception of HA, exist *in vivo* as components of PGs.

Glycosaminoglycan	Uronic acid	Galactose	Hexosamine
Hyaluronan	Glucuronic	-	N-acetylglucosamine
Heparin	Glucuronic	-	N-acetylglucosamine
	Iduronic		
Heparan sulfate	Glucuronic	-	N-acetylglucosamine
	Iduronic		
Chondroitin sulfate	Glucuronic	-	N-acetylgalactosamine
Dermatan sulfate	Glucuronic	-	N-acetylgalactosamine
	Iduronic		
Keratan sulfate	-	+	N-acetylglucosamine

Table 2. List of glycosaminoglycans and their composition [59]

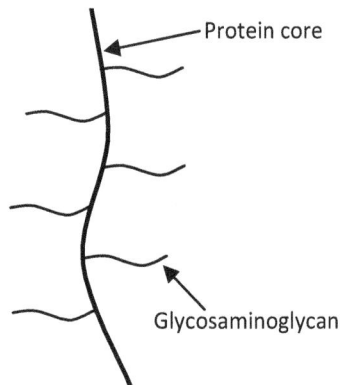

Figure 2. Proteoglycan structure

PGs are formed when GAGs are added to a protein core through a covalent linkage (Figure 2). During PG synthesis, a protein core moves from the endoplasmic reticulum of a cell to the Golgi apparatus, where GAGs are then added to the protein core [55]. PGs can be found in intracellular organelles, on the cell surface, and in the extracellular matrix (ECM) [59]. PGs found in the ECM can be divided into three categories: PGs found within the basement membrane, hyalectans or PGs that interact with HA and lectins, and small leucine-rich PGs (SLRPs) or PGs that contain a leucine motif and have considerably low molecular weights. These PGs can be further classified by the type of protein backbone they contain, as well as the amount, type, and sulfation pattern of the GAGs that are attached to the backbone. More than thirty PGs have been characterized [61]. For example, well-characterized PGs that exist in cardiovascular tissue include decorin, biglycan, and versican. Decorin and biglycan have a core protein size of 40 kDa and are a part of the SLRP family of PGs. They contain CS and DS GAG chains [61]. Versican is a large, chondroitin sulfate proteoglycan. It interacts with HA, and therefore is a hyalectan PG [62]. Other significant PGs in mammalian tissues include perlecan—a basement membrane protein that contains HS and CS, aggrecan—a hyalectan containing CS, and syndecans—a family of cell surface heparan sulfate proteoglycans containing HS and CS [61].

GAGs, and in turn PGs, have a significant role in aortic valve tissue behavior. GAGs have been shown to enhance the viscoelastic properties of the valve leaflets through binding of water molecules [63]. The sulfation and carboxylation on the GAGs make them highly negatively-charged polysaccharides. This negative charge draws in water molecules. Once the tissue becomes hydrated, it acts like a sponge for the valve leaflets. As noted previously, GAGs and PGs are highly abundant in the middle layer of the aortic valve leaflet. One of the main functions of this cushioned layer, the spongiosa, is to provide a barrier between two other layers, the ventricularis and fibrosa, of the valve. This barrier allows for proper shearing between the layers as well as compressibility of the leaflet without compromising the leaflet's overall structural or biological integrity when mechanical stimuli are applied to aortic valve leaflets [63,64]. The mechanical competency that GAGs provide is crucial to the aortic valve leaflets. The aortic valve leaflets serve to ensure unidirectional blood flow from the left ventricle to the aorta. In order to guarantee normal blood flow, the leaflets must open and close properly. Therefore, the flexibility that GAGs provide to the leaflet is crucial to the normal valve's function. In addition, the space that GAGs occupy and form in the matrix serve to organize other molecules within the structure. The structure and hydration that GAGs provide also allow for biological cues to occur within the valve. Moreover, GAGs are known to aid in cell migration, proliferation, act as receptors for signaling molecules, bind growth factors, and serve in the recruitment of various cell types [54].

It is believed that GAGs/PGs likely play an active role in aortic valve tissue disease. Research has shown regional variation of decorin, biglycan, versican and HA in, near, and distal to regions of calcification in diseased aortic valves, suggesting the occurrence of remodeling in the tissue during an unhealthy state [65]. In addition, although the exact causation of calcific aortic valve disease is unknown, it is speculated that it may be due, at least in part, to an inflammatory process [17]. Interestingly, GAGs are thought to play an active role, quite often in the case of cellular injury, in many inflammatory processes for a variety of cell types and have shown to alter in structure and localization in these processes [66]. In addition, some researchers believe that lipid binding due to the unique structure of GAGs may be critical to the accumulation of lipids in calcified aortic valves, a characteristic that is hypothesized to aid in valvular calcification [67]. Although the specific mechanisms underlying calcific aortic valve disease are not quite understood, the complex nature and distinguishable differences of GAGs in both healthy and diseased tissue give rise to the possibility of GAGs being a key factor in valve calcification.

GAGs are very complex disaccharides that highly dictate the behavior of PGs. These polysaccharides are vital in maintaining mechanical, structural, and biological integrity of the aortic valve. Although there is growing interest in further elucidating the role of GAGs in healthy tissues, the exact role of GAGs in diseased aortic valves needs further investigation, as well.

6. Minor ECM components in heart valves also play significant roles in normal valve function and in pathological states

The extracellular matrix of heart valves contain a number of minor components that perform a variety of functions. They are important in valve development, function, and pathology. The study and further characterization of these minor ECM components not only facilitates the development of targeted therapies but would also aid in the microenvironmental mimicry needed for potential tissue engineering applications.

Vitronectin is a glycoprotein that is approximately 75 kDa in size and is present in both serum and the ECM as an adhesive substrate [68]. It is involved in the inhibition of the complement system [68] and is associated with the regulation of hemostasis [69]. Vitronectin also promotes cellular attachment to ECM and is involved in cellular migration [68]. This glycoprotein, along with fibronectin, is found in moderate amounts in aortic, pulmonary, and mitral valves, localizing around valve endothelial cells (VEC) on the inflow layer [25]. In addition, both fibronectin and vitronectin have been shown to associate with collagen fibers in chordae tendinae [70].

Fibronectin is a dimer glycoprotein which consists of two ~250 kDa subunits and is a component of the extracellular matrix [71]. There are many various isoforms of fibronectin, which is the result of alternative mRNA splicing [71]. In addition to being an insoluble ECM component secreted primarily by fibroblasts, soluble fibronectin is also found in the plasma [71]. Fibronectin acts by binding to integrins, collagens, fibrin, and heparin sulfate proteoglycans [71], which allows it to participate in wound healing [72,73] and act as a critical player in embryogenesis [74]. Although not a major ECM component in heart valves, valve interstitial cells (VIC) secrete fibronectin in response to valve damage, providing a means for cell migration [75].

Additionally, fibronectin, along with osteonectin and periostin, confers stiffness to the fibrosa layer [76]. Periostin is a component of the ECM that acts as a ligand for α-V/β-3 and α-V/β-5 integrins and is known to support adhesion and epithelial migration [77]. It is present in the extracellular matrix of several types of tissues and is upregulated in several types of cancers [78]. Recombinant periostin has been shown to promote cardiomyocyte proliferation and angiogenesis after a myocardial infarction [79]. It has been shown previously that periostin plays a role in murine embryonic valve development and remains present in the valves throughout the lifespan even when there is no pathological calcification [80]. A recent study involving chick cardiac development suggests that the presence of periostin in the developing heart may provide a means of organizing other ECM molecules in order to facilitate early epithelial-mesenchymal transition (EMT) [81]. However, the overexpression of periostin and osteopontin can lead to valve calcification.

Osteopontin is a phosphoprotein, meaning that it contains chemically bound phosphoric acid. Originally found in bone, it also contains the arginine-glycine-aspartate (RGD) motif more commonly attributed to fibronectin and is also a constituent of ECM in other tissues [82]. It is secreted by various tissues such as fibroblasts [82] and immune cells, including dendritic cells, macrophages, and neutrophils [83]. Osteopontin is known to interact with various surface receptors that make it a crucial player in bone remodeling [84], wound healing, inflammation, and immune responses [83]. It is also known to be involved in vascular remodeling during endothelial injury [82]. Osteopontin is present in valves calcified as a result of disease as well as in calcified bioprosthetic heart valves [85]. The calcification process of aortic valves closely resembles osteoblast differentiation in regards to expression of genes characteristic of bone formation, such as osteopontin and osteocalcin [86].

Osteocalcin is a small, non-collagenous protein that is considered a late-stage marker for bone formation and is one of a small group of proteins that are osteoblast-specific [87,88]. It is present in general circulation [87] and its capacity for binding hydroxyapatite and calcium suggests that it is largely involved in mineral deposition [88], but it also has recently been shown to act in a hormone-like manner by enhancing insulin secretion [87]. Its traditional role as a product of bone indicates that valve calcification may actually be a result of active bone formation in the valve tissue [86]. This bone formation may be the result of VEGF secretion by endothelial cells during neoangiogenesis occurring in response to inflammation, as seen in rheumatic valve calcification [89]. Additionally, increased serum levels of osteocalcin were shown to be indicative of aortic valve disease in patients [90].

In addition to the matrix proteins, matrix metalloproteinases (MMPs) and their inhibitors (TIMPs) are also found in heart valves. They assist in tissue development and remodeling and can be used as indicators of disease. It is also believed that the ECM degradation resulting from MMP activity serves to release growth factors bound to ECM components and thus alter the microenvironment chemically, as well as structurally [91]. Calcified leaflets from stenotic valves have been shown to express levels of MMP-2 that are similar to those of normal valves but express higher levels of MMP-3, MMP-9, and TIMP-1 [14]. MMP-1, produced by activated myofibroblasts and macrophages, is also prevalent in calcific aortic valve stenosis and may be related to high TNF-α levels resulting from inflammation [92].

7. The basement membrane supports valve endothelial cells and acts as a barrier between circulating blood and subendothelial components

The basement membrane is a myriad of proteins, proteoglycans, and glycoproteins that not only supply a substrate to anchor the valve endothelial cells, but also has a large array of biological activities that regulate spatial organization, sequester growth factors, modulate angiogenesis and migration, and regulate the diffusion of nutrients through it towards the underlying valve interstitial cells [93]. The major constituents of the basement membrane are laminin, perlecan, collagen type IV and VIII, nidogen, and the glycoprotein SPARC (secreted protein, acidic and rich in cysteine). Each of these constituents play a role in the overall function of the basement membrane. In addition, MMPs contribute to the biological activity that occurs within the basement membrane. Understanding basement membrane composition and behavior, during both healthy and diseased states of the aortic valve, may lead to a better understanding of calcific aortic valve disease.

Laminins belong to a family of heterotrimeric glycoproteins composed of combinations of α, β, and γ chains that form a cross-like structure averaging between 400-900 kDa in size [94,95]. Laminins play an integral role in the formation of the supportive ECM network. The unique cross-like shape allows laminin molecules to bind with neighboring laminins and ECM via the three short chains, and use the long alpha chain as a cell anchoring site [96]. In addition to their structural contributions to the basement membrane, laminins are essential for proper biological activity. These glycoproteins have been shown to promote cell adhesion, migration, differentiation, and maintenance of cellular phenotype [94,97,98]. Dysfunction in laminin expression has been linked to diseases with improper tissue formation such as muscular dystrophy, epidermolysis bullosa, and various nephritic syndromes [94,99].

Although laminin is not as ubiquitous as collagen, this basement membrane component has been highly investigated as an ECM substrate for *in vitro* cultures. However, this glycoprotein may influence valve cell types differently. *In vivo* and *in vitro* studies have shown that laminin interacts with endothelial and epithelial cells, and can help maintain physiological functionality of the cells [97,100,101]. However, VICs cultured on laminin have been found to support high quantities of calcific nodule formation in the presence of TGF-β, when compared to subendothelial ECM components collagen type I and fibronectin [19,102]. The various regions of laminin protein have been reported to mediate specific cell responses. The G-domains of laminin α chains are associated with heparin binding and cell adhesion, whereas regions along the laminin β chains promote cell differentiation [98,100,101]. The peptide sequence YIGSR from the laminin β-1 chain has been shown to promote endothelial cell adhesion and proliferation, however, it also influences other cell types including smooth muscle and tumor cells [98,101]. VICs cultured on YIGSR were also shown to promote calcific nodule formation, although less than those seeded on fibronectin derived RGDS peptides. However, when the 67-kDa laminin cell receptor was blocked, the YIGSR seeded VIC cultures significantly increased in nodule formation and gene expression for various myogenic and osteogenic markers, suggesting that disruption in laminin binding may be linked to valve calcification [103]. IKVAV, another peptide sequence derived from the laminin α1-chain, has been linked to promoting angiogenesis, cell migration and spreading [97,98,104]. Though most work with this peptide has been done with endothelial and tumor cells, its ability to promote angiogenesis may also be a future area of interest in studying how angiogenesis mediates valve tissue calcification. Furthermore, laminin influence on cell activity varies between cell types, and may promote VIC activation and tissue calcification in diseased states.

Perlecan (Pln) is one of the more abundant heparan sulfate proteoglycans and is found in several tissues including in the endochondral barrier in bones [105]; however, it is primarily localized in vascular basement membranes. It has a major role in regulating the development of blood vessels, the heart, cartilage, and the nervous system. Physiologically, perlecan plays a prominent role in regulating cellular proliferation, differentiation, organization, and mediating inflammation [106]. Perlecan derives its functionality from five protein subdomains which share their sequence homology with several other proteins [107]. Domain 1 contains an SEA (Sperm protein, Enteokinase, Agrin) module and three SGD (Ser-Gly-Asp) tripeptide sequences to which three heparan sulfate (HS) glycosaminoglycans attach. These HS can bind and sequester several important growth factors for determining endothelial quiescence in a process known as matricrine signaling. The SEA section is unique to perlecan, and it has no known function other than to influence the O-linked glycosylation of the SGD domain. Interestingly, it has been shown that several factors that determine the activity of these sugar chains vary greatly by the cell source that is producing them [108]. These factors can include the ratio of heparan sulfate to chondroitin sulfate, the length of the chains, and the sulfation level of the chains which all affect how the chains modulate the bioactivity of nearby growth factors. Domain II contains 4 low-density lipoprotein receptor sequences and one immunoglobulin-like repeat. Domain III contains three laminin-like domain modules and eight epidermal growth factor-like repeats. Domain IV, the largest domain, contains many N-CAM-like Ig repeats. Domain V has been demonstrated to be the major cell-binding domain of perlecan due to the laminin and agrin homologies that it contains. Domain V can also be glyocosylated, which can contribute along with domain I to the matricrine signaling capabilities of perlecan, which could potentially contribute to the development of CAVD [109].

Matricrine signaling occurs when the ECM modulates cell behavior by controlling the local levels of growth factor concentrations by sequestering or releasing them when the underlying matrix is intact or degraded, respectively [109]. Proteoglycans, like perlecan, and their GAG chains are the major sites for matricrine signaling due to their heparan sulfate and chondroitin sulfate chains electrostatically binding free growth factors. Their role in the pathology of CAVD is widely unexplored despite their presence in normal valves and their increased production in diseased valves [67]. It is known that PGs and GAGs play an integral role in the progression of atherosclerosis via sequestering of inflammatory molecules and lipids [110–113] and mediating angiogenesis into the vessel supplying an entry way for additional inflammatory entities. Both of these factors are seen histologically in CAVD, but their role is merely speculative at this moment.

Collagens in the basement membrane can form lateral, axial, and linear connections with surrounding ECM. Of the basement membrane collagens, collagen IV (COL IV) is the most abundant and essential for network formation. Only found in basement membrane tissues, COL IV molecules are approximately 400 kDa, and composed of two α_1, and one α_2 [115–117]. COL IV proteins have many biologically active domains that can influence specific cellular responses, as well as have specific affinities to other molecules such as BMP-4, fibronectin, Von Hippel Lindau protein, and factor IX [115,117]. Mapping of COL IV protein reveals 3 major integrin motifs that are located in strategic regions to promote cell activity or protein degradation when activated [115]. During angiogenesis and tumor invasion, COL IV is degraded by MMP-2 and MMP-9 enzymes to allow for cell migration and infiltration into the matrix. Studies have found that the cleavage sites also overlap with many integrin binding domains such as $\alpha_1\beta_1$, resulting in the availability of $\alpha_v\beta_3$ integrin binding sites known to promote neutrophil binding [115,118]. Collagen IV networks are highly adhesive to all cells types except erythrocytes [115,119]. Furthermore, cell binding has been found to be enhanced in the presence of various ECM molecules such as perlecan, SPARC, and von Willebrand factor (vWF) [115,118,119]. Interestingly, COL IV also has numerous anti-angiogenic domains that are activated after MMP degradation at the non-collagenous (NC) 1 domain, thereby limiting angiogenesis or migration of endothelial and tumor cells [115]. The changes in COL IV bioactivity depending on the domain region and cleavage state can greatly affect the functionality of surrounding cells. Dysfunctional COL IV expression or mutations in the heterotrimer formation have been found to be extremely detrimental and cause matrix disorders such as Goodpasture's syndrome or Alport syndrome [94,115]. Therefore, additional studies should be done to investigate how the highly bioactive COL IV meshworks may promote the onset of calcification in valve tissues.

COL VIII has also been found to play a network forming role, maintaining the sheet-like structure ECM, while sequestering various integrin binding sites and growth factors. COL VIII is smaller than COL IV, and can form tetrahedral and hexagonal assemblies [117,118]. Though work on COL VIII in regards to valve tissues has been limited, vascular basement membrane studies have found that COL VIII plays a large role in interacting with subendothelial cells such as smooth muscle cells and fibroblasts. In vitro, COL VIII promotes fibroblast proliferation and migration [114]. Furthermore, COL VIII may be linked to atherogenesis, a pathology similar to CAVD, as its expression in cells is upregulated during vessel injury [114,120]. This collagen has even been found to interact with elastic fibers in liver tissues, suggesting it may have a bridging function between the basement membrane components and subendothelial ECM [118]. Therefore, COL VIII could play an integral role in mediating valve interstitial and endothelial cell communication. Recent studies have found after enzyme cleavage at the NC1 domain, the resulting C-terminal fragment known as vastatin will prevent endothelial cell proliferation and induce cell apoptosis [120]. While some work has investigated using vastatin as an anti-angiogenic agent, further studies are needed to elucidate how it may affect the functionality of surrounding cells and ECM, especially in older valve tissue.

Similar to perlecan, nidogen is a 150 kDa glycoprotein that has sequence homologies with other basement membrane proteins. It consists of two amino (G1, G2) and one carboxyl (G3) terminal globular domains that are connected by a rod domain composed primarily of endothelial growth factor repeats [121]. Nidogen binds collagen type IV, perlecan, and laminin. This binding contributes to the hypothesis that nidogen is important in basement membrane assembly; although some recent animal studies have demonstrated that nidogen may not be necessary for basement membrane formation [121]. The role of nidogen in CAVD is unexplored, but it may play a role in maintaining valvular basement membrane functionality by regulating infiltration of inflammatory agents [93].

SPARC positive neovascularisation is a documented histological change in CAVD [122]. Secreted protein acidic and rich in cysteine (SPARC), also known as osteonectin, is a small basement membrane protein. It interacts with cells, binds to other members of the basement membrane, growth factors, various proteases, and is found in newly developing neovessels.

Intact SPARC protein inhibits cellular proliferation and has anti-angiogenic activity in vitro [123]. However, enzymatic degradation of SPARC can release matricryptic fragments with the KGHK motif that may induce angiogenic activity both *in vitro* and *in vivo* [124]. SPARC has been observed lining blood vessels in early to mid stage calcified valves suggesting the presence of a fully formed basement membrane lining these vessels [125]. However, the presence of the other constituents of the basement membrane is merely speculative at this point as the studies investigating their presence during CAVD have not been completed.

8. Summary

In conclusion, the last several years have witnessed significant acceleration in the number of studies characterizing specific types of extracellular matrix in heart valves, although there is still much to be learned. The basement membrane of heart valves, and its role in regulating valvular endothelial cell function, are particularly understudied. The broad scope of cell-matrix and matrix-matrix interactions within heart valves, and how these are regulated by the local, dynamic signaling environment, is another subject that merits further investigation. We expect that insights gained from these research endeavors will lead to novel treatments for valve diseases in the future.

Author details

Dena Wiltz, C. Alexander Arevalos, Liezl R. Balaoing, Alicia A. Blancas, Matthew C. Sapp, Xing Zhang and K. Jane Grande-Allen

Department of Bioengineering, Rice University, Houston, TX, USA

References

[1] Nemir S, West JL. Synthetic materials in the study of cell response to substrate rigidity. *Annals of Biomedical Engineering*. 2010 Jan;38(1):2–20.

[2] Sacks MS, Schoen FJ, Mayer, Jr. JE. Bioengineering challenges for heart valve tissue engineering. *Annual Review of Biomedical Engineering*. 2009 Jan;11:289–313.

[3] Schoen FJ, Levy RJ. Founder's Award, 25th Annual Meeting of the Society for Biomaterials, perspectives. Providence, RI, April 28-May 2, 1999. Tissue heart valves: current challenges and future research perspectives. *Journal of Biomedical Materials Research*. 1999 Dec 15;47(4):439–65.

[4]   Vesely I, Lozon A. Natural preload of aortic valve leaflet components during gluta-raldehyde fixation: effects on tissue mechanics. *Journal of Biomechanics*. 1993 Feb;26(2): 121–31.

[5]   Schoen FJ. Aortic valve structure-function correlations: role of elastic fibers no longer a stretch of the imagination. *Journal of Heart Valve Disease*. 1997 Jan;6(1):1–6.

[6]   Scott MJ, Vesely I. Aortic valve cusp microstructure: the role of elastin. *Annals of Thoracic Surgery*. 1995;60(Fig 2):S391–S394.

[7]   Filion RJ, Ellis CG. A finite difference model of O2 transport in aortic valve cusps: importance of intrinsic microcirculation. *American Journal of Physiology. Heart and Circulatory Physiology*. 2003 Nov;285(5):H2099–104.

[8]   Tseng H, Grande-Allen KJ. Elastic fibers in the aortic valve spongiosa: A fresh per-spective on its structure and role in overall tissue function. *Acta Biomaterialia*. 2011 Jan 19;7(5):2101–8.

[9]   Missirlis YF, Chong M. Aortic valve mechanics–Part I: material properties of natural porcine aortic valves. *Journal of Bioengineering*. 1978;2(3-4):287.

[10] Sauren AAHJ, van Hout MC, van Steenhoven AA, Veldpaus FE, Janssen JD. The me-chanical properties of porcine aortic valve tissues. *Journal of Biomechanics*. 1983 Jan; 16(5):327–37.

[11] Lee JM, Courtman DW, Boughner DR. The glutaraldehyde-stabilized porcine aortic valve xenograft. I. Tensile viscoelastic properties of the fresh leaflet material. *Journal of Biomedical Materials Research*. 1984 Jan;18(1):61–77.

[12] Hinton RB, Lincoln J, Deutsch GH, Osinska H, Manning PB, Benson DW, et al. Ex-tracellular matrix remodeling and organization in developing and diseased aortic valves. *Circulation Research*. 2006 Jun 9;98(11):1431–8.

[13] Chen WLK, Simmons CA. Lessons from (patho)physiological tissue stiffness and their implications for drug screening, drug delivery and regenerative medicine. *Advanced Drug Delivery Reviews*. 2011 Apr 30;63(4-5):269–76.

[14] Fondard O, Detaint D, Iung B, Choqueux C, Adle-Biassette H, Jarraya M, et al. Ex-tracellular matrix remodelling in human aortic valve disease: the role of matrix met-alloproteinases and their tissue inhibitors. *European Heart Journal*. 2005 Jul;26(13): 1333–41.

[15] Edep ME, Shirani J, Wolf P, Brown DL. Matrix metalloproteinase expression in non-rheumatic aortic stenosis. *Cardiovascular Pathology*. 9(5):281–6.

[16] Aikawa E, Aikawa M, Libby P, Figueiredo J-L, Rusanescu G, Iwamoto Y, et al. Arteri-al and aortic valve calcification abolished by elastolytic cathepsin S deficiency in chronic renal disease. *Circulation*. 2009 Apr 7;119(13):1785–94.

[17] Mohler, III ER, Gannon FH, Reynolds C, Zimmerman R, Keane MG, Kaplan FS. Bone formation and inflammation in cardiac valves. *Circulation*. 2001 Mar 20;103(11):1522–8.

[18] Simionescu A, Simionescu DT, Vyavahare NR. Osteogenic responses in fibroblasts activated by elastin degradation products and transforming growth factor-beta1: role of myofibroblasts in vascular calcification. *American Journal of Pathology*. 2007 Jul; 171(1):116–23.

[19] Rodriguez KJ, Masters KS. Regulation of valvular interstitial cell calcification by components of the extracellular matrix. *Journal of Biomedical Materials Research. Part A*. 2009 Sep 15;90(4):1043–53.

[20] Bailey AJ, Paul RG, Knott L. Mechanisms of maturation and ageing of collagen. *Mechanisms of Ageing and Development*. 1998 Dec 1;106(1-2):1–56.

[21] Ottani V, Martini D, Franchi M, Ruggeri A, Raspanti M. Hierarchical structures in fibrillar collagens. *Micron*. 2002 Jan;33(7-8):587–96.

[22] Doehring TC, Kahelin M, Vesely I. Mesostructures of the aortic valve. *Journal of Heart Valve Disease*. 2005 Sep;14(5):679–86.

[23] Eriksen HA, Satta J, Risteli J, Veijola M, Väre P, Soini Y. Type I and type III collagen synthesis and composition in the valve matrix in aortic valve stenosis. *Atherosclerosis*. 2006 Nov;189(1):91–8.

[24] Kunzelman KS, Cochran RP, Murphree SS, Ring WS, Verrier ED, Eberhart RC. Differential collagen distribution in the mitral valve and its influence on biomechanical behaviour. *Journal of Heart Valve Disease*. 1993 Mar;2(2):236–44.

[25] Latif N, Sarathchandra P, Taylor PM, Antoniw J, Yacoub MH. Localization and pattern of expression of extracellular matrix components in human heart valves. *Journal of Heart Valve Disease*. 2005 Mar;14(2):218–27.

[26] Cole WG, Chan D, Hickey AJ, Wilcken DEL. Collagen composition of normal and myxomatous human mitral heart valves. *Biochemical Journal*. 1984 Apr 15;219(2):451–60.

[27] Ku C-H, Johnson PH, Batten P, Sarathchandra P, Chambers RC, Taylor PM, et al. Collagen synthesis by mesenchymal stem cells and aortic valve interstitial cells in response to mechanical stretch. *Cardiovascular Research*. 2006 Aug 1;71(3):548–56.

[28] de Hart J, Peters GWM, Schreurs PJG, Baaijens FPT. Collagen fibers reduce stresses and stabilize motion of aortic valve leaflets during systole. *Journal of Biomechanics*. 2004 Mar;37(3):303–11.

[29] Sacks MS, Smith DB, Hiester ED. The aortic valve microstructure: effects of transvalvular pressure. *Journal of Biomedical Materials Research*. 1998 Jul;41(1):131–41.

[30] Vesely I, Noseworthy R. Micromechanics of the fibrosa and the ventricularis in aortic valve leaflets. *Journal of Biomechanics*. 1992 Jan;25(1):101–13.

[31] Balguid A, Rubbens MP, Mol A, Bank RA, Bogers AJJC, van Kats JP, et al. The role of collagen cross-links in biomechanical behavior of human aortic heart valve leaflets-- relevance for tissue engineering. *Tissue Engineering*. 2007 Jul;13(7):1501–11.

[32] Stephens EH, de Jonge N, McNeill MP, Durst CA, Grande-Allen KJ. Age-related changes in material behavior of porcine mitral and aortic valves and correlation to matrix composition. *Tissue Engineering. Part A*. 2010 Mar;16(3):867–78.

[33] Dreger SA, Thomas PS, Sachlos E, Chester AH, Czernuszka JT, Taylor PM, et al. Potential for synthesis and degradation of extracellular matrix proteins by valve interstitial cells seeded onto collagen scaffolds. *Tissue Engineering*. 2006 Sep;12(9):2533–40.

[34] Stephens EH, Grande-Allen KJ. Age-related changes in collagen synthesis and turnover in porcine heart valves. *Journal of Heart Valve Disease*. 2007 Nov;16(6):672–82.

[35] Masters KS, Shah DN, Walker GA, Leinwand LA, Anseth KS. Designing scaffolds for valvular interstitial cells: cell adhesion and function on naturally derived materials. *Journal of Biomedical Materials Research. Part A*. 2004 Oct 1;71(1):172–80.

[36] Taylor PM, Sachlos E, Dreger SA, Chester AH, Czernuszka JT, Yacoub MH. Interaction of human valve interstitial cells with collagen matrices manufactured using rapid prototyping. *Biomaterials*. 2006 May;27(13):2733–7.

[37] Yip CYY, Chen J-H, Zhao R, Simmons CA. Calcification by valve interstitial cells is regulated by the stiffness of the extracellular matrix. *Arteriosclerosis, Thrombosis, and Vascular Biology*. 2009 Jun;29(6):936–42.

[38] Wagenseil JE, Mecham RP. New insights into elastic fiber assembly. *Birth Defects Research Part C: Embryo Today: Reviews*. 2007 Dec;81(4):229–40.

[39] Mecham RP, Davis EC. Elastic fiber structure and assembly. In: Yurchenco PD, Birk DE, Mecham RP, editors. *Extracellular Matrix Assembly and Structure*. 1994. p. 281–314.

[40] Haston JL, Engelsen SB, Roessle M, Clarkson J, Blanch EW, Baldock C, et al. Raman microscopy and X-ray diffraction, a combined study of fibrillin-rich microfibrillar elasticity. *Journal of Biological Chemistry*. 2003 Oct 17;278(42):41189–97.

[41] Bax DV, Mahalingam Y, Cain S, Mellody K, Freeman L, Younger K, et al. Cell adhesion to fibrillin-1: identification of an Arg-Gly-Asp-dependent synergy region and a heparin-binding site that regulates focal adhesion formation. *Journal of Cell Science*. 2007 Apr 15;120(Pt 8):1383–92.

[42] Stephens EH, Kearney DL, Grande-Allen KJ. Insight into pathologic abnormalities in congenital semilunar valve disease based on advances in understanding normal valve microstructure and extracellular matrix. *Cardiovascular Pathology*. 2011 Feb 22.

[43] Schoen FJ. Cardiac valve prostheses: pathological and bioengineering considerations. *Journal of Cardiac Surgery*. 1987 Mar;2(1):65–108.

[44] Klövekorn WP, Meisner H, Paek SU, Sebening F. Long-term results after right ventricular outflow tract reconstruction with porcine and allograft conduits. *Thoracic and Cardiovascular Surgeon*. 1991 Dec;39 Suppl 3:225–7.

[45] Misfeld M, Sievers H-H. Heart valve macro- and microstructure. *Philosophical Transactions of the Royal Society of London. Series B, Biological Sciences*. 2007 Aug 29;362(1484):1421–36.

[46] Scott MJ, Vesely I. Morphology of porcine aortic valve cusp elastin. *Journal of Heart Valve Disease*. 1996 Sep;5(5):464–71.

[47] Vesely I. The role of elastin in aortic valve mechanics. *Journal of Biomechanics*. 1998 Feb;31(2):115–23.

[48] Stella JA, Sacks MS. On the biaxial mechanical properties of the layers of the aortic valve leaflet. *Journal of Biomechanical Engineering*. 2007 Oct;129(5):757–66.

[49] Konig K, Schenke-Layland K, Riemann I, Stock UA. Multiphoton autofluorescence imaging of intratissue elastic fibers. *Biomaterials*. 2005;26(5):495–500.

[50] Christov AM, Liu L, Lowe S, Icton C, Dunmore-Buyze J, Boughner DR, et al. Laser-induced fluorescence (LIF) recognition of the structural composition of porcine heart valves. *Photochemistry and Photobiology*. 1999 Mar;69(3):382–9.

[51] Talman EA, Boughner DR. Glutaraldehyde fixation alters the internal shear properties of porcine aortic heart valve tissue. *Annals of Thoracic Surgery*. 1995 Aug;60(2 Suppl):S369–73.

[52] Talman EA, Boughner DR. Effect of altered hydration on the internal shear properties of porcine aortic valve cusps. *Annals of Thoracic Surgery*. 2001 May;71(5 Suppl):S375–8.

[53] Vesely I, Boughner DR, Song T. Tissue buckling as a mechanism of bioprosthetic valve failure. *Annals of Thoracic Surgery*. 1988;46(3):302–8.

[54] Esko JD, Kimata K, Lindahl U. Proteoglycans and Sulfated Glycosaminoglycans. In: Varki A, Cummings RD, Esko JD, editors. *Essentials of Glycobiology*. 2nd editio. 2009.

[55] Silbert JE, Sugumaran G. Biosynthesis of chondroitin/dermatan sulfate. *IUBMB Life*. 2002 Oct;54(4):177–86.

[56] Bodevin-Authelet S, Kusche-Gullberg M, Pummill PE, DeAngelis PL, Lindahl U. Biosynthesis of hyaluronan: direction of chain elongation. *Journal of Biological Chemistry*. 2005 Mar 11;280(10):8813–8.

[57] Sasisekharan R, Venkataraman G. Heparin and heparan sulfate: biosynthesis, structure and function. *Current Opinion in Chemical Biology*. 2000 Dec;4(6):626–31.

[58] Funderburgh JL. Keratan sulfate: structure, biosynthesis, and function. *Glycobiology.* 2000 Oct;10(10):951–8.

[59] Prydz K, Dalen KT. Synthesis and sorting of proteoglycans. *Journal of Cell Science.* 2000 Jan;113 Pt 2:193–205.

[60] Murata K. Acidic glycosaminoglycans in human heart valves. *Journal of Molecular and Cellular Cardiology.* 1981 Mar;13(3):281–92.

[61] Iozzo RV. Matrix proteoglycans: from molecular design to cellular function. *Annual Review of Biochemistry.* 1998 Jan;67:609–52.

[62] Wight TN. Versican: a versatile extracellular matrix proteoglycan in cell biology. *Current Opinion in Cell Biology.* 2002 Oct;14(5):617–23.

[63] Bhatia A, Vesely I. The effect of glycosaminoglycans and hydration on the viscoelastic properties of aortic valve cusps. *Conference Proceedings: Annual International Conference of the IEEE Engineering in Medicine and Biology Society.* 2005 Jan;3:2979–80.

[64] Lincoln J, Lange AW, Yutzey KE. Hearts and bones: shared regulatory mechanisms in heart valve, cartilage, tendon, and bone development. *Developmental Biology.* 2006 Jun 15;294(2):292–302.

[65] Stephens EH, Saltarrelli JG, Baggett LS, Nandi I, Kuo JJ, Davis AR, et al. Differential proteoglycan and hyaluronan distribution in calcified aortic valves. *Cardiovascular Pathology.* 2010 Dec 23;

[66] Taylor KR, Gallo RL. Glycosaminoglycans and their proteoglycans: host-associated molecular patterns for initiation and modulation of inflammation. *FASEB Journal.* 2006 Jan;20(1):9–22.

[67] Grande-Allen KJ, Osman N, Ballinger ML, Dadlani HM, Marasco S, Little PJ. Glycosaminoglycan synthesis and structure as targets for the prevention of calcific aortic valve disease. *Cardiovascular Research.* 2007 Oct 1;76(1):19–28.

[68] Felding-Habermann B, Cheresh DA. Vitronectin and its receptors. *Current Opinion in Cell Biology.* 1993 Oct;5(5):864–8.

[69] Preissner KT, Seiffert D. Role of vitronectin and its receptors in haemostasis and vascular remodeling. *Thrombosis Research.* 1998 Jan 1;89(1):1–21.

[70] Akhtar S, Meek KM, James V. Immunolocalization of elastin, collagen type I and type III, fibronectin, and vitronectin in extracellular matrix components of normal and myxomatous mitral heart valve chordae tendineae. *Cardiovascular Pathology.* 1999;8(4):203–11.

[71] Pankov R, Yamada KM. Fibronectin at a glance. *Journal of Cell Science.* 2002 Oct 15;115(Pt 20):3861–3.

[72] Valenick LV, Hsia HC, Schwarzbauer JE. Fibronectin fragmentation promotes al-pha4beta1 integrin-mediated contraction of a fibrin-fibronectin provisional matrix. *Experimental Cell Research*. 2005 Sep;309(1):48–55.

[73] Ffrench-Constant C, Van de Water L, Dvorak HF, Hynes RO. Reappearance of an embryonic pattern of fibronectin splicing during wound healing in the adult rat. *The Journal of Cell Biology*. 1989 Aug;109(2):903–14.

[74] George EL, Georges-Labouesse EN, Patel-King RS, Rayburn H, Hynes RO. Defects in mesoderm, neural tube and vascular development in mouse embryos lacking fibro-nectin. *Development*. 1993 Dec;119(4):1079–91.

[75] Fayet C, Bendeck MP, Gotlieb AI. Cardiac valve interstitial cells secrete fibronectin and form fibrillar adhesions in response to injury. *Cardiovascular Pathology*. 2007;16(4):203–11.

[76] Combs MD, Yutzey KE. Heart valve development: regulatory networks in develop-ment and disease. *Circulation Research*. 2009 Aug 28;105(5):408–21.

[77] Gillan L, Matei D, Fishman DA, Gerbin CS, Karlan BY, Chang DD. Periostin secreted by epithelial ovarian carcinoma is a ligand for alpha(V)beta(3) and alpha(V)beta(5) integrins and promotes cell motility. *Cancer Research*. 2002 Sep 15;62(18):5358–64.

[78] Tilman G, Mattiussi M, Brasseur F, van Baren N, Decottignies A. Human periostin gene expression in normal tissues, tumors and melanoma: evidences for periostin production by both stromal and melanoma cells. *Molecular Cancer*. 2007 Jan;6:80.

[79] Polizzotti BD, Arab S, Kühn B. Intrapericardial delivery of gelfoam enables the tar-geted delivery of Periostin peptide after myocardial infarction by inducing fibrin clot formation. *PloS One*. 2012 Jan;7(5):e36788.

[80] Kruzynska-Frejtag A, Machnicki M, Rogers R, Markwald RR, Conway SJ. Periostin (an osteoblast-specific factor) is expressed within the embryonic mouse heart during valve formation. *Mechanisms of Development*. 2001 May;103(1-2):183–8.

[81] Kern CB, Hoffman S, Moreno R, Damon BJ, Norris RA, Krug EL, et al. Immunolocali-zation of chick periostin protein in the developing heart. *The Anatomical Record. Part A, Discoveries in Molecular, Cellular, and Evolutionary Biology*. 2005 May;284(1):415–23.

[82] Ashizawa N, Graf K, Do YS, Nunohiro T, Giachelli CM, Meehan WP, et al. Osteopon-tin is produced by rat cardiac fibroblasts and mediates A(II)-induced DNA synthesis and collagen gel contraction. *Journal of Clinical Investigation*. 1996 Nov;98(10):2218–27.

[83] Wang KX, Denhardt DT. Osteopontin: role in immune regulation and stress respons-es. *Cytokine & Growth Factor Reviews*. 2008;19(5-6):333–45.

[84] Choi ST, Kim JH, Kang E-J, Lee S-W, Park M-C, Park Y-B, et al. Osteopontin might be involved in bone remodelling rather than in inflammation in ankylosing spondylitis. *Rheumatology*. 2008 Dec;47(12):1775–9.

[85] Srivatsa SS, Harrity PJ, Maercklein PB, Kleppe L, Veinot J, Edwards W, et al. Increased cellular expression of matrix proteins that regulate mineralization is associated with calcification of native human and porcine xenograft bioprosthetic heart valves. *Journal of Clinical Investigation*. 1997 Mar 1;99(5):996–1009.

[86] Rajamannan NM, Subramaniam M, Rickard D, Stock SR, Donovan J, Springett M, et al. Human aortic valve calcification is associated with an osteoblast phenotype. *Circulation*. 2003 May 6;107(17):2181–4.

[87] Lee NK, Sowa H, Hinoi E, Ferron M, Ahn JD, Confavreux C, et al. Endocrine regulation of energy metabolism by the skeleton. *Cell*. 2007 Aug 10;130(3):456–69.

[88] Gundberg CM, Hauschka PV, Lian JB, Gallop PM. Osteocalcin: isolation, characterization, and detection. *Methods in Enzymology*. 1984 Jan;107(1975):516–44.

[89] Rajamannan NM, Nealis TB, Subramaniam M, Pandya S, Stock SR, Ignatiev CI, et al. Calcified rheumatic valve neoangiogenesis is associated with vascular endothelial growth factor expression and osteoblast-like bone formation. *Circulation*. 2005 Jun 21;111(24):3296–301.

[90] Levy RJ, Zenker JA, Lian JB. Vitamin K-dependent calcium binding proteins in aortic valve calcification. *Journal of Clinical Investigation*. 1980 Feb;65(2):563–6.

[91] Nagase H, Visse R, Murphy G. Structure and function of matrix metalloproteinases and TIMPs. *Cardiovascular Research*. 2006 Feb;69(3):562–73.

[92] Kaden JJ, Dempfle C-E, Grobholz R, Fischer CS, Vocke DC, Kiliç R, et al. Inflammatory regulation of extracellular matrix remodeling in calcific aortic valve stenosis. *Cardiovascular Pathology*. 2005;14(2):80–7.

[93] Yip CYY, Simmons CA. The aortic valve microenvironment and its role in calcific aortic valve disease. *Cardiovascular Pathology*. 2011;20(3):177–82.

[94] Kreis T, Vale R. Guidebook to the Extracellular Matrix, Anchor, and Adhesion Proteins. 2nd ed. Kreis T, Vale R, editors. 1999.

[95] Timpl R, Rohde H, Robey PG, Rennard SI, Foidart J-M, Martin GR. Laminin--a glycoprotein from basement membranes. *Journal of Biological Chemistry*. 1979 Oct 10;254(19):9933–7.

[96] Durbeej M. Laminins. *Cell and Tissue Research*. 2010 Jan;339(1):259–68.

[97] Okazaki I, Suzuki N, Nishi N, Utani A, Matsuura H, Shinkai H, et al. Identification of biologically active sequences in the laminin alpha 4 chain G domain. *Journal of Biological Chemistry*. 2002 Oct;277(40):37070–8.

[98] Pradhan S, Farach-Carson MC. Mining the extracellular matrix for tissue engineering applications. *Regenerative Medicine*. 2010 Nov;5(6):961–70.

[99]   McGowan KA, Marinkovich MP. Laminins and human disease. *Microscopy Research and Technique*. 2000 Nov 1;51(3):262–79.

[100] Hozumi K, Suzuki N, Nielsen PK, Nomizu M, Yamada Y. Laminin alpha1 chain LG4 module promotes cell attachment through syndecans and cell spreading through integrin alpha2beta1. *Journal of Biological Chemistry*. 2006 Oct;281(43):32929–40.

[101] Ponce ML, Nomizu M, Delgado MC, Kuratomi Y, Hoffman MP, Powell S, et al. Identification of endothelial cell binding sites on the laminin gamma 1 chain. *Circulation Research*. 1999 Apr;84(6):688–94.

[102] Gwanmesia P, Ziegler H, Eurich R, Barth M, Kamiya H, Karck M, et al. Opposite effects of transforming growth factor-β1 and vascular endothelial growth factor on the degeneration of aortic valvular interstitial cell are modified by the extracellular matrix protein fibronectin: implications for heart valve engineering. *Tissue Engineering. Part A*. 2010 Dec;16(12):3737–46.

[103] Gu X, Masters KS. Regulation of valvular interstitial cell calcification by adhesive peptide sequences. *Journal of Biomedical Materials Research. Part A*. 2010 Jun 15;93(4):1620–30.

[104] Genové E, Shen C, Zhang S, Semino CE. The effect of functionalized self-assembling peptide scaffolds on human aortic endothelial cell function. *Biomaterials*. 2005 Jun;26(16):3341–51.

[105] Ishijima M, Suzuki N, Hozumi K, Matsunobu T, Kosaki K, Kaneko H, et al. Perlecan modulates VEGF signaling and is essential for vascularization in endochondral bone formation. *Matrix Biology*. 2012 May;31(4):234–45.

[106] Knox SM, Whitelock JM. Perlecan: how does one molecule do so many things? *Cellular and Molecular Life Sciences*. 2006 Nov;63(21):2435–45.

[107] Farach-Carson MC, Carson DD. Perlecan--a multifunctional extracellular proteoglycan scaffold. *Glycobiology*. 2007 Sep;17(9):897–905.

[108] Ellis AL, Pan W, Yang G, Jones K, Chuang C, Whitelock JM, et al. Similarity of recombinant human perlecan domain 1 by alternative expression systems bioactive heterogenous recombinant human perlecan D1. *BMC Biotechnology*. 2010 Jan;10:66.

[109] Chen J-H, Simmons CA. Cell-matrix interactions in the pathobiology of calcific aortic valve disease: critical roles for matricellular, matricrine, and matrix mechanics cues. *Circulation Research*. 2011 Jun;108(12):1510–24.

[110] Wilkinson TS, Bressler SL, Evanko SP, Braun KR, Wight TN. Overexpression of hyaluronan synthases alters vascular smooth muscle cell phenotype and promotes monocyte adhesion. *Journal of Cellular Physiology*. 2006 Feb;206(2):378–85.

[111] Nakashima Y, Fujii H, Sumiyoshi S, Wight TN, Sueishi K. Early human atherosclerosis: accumulation of lipid and proteoglycans in intimal thickenings followed by mac-

rophage infiltration. *Arteriosclerosis, Thrombosis, and Vascular Biology*. 2007 May;27(5): 1159–65.

[112] Wight TN. Cell biology of arterial proteoglycans. *Arteriosclerosis*. 1989;9(1):1–20.

[113] Yan J, Stringer SE, Hamilton A, Charlton-Menys V, Götting C, Müller B, et al. Decorin GAG synthesis and TGF-β signaling mediate Ox-LDL-induced mineralization of human vascular smooth muscle cells. *Arteriosclerosis, Thrombosis, and Vascular Biology*. 2011 Mar;31(3):608–15.

[114] Plenz GAM, Deng MC, Robenek H, Völker W. Vascular collagens: spotlight on the role of type VIII collagen in atherogenesis. *Atherosclerosis*. 2003 Jan;166(1):1–11.

[115] Parkin JD, San Antonio JD, Pedchenko V, Hudson B, Jensen ST, Savige J. Mapping structural landmarks, ligand binding sites, and missense mutations to the collagen IV heterotrimers predicts major functional domains, novel interactions, and variation in phenotypes in inherited diseases affecting basement membranes. *Human Mutation*. 2011 Feb;32(2):127–43.

[116] Soininen R, Haka-Risku T, Prockop DJ, Tryggvason K. Complete primary structure of the alpha 1-chain of human basement membrane (type IV) collagen. *FEBS Letters*. 1987 Dec;225(1-2):188–94.

[117] Shuttleworth CA. Type VIII collagen. *International Journal of Biochemistry & Cell Biology*. 1997 Oct;29(10):1145–8.

[118] Wells RG. Function and metabolism of collagen and other extracellular matrix proteins. In: Rodés J, Benhamou J-P, Blei A, Reichen J, Rizzetto M, editors. *Textbook of Hepatology*. 3rd ed. 2002. p. 264–73.

[119] Tsilibary EC, Reger LA, Vogel AM, Koliakos GG, Anderson SS, Charonis AS, et al. Identification of a multifunctional, cell-binding peptide sequence from the a1(NC1) of type IV collagen. *Journal of Cell Biology*. 1990 Oct;111(4):1583–91.

[120] Xu R, Yao Z-Y, Xin L, Zhang Q, Li T-P, Gan R-B. NC1 domain of human type VIII collagen (alpha 1) inhibits bovine aortic endothelial cell proliferation and causes cell apoptosis. *Biochemical and Biophysical Research Communications*. 2001 Nov 23;289(1): 264–8.

[121] Kang SH, Kramer JM. Nidogen is nonessential and not required for normal type IV collagen localization in Caenorhabditis elegans. *Molecular Biology of the Cell*. 2000 Nov;11(11):3911–23.

[122] Charest A, Pépin A, Shetty R, Côté C, Voisine P, Dagenais F, et al. Distribution of SPARC during neovascularisation of degenerative aortic stenosis. *Heart*. 2006 Dec; 92(12):1844–9.

[123] Chlenski A, Liu S, Crawford SE, Volpert OV, DeVries GH, Evangelista A, et al. SPARC is a key Schwannian-derived inhibitor controlling neuroblastoma tumor angiogenesis. *Cancer Research*. 2002 Dec 15;62(24):7357–63.

[124] Sage H. Pieces of eight: bioactive fragments of extracellular proteins as regulators of angiogenesis. *Trends in Cell Biology*. 1997 May;7(5):182–6.

[125] Kalluri R, Zeisberg E. Controlling angiogenesis in heart valves. *Nature Medicine*. 2006 Oct;12(10):1118–9.

Mechanisms of Calcific Aortic Valve Disease

Chapter 3

Developmental Pathways in CAVD

Elaine E. Wirrig and Katherine E. Yutzey

Additional information is available at the end of the chapter

1. Introduction

Calcific Aortic Valve Disease (CAVD) occurs in >2% of the population over 65 years of age and often leads to valvular stenosis that necessitates valve replacement [1]. CAVD is a progressive disease, often manifesting first as aortic valve sclerosis and later developing into stenosis and valve dysfunction [2]. The specific molecular and cellular mechanisms of CAVD initiation and advancement are not well defined, and inhibitors of CAVD progression have not been identified. The current standard of treatment for CAVD is aortic valve replacement [3]. Presently, there are no pharmacologic-based treatments for CAVD, and new therapeutic approaches for CAVD are needed. The majority of aortic valves that are replaced have congenital malformations, such as bicuspid aortic valve (BAV), establishing a link between valve development and disease mechanisms [4].

The molecular mechanisms of CAVD include activation of signaling pathways implicated in both heart valve development (valvulogenesis) and bone development (osteogenesis) [5-8]. These include activation of regulators of progenitor specification, cell proliferation, and differentiation. Heart valves and bone are complex connective tissues with compartmentalized ECM produced by specialized cell types. Over the past several years, extensive progress has been made in defining molecular regulatory mechanisms in heart valve and bone development (Reviewed in [8-10]). Strikingly, regulatory pathways that control development of cartilage, tendon and bone also are active in developing valves [8, 11]. In addition, recent studies have reported induction of molecular regulators of valvulogenesis and osteogenesis in CAVD [7, 12-14]. However, it is not known if these developmental mechanisms have reparative functions or contribute to the progression of CAVD.

Here we review molecular mechanisms of valve and bone development as they relate to molecular mechanisms of CAVD. Recent studies have provided evidence for the involvement of specific regulatory pathways in CAVD as activators or inhibitors of disease progression.

Additional research in animal models and human patient specimens is necessary to determine the detrimental molecular regulatory pathways that promote CAVD progression and
also beneficial pathways that potentially inhibit CAVD. In the future, manipulation of these
pathways could be exploited therapeutically in the treatment of patients with CAVD or with
aortic valve sclerosis that precedes calcification.

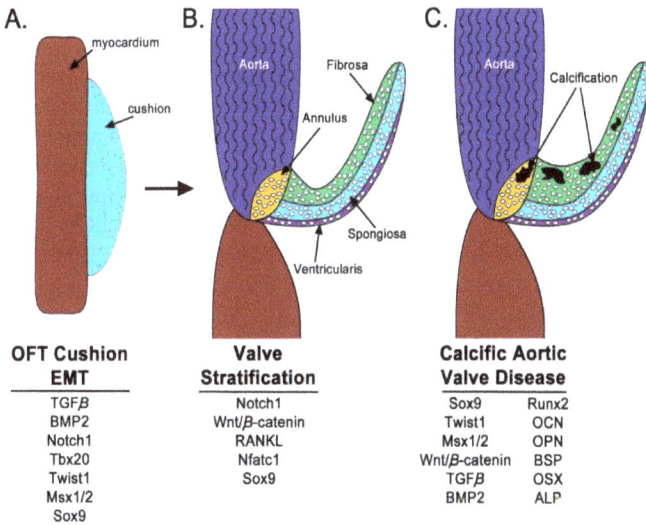

Figure 1. Molecular pathways active during endocardial cushion development and valve stratification are reactivated in CAVD. (A) Early stages of OFT cushion development are marked by ECM deposition, EMT, and neural crest cell infiltration. Factors necessary for EMT and mesenchymal cell function are expressed. (B) During late embryonic development
and early postnatal development, the aortic valve becomes stratified and possesses three ECM layers. Factors necessary for
ECM remodeling are active at this stage. (C) In CAVD, the ECM remodels and the valve becomes thickened. Calcification
(black nodules) is typically observed in the collagen-rich fibrosa layer. Many factors expressed during OFT cushion development and valve stratification are reactivated during disease. Furthermore, osteogenic factors involved in bone development are also observed in CAVD. Please see text for details and references. OFT = outflow tract, EMT = epithelial-to-
mesenchymal transition, ECM = extracellular matrix, CAVD = calcific aortic valve disease.

2. The cellular and molecular regulation of valve development

2.1. Overview of valve development

Valve development begins with the formation of endocardial cushions in the atrioventricular (AV) canal and outflow tract (OFT) of the primitive heart tube, which occurs at embryonic day (E)9-10 in mice, E3 in chickens, and E31-35 in humans [8]. The first evidence of
endocardial cushion formation is the separation of the endocardium and overlying myocardium in the AV canal by expansion of the cardiac jelly through increased expression of hya-

luronan (Figure 1) [15]. These swellings are invested with mesenchymal cells that arise from endothelial-to-mesenchymal transformation (EMT) of the endocardium [16]. Similar swelling and induction of EMT occur approximately a day later in the cardiac OFT cushions that will contribute to the semilunar valves [17]. Endocardial EMT is induced by signaling molecules, including bone morphogenetic proteins (BMPs), emanating from the adjacent myocardium in the AVC and OFT [8, 18-20]. Once established, the endocardial cushions expand through increased extracellular matrix (ECM) production and cell proliferation of mesenchymal and endothelial cells. The AV cushions subsequently fuse to separate right and left cardiac channels. In addition, lateral cushions are induced in the AV sulcus that will give rise to the mural leaflets of the mitral and tricuspid valves [21]. Neural crest cells (NCCs) migrate into the cushions of the cardiac OFT, contributing to the septum between the aortic and pulmonic roots and also to the morphogenesis of individual semilunar valve leaflets [21, 22]. At this point, distinct primordia of individual valve leaflets become apparent and proliferation of valve interstitial cells (VICs) is reduced [23]. Valve morphogenesis occurs with elongation and thinning of the valve primordia, in addition to ECM remodeling and stratification. In general, the development of the AV and semilunar (SL) valves is similar, but there are some differences in the sources of cells and structure of the resulting leaflets [8, 10, 11, 24]. In mature SL and AV valves, the ECM is stratified into collagen-rich fibrosa, proteoglycan-rich spongiosa, and elastin-rich (atrialis-ventricularis) layers oriented relative to blood flow [24].

2.2. Embryonic origins of valve cell lineages

The primary embryonic source of adult semilunar valve interstitial cells is the endothelial-derived cells of the endocardial cushions, that arise as a result of EMT as determined by Tie2-Cre lineage tracing in mice [23, 25]. Since the cardiac OFT is derived from the secondary heart field (SHF), semilunar VICs derived from OFT endocardium also are SHF-derived [20, 26]. NCC-derived cells are present in adult mouse semilunar valve leaflets as demonstrated by cell lineage tracing with Wnt1-Cre [27]. These cells are predominant throughout the aortic and pulmonic valve leaflets, but are enriched in the leaflets adjacent to the aorticopulmonary septum, which also is derived from NCCs [21, 28]. NCCs are required for semilunar valve morphogenesis and remodeling, likely by providing signals necessary for cell lineage differentiation and leaflet maturation [29, 30]. Another potential source of VICs is the epicardium, which contributes cells to the parietal leaflets of AV valves [31]. However, epicardial-derived cells (EPDCs) have not been not reported to contribute to the semilunar valves, based on Wt1-Cre fatemapping studies [31, 32]. Recent studies have reported that bone marrow-derived stem cells (BMSCs) are present in the developing and mature semilunar valves [33, 34]. Additional work is necessary to determine if these cells have lineages and functions distinct from the predominant endocardial cushion-derived or neural crest-derived VICs. It is possible that valve cell lineages derived from different developmental sources have distinct functions in normal and diseased aortic valves, but this has not yet been demonstrated. The sources of increased proliferative cells in diseased valves are relatively unknown, but could be any of these embryonic sources or, alternatively, an infiltrating cell type.

2.3. Transcription factors involved in valve development

Several transcription factors have been implicated in various processes of endocardial cushion formation and EMT (reviewed in [8, 35]). Notch pathway function in EMT is dependent on the transcription factor RBPJ, which activates expression of the bHLH transcription factor *snail1* (Snai1) in endothelial cells [36]. Snai1 represses *ve-cadherin* gene expression, and loss of Snai1 in endothelial cells inhibits endocardial cushion formation [36, 37]. The mesenchymal valve progenitor cells of the endocardial cushions express several transcription factors characteristic of a variety of embryonic mesenchymal progenitor populations. These factors include, Twist1, Msx1/2, Tbx20, and Sox9 [18, 38-41]. Gain and loss of function studies have demonstrated critical roles for Tbx20, Twist1, and Sox9 in endocardial cushion mesenchymal cell proliferation [38-40]. Twist1 promotes *tbx20* expression directly and also regulates several genes associated with cell proliferation and migration [38, 42]. After endocardial cushion fusion and formation of valve primordia, mesenchymal genes, notably *twist1* [43], are down-regulated and cell proliferation is decreased [23, 24, 44]. In normal adult valves, there is little to no cell proliferation [24, 44], and expression of valve developmental transcription factors including Twist1, Sox9, and Msx2 is not detectable [13]. However, all of these factors are predominantly expressed in adult human CAVD (see below).

Additional regulatory pathways control heart valve ECM remodeling and compartmentalization. Loss of NFATc1 results in defective remodeling of the AV and SL valves in mice, with embryonic lethality by E14.5 [45, 46]. EMT occurs with loss of NFATc1, but valve primordia fail to remodel and mature ECM molecules are not expressed in null mice or in cultured VICs with inhibition of receptor activator of nuclear factor κ-B ligand (RANKL) or calcineurin signaling upstream of NFATc1 activation [45, 47]. In addition to being required for endocardial cushion mesenchymal proliferation, Sox9 also promotes cartilage-like ECM gene expression in valve progenitor cells [48]. In late stage mouse embryos, loss of Sox9 in remodeling valves results in reduced proteoglycan expression, and Sox9 haploinsufficiency in adults leads to valve calcification [40, 49]. Conversely, the bHLH transcription factor Scleraxis, critical for tendon development, promotes expression of elastic/tendon-like matrix genes in cultured valve progenitor cells [48]. Loss of Scleraxis in mice is not lethal, but heart valve defects similar to myxomatous valve disease occur in these animals [50]. Little is known of the transcriptional regulatory mechanisms that control the development of the valve fibrosa layer, which is most critically involved in CAVD.

2.4. Signaling pathways in valve development

Several essential embryonic signaling pathways have been implicated in endocardial cushion formation and EMT (Table 1) (reviewed in [8]). Transforming growth factor (TGF)β signaling was the first pathway implicated in endocardial cushion formation and is required for EMT in chicken and mouse embryonic systems (reviewed in [16]). BMP signaling from the myocardium is required in endothelial cells for the initiation of EMT in the AV canal, and BMP2 and 4 are the predominant ligands involved in endocardial cushion development [18-20]. Notch signaling also is required for EMT as described above. Moreover, Notch signaling is required for expression of TGFβ ligands and receptors, in addition to activating

BMP signaling, which promotes mesenchymal cell invasion [36, 51]. Likewise, vascular endothelial growth factor (VEGF) signaling promotes endocardial cushion endothelial cell proliferation and EMT [47, 52]. Furthermore, targeted mutagenesis of β-catenin has implicated Wnt/β-catenin signaling in endocardial cushion EMT and mesenchymal proliferation [53, 54]. Thus multiple pathways are involved in endocardial cushion EMT and mesenchymal cell proliferation. However, the intersection and specific cellular functions of these pathways have not been fully determined.

A. Signaling pathways			
	Role in valvulogenesis	Role in osteogenesis	Role in CAVD
VEGF	EMT, endothelial proliferation	angiogenesis	angiogenesis
Notch	EMT	Inhibit OB differentiation	represses calcification
TGFβ	EMT	bone homeostasis	promotes VIC calcification
FGF	promotes tenascin expression	OB proliferation, differentiation	blocks VIC calcification
BMP	EMT, PG expression	promotes OB specification	active in CAVD
Wnt/β-catenin	EMT, fibrosa expression	promotes OB differentiation	active in CAVD
RANKL	ECM remodeling	OC differentiation	promotes VIC calcification
B. Transcription factors			
	Role in valvulogenesis	Role in osteogenesis	Role in CAVD
Twist1	ECC proliferation, migration	represses differentiation	active in CAVD
Msx2	EMT, proliferation	present in progenitors, OB	active in CAVD
Sox9	proliferation, PG expression	progenitor proliferation, cartilage differentiation	active in CAVD inhibits calcification
NFATc1	endothelial proliferation, ECM remodeling	promotes OC differentiation promotes OB differentiation	reported in CAVD
Runx2	not present	promotes OB differentiation	active in CAVD
Osterix	not present	promotes OB differentiation	reported in CAVD

[a]Please see text for details and references. [b]Abbreviations used: CAVD=calcific aortic valve disease; ECM=extracellular matrix; EMT=endothelial to mesenchymal transition; OB=osteoblast; OC=osteoclast; PG=proteoglycan; VIC=valve interstitial cell.

Table 1. Signaling pathways and transcription factors involved in valvulogenesis, osteogenesis, and CAVD[a, b]

Many of the signaling pathways important for endocardial cushion formation also have later functions in valve lineage diversification, remodeling, and stratification. However, these functions have been difficult to elucidate due to limitations of available genetic tools and critical requirements for these same regulatory pathways in endocardial cushion formation. BMP signaling, as indicated by phosphorylation of the intermediate signaling molecules Smad1/5/8, is active throughout endocardial cushion mesenchymal cells, is associated with mesenchymal cell proliferation [55], and also is active later in valve cell lineage diversification [48]. *BMP Receptor II* mutations and conditional mutagenesis results in thickening of semilunar valve leaflets at late fetal stages [56, 57]. Loss of inhibitory Smad6 leads to increased BMP signaling, in addition to thickening of valve leaflets and CAVD in adult animals [58]. Studies in explanted avian valve progenitors have revealed antagonistic regulatory roles for BMP and fibroblast growth factor (FGF) signaling in promoting diversified ECM gene expression, conserved with mechanisms that control cartilage and tendon lineage development [11, 48, 59]. Wnt pathway activation is evident throughout the remodeling AV and semilunar valve primordia, as indicated in TopGal reporter mice [60]. Multiple Wnt ligands are expressed during valvulogenesis, but the function of Wnt signaling in heart valve remodeling has not yet been determined [60]. Thus, additional in vivo studies are necessary to determine the specific functions and intersecting regulatory mechanisms of these critical signaling pathways in valve leaflet development and also to determine specific contributions to valve degeneration and disease.

The later stages of heart valve development are characterized by leaflet elongation, ECM remodeling, and stratification, all of which are critical for mature valve structure and function [24]. Limited information is available on the regulation of these processes, but several regulatory pathways have been implicated in late valve remodeling and morphogenesis. Strikingly these same pathways have been implicated in adult CAVD (see below). RANKL, expressed by valve endothelial cells, promotes ECM remodeling and Cathepsin K (Ctsk) expression by NFATc1 in a mechanism partially conserved with osteoclast differentiation and function [11, 47, 61]. The signaling mechanisms that control stratification and ECM organization of the valve leaflets are relatively unknown. Notch signaling is localized on the ventricularis surface of the remodeling aortic valve in mice [62], and Wnt/β-catenin signaling is active throughout aortic valve primordia at late gestation and in a subpopulation of VICs after birth [60]. Likewise, Wnt signaling promotes expression of fibrosa genes *periostin* and *matrix gla-protein (mgp)* in cultured chicken embryo aortic VICs, but a role in valve stratification or lineage diversification has not yet been established in vivo [60]. Additional studies are necessary to demonstrate the specific functions and potential biomechanical stimulation of these pathways in an in vivo context. Since, both Notch and Wnt signaling pathways are required for initial stages of endocardial cushion formation, it has been difficult to establish their roles in the later stages of valvulogenesis in vivo using available conditional targeting approaches.

Bicuspid aortic valve is arguably the most common congenital heart malformation with an incidence of 1-2% in the US adult population [63]. BAV often does not often manifest in valve dysfunction in early life, but malformed aortic valves are predisposed to calcification. Strikingly, the majority of stenotic aortic valves that are replaced in adults are congenitally malformed [4]. However, the molecular and cellular mechanisms of BAV are not well defined. In humans, mutations in *NOTCH1* are associated with BAV, but the mechanisms by which valve leaflet number is regulated by Notch signaling have not yet been identified [64]. Likewise, Notch1 haploinsufficiency in mice leads to BAV at very low penetrance and there are likely to be additional factors necessary for congenital malformation of the aortic valve leaflets [65]. Loss of the zinc finger transcription factor GATA5 in mice [66] and mutations in human *GATA5* [67] are associated with BAV with incomplete penetrance. Likewise eNOS haploinsufficiency also leads to BAV, albeit with incomplete penetrance [68]. The mechanisms by which these genetic lesions lead to BAV in some individuals and not others are not known. However, based on the expression and function of Notch1, GATA5, and eNOS in endothelial cells, it is likely that these cells contribute to development of BAV in these models. The link between BAV and CAVD could be due to similar regulatory mechanisms in development and disease or could, alternatively, result from induction of calcification in a hemodynamically compromised congenitally malformed aortic valve (see other chapters for a more complete discussion of BAV and CAVD).

2.5. Extracellular matrix composition and stratification of the developing valves

The mature valve leaflets are composed of stratified ECM with layered compartments of fibrillar collagen, proteoglycan, and elastin (Figure 1) (reviewed in [10, 69]). During heart valve remodeling, there is little proliferation of VICs, but the cells are highly synthetic and produce multiple ECM proteins of the mature leaflets [24, 44]. The distinct layers of matrix are integral to heart valve function and confer specific biomechanical properties to the valve leaflets [69]. The regulatory mechanisms for ECM remodeling and stratification are not well defined but are relevant to heart valve disease mechanisms. Periostin is required for collagen remodeling, and loss of periostin in mice leads to adult valve malformations and cardiac dysfunction [70, 71]. Likewise, mutations in *Collagen 1a2* or elastin haploinsufficiency also result in aortic valve dysmorphogenesis and adult disease [72, 73]. Gene expression of *CtsK*, a matrix remodeling enzyme expressed during heart valve elongation, is regulated by the RANKL/NFATc1 regulatory pathway [47, 61]. Additional ECM remodeling enzymes, including matrix metalloproteinase (MMP)13, a collagenase, and Adam-TS5 and 9 proteoglycan proteases, also are expressed during late valve morphogenesis and have been implicated in ECM maturation and organization [39, 74, 75]. Several ECM molecules required for normal valve structure/function also are expressed during osteogenesis, and valve progenitors have gene expression profiles similar to bone progenitors [43]. *Osteopontin, osteonectin,* and *periostin* gene expression and collagen fiber deposition are increased during heart valve remodeling [24, 43, 60]. However, the regulatory mechanisms for expression of these genes in valve development are not well defined. These proteins also are induced and mislocalized in pediatric and adult heart valve disease [13, 24, 70], but the pathways leading to their dysregulation have not yet been fully characterized.

3. Molecular mechanisms of osteogenesis

3.1. Overview of skeletal development

Many osteogenic regulatory interactions identified in developing bone also are active in CAVD (Table 1). The regulatory hierarchies and ECM composition of the developing valves, most notably the collagen rich fibrosa layer, are similar to those observed in osteoblast precursor cells [43]. Both the bone substratum and valve ECM are composed primarily of fibrillar collagen. Thus, it is not surprising that there are extensive similarities in their composition and developmental regulation. Normally, heart valves do not progress to mineralization, but striking similarities have been identified between osteogenic pathways that regulate bone mineralization and CAVD mechanisms [7]. Thus the molecular understanding of normal development of bone has clear implications for pathogenic mechanisms of connective tissue mineralization, including CAVD.

The osteogenic precursors of the developing axial skeleton and long bones of the limbs are derived primarily from paraxial mesoderm of the developing somites and also lateral plate mesoderm, the main source of cardiac precursor cells [76, 77]. Additional progenitors of the craniofacial skeleton are derived from cranial neural crest [78]. Most axial skeletal elements develop by endochondral bone formation that occurs through a cartilage intermediate [76, 77]. Alternatively, the craniofacial bones of the skull form through membranous ossification in which condensed osteogenic progenitors differentiate directly into bone and do not go through a cartilage intermediate [76]. The osteochondroprogenitors present in the axial and appendicular skeletal elements develop into both bone and cartilage lineages [77, 79, 80]. Extensive research over the past several years has defined transcriptional regulatory mechanisms and signaling events that control the development of cartilage and bone (Figure 2) [79, 80].

Mature cartilage is composed predominantly of chondroitin sulfate proteoglycans that provides cushioning and flexibility to cartilaginous structures [77, 81]. In addition, the proteoglycan-rich ECM is angiostatic and mature cartilage is avascular [81]. Interestingly, the predominant proteoglycan composition and lack of vasculature also are features of the mature aortic valve leaflet spongiosa layer [82]. Likewise, the cartilage ECM inhibits mineralization, and a similar role has been hypothesized for the proteoglycan-rich matrix of the aortic valve [49]. During normal axial bone development, osteoblasts from the laterally placed periostium differentiate into trabecular bone, and secondary ossification centers at the ends of the bone displace the growth plate hypertrophic cartilage [79, 80]. During bone differentiation, hypertrophic cartilage cells must die for mineralization to occur in a process of endochondral ossification, which could be related to dystrophic mechanisms of CAVD [79, 80].

Bone cell lineage maturation goes through multiple stages defined by molecular regulatory mechanisms that also are active in valve development and disease processes [80]. Osteochondroprogenitor cells express several mesenchymal transcription factors, including Twist1, Msx2, and Sox9, that also are predominant in valve progenitor cells and diseased aortic valves [79]. Immature pre-osteoblasts express high levels of fibrillar type 1 collagen, in addition to periostin, osteonectin, and osteopontin, similar to normal differentiated VICs [43, 60]. Differentiated osteoblasts are not yet mineralized but express the transcription factor Runx2, in addition to osteocalcin and bone sialoprotein involved in bone mineralization and also in valve calcification, [7, 80]. Later stage osteoblasts and osteocytes express the transcription factor Osterix (Osx), which is regulated by Runx2 and is required for mature bone formation [83]. Bone mineralization occurs with the deposition of calcium phosphate and hydroxyapatite by osteocytes and is dependent on Runx2 and Osx function [80]. Bone homeostasis is maintained throughout life by the osteogenic activity of osteocytes and bone resorption activity of osteoclasts [80].

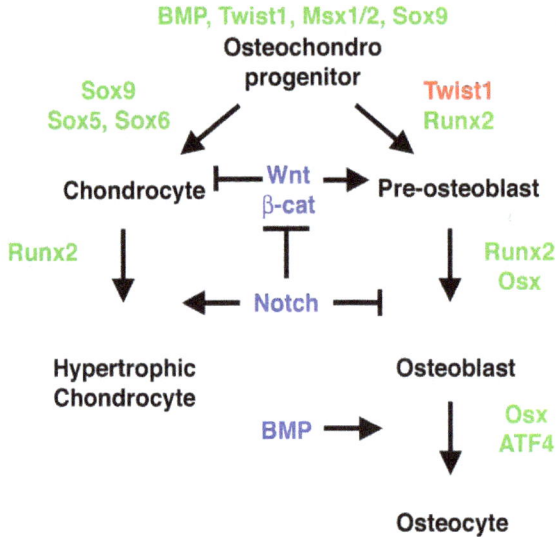

Figure 2. Hierarchies of signaling pathways and transcription factors regulate the differentiation of chondrogenic and osteogenic progenitor cells during skeletal development. Early osteochondrogenic progenitor cells express BMPs, Twist1, Msx1/2, and Sox9. Wnt/β-catenin signaling promotes pre-osteoblast differentiation while inhibiting chondrocyte differentiation. In contrast, Notch signaling promotes cartilage differentiation and inhibits osteoblast differentiation. BMP signaling is further required for osteocyte differentiation in the final stages of bone maturation. Sox5, 6, and 9 are transcription factors crucial for maintaining the chondrogenic lineage, whereas, Runx2, Osx, and ATF4 are transcription factors necessary for osteoblast and osteocyte differentiation and maturation. Many of these factors are also expressed during calcific aortic valve disease and have been implicated in pathologic calcification. Please see text for details and references. Activating factors are shown in green, inhibitory factors are shown in red, and signaling pathways are indicated in blue.

3.2. Transcriptional regulation of osteoblast lineage development and bone differentiation

Twist1 is expressed early in the osteochondroprogenitor lineage and inhibits terminal differentiation of cartilage and bone [84]. In preosteoblasts, Twist1 binds to Runx2 and inhibits its transcriptional activation of bone differentiation genes including *osteocalcin* [84]. Similarly, Twist1 can inhibit cartilage differentiation by binding to Sox9 and preventing activation of cartilage-specific gene expression [85]. Mutations in human *TWIST1* cause Saethre-Chotzen syndrome, characterized by premature bone differentiation evident in premature fusion of cranial sutures of the skull [86]. Msx2 also is involved in early mesenchymal stages of osteo-chondroprogenitor development and is down regulated during osteoblast differentiation [79]. Persistent Msx2 expression in osteoblasts prevents differentiation and mineralization, while antisense mRNA-mediated loss of Msx2 accelerates these processes [87]. Thus Msx2 is expressed in osteoblast progenitor cells but has an inhibitory role in osteogenic differentiation. Together Twist1 and Msx2 act to maintain undifferentiated osteochondroprogenitors during development.

Sox9 functions in the expansion of cartilage progenitors and promotes cartilage differentiation, while inhibiting bone differentiation [77, 80]. Sox9 is required for osteochondroprogenitor lineage specification but is not expressed in differentiated osteoblasts [88]. At early stages of cartilage lineage development, Sox9 promotes cell proliferation and later is required for cartilage lineage differentiation [88]. BMP signaling induces Sox9 gene expression in cartilage progenitor cells [89], and Sox9 regulates expression of cartilage marker genes Col2a1 and aggrecan [90, 91]. Sox9 transcriptional activity can be inhibited by binding to Twist1, thus inhibiting differentiation of early stage osteochondroprogenitor cells [85]. At later stages of cartilage maturation, Sox9 inhibits Runx2 transcriptional activity, thus promoting hypertrophic cartilage and inhibiting osteogenic differentiation [92]. Thus downregulation of Sox9 is required in osteoblasts for differentiation and mineralization of bone.

Runx2, originally called Cbfa1, has been defined as a master regulatory gene in bone formation [79, 93]. Gain and loss of function studies in mice demonstrate that Runx2 is both necessary and sufficient for osteoblast differentiation [93]. During bone development, Runx2 directly regulates osteocalcin gene expression [93]. Runx2 transcriptional function can be inhibited by interaction with Twist1 and also by Hey1, downstream of Notch signaling [84, 94]. Mice lacking Runx2 lack mineralized bone, and haploinsufficiency of Runx2 results in reduced bone formation in mice and humans [80]. Induction of a dominant negative form of Runx2 in differentiated osteoblasts after birth also leads to reduced bone mineralization, demonstrating a role for Runx2 in bone homeostasis and mineralization throughout life [95]. Runx2 has not been implicated in normal heart valve development, and its expression in developing valves has not been reported, consistent with the lack of calcification in normal valves. Likewise, in adult valves Runx2 is not normally expressed, but its expression is induced in CAVD in both humans and mice [13, 73]. The presence of Runx2 in diseased aortic valves and association with calcification is consistent with a role in mineralization, as has been established for bone cell lineages.

NFATc1 is a critical transcription factor in osteoclast differentiation and also has been implicated in osteoblast development [80, 96]. Osteoclasts, derived from a macrophage lineage, have bone resorptive activity and are necessary for bone homeostasis [96]. During osteoclast development, RANKL signaling induces activation of NFATc1, which promotes the transcription of bone matrix remodeling genes including CtsK and mmp9 [97, 98]. RANKL activity in bone is antagonized by the receptor decoy osteoprotegerin (OPG) that promotes bone calcification [99, 100]. In osteoblasts, NFATc1 promotes cell proliferation and also enhances differentiation by cooperating with Osx to promote Col1a1 gene expression [101, 102]. Thus, the balance of RANKL and OPG signaling acting on NFATc1 transcriptional function is a critical mediator of bone calcification and resorption [96]. A similar balance of OPG and RANKL signaling in CAVD has been proposed [103]. While NFATc1 is a critical regulator of heart valve remodeling during development and activates valvular *CtsK* expression [47, 61], its role in CAVD and adult valve homeostasis has not been determined.

Additional transcription factors involved in bone differentiation are not generally found in CAVD, although there are conflicting reports. Most notable is Osx, which is required for terminal differentiation of osteoblasts and mineralization of bone [83]. Osx, promotes expression of *collagen 1a1* and the matrix metalloproteinase *mmp13*, which also are upregulated in aortic valve disease [73, 101, 104, 105]. Studies based on antibody staining demonstrate Osx expression in Notch signaling-deficient calcified mouse valves [65] and human CAVD [106]. ATF4 is an additional transcription factor critical for bone differentiation, mineralization, and homeostasis that has not been found in developing or diseased valves [79]. Further studies are necessary to determine if *ATF4* or *Osx* gene expression is induced or if they contribute to valve mineralization in CAVD.

3.3. Signaling pathways involved in bone development

Multiple signaling pathways control the stages of bone cell lineage determination, differentiation and maturation [80, 107]. These include BMP, Wnt, and Notch pathways, also active in developing and diseased heart valves, as well as FGF, hedgehog, insulin-like growth factor (IGF), and retinoic acid (RA) pathways, not yet characterized in heart valve pathogenesis [80]. BMP, Wnt, and Notch pathways are required at multiple stages of osteogenesis and have distinct regulatory interactions that control transcription factor function and cell type-specific gene expression in cartilage and bone cell lineages (Figure 2). In addition, these pathways crosstalk with each other in synergistic and antagonistic regulatory interactions. Strikingly many of these same regulatory interactions occur in heart valve development and pathogenesis (Table 1) [8].

Bone morphogenetic proteins were originally identified based on their ability to induce ectopic bone formation [108]; however, in vivo functions in normal bone development are less clear [109]. In the developing limb buds, BMP signaling has a critical role in mesenchymal condensation, Sox9 activation, and cartilage lineage differentiation [89]. Thus BMP signaling is an important regulator of the earliest stages of skeletal development. Later in differentiating osteoblasts, BMP signaling through Smad1/5/8 phosphorylation (pSmad1/5/8) promotes osteogenic differentiation and calcification [110]. Runx2 directly binds to activated Smads1 and 5 to cooperatively activate osteoblast gene expression in response to BMP signaling [109]. Conditional loss of BMP2 and BMP4 in the osteoblast lineage in mice inhibits late stage differentiation into Osx1-positive osteocytes, and BMP signaling is required for bone homeostasis after birth [80, 109]. Surprisingly, earlier stages of bone lineage development are apparently unaffected with conditional loss of these ligands.

Wnt/β-catenin signaling is required for osteoblast differentiation as demonstrated by loss of osteoblast differentiation with conditional loss of β-catenin in osteochondroprogenitor cells in mice [80]. In addition, loss of β-catenin in pre-osteoblasts leads to ectopic cartilage formation, thus implicating Wnt signaling in osteogenic versus chondrogenic cell fate determination. At a molecular level, Wnt/β-catenin signaling promotes osteoblast lineage differentiation, while inhibiting chondrogenesis, by activating Runx2, while inhibiting Sox9 [77]. In bone lineages, BMP and Wnt signaling act synergistically to promote calcification, although neither pathway alone is sufficient to induce a full osteogenic response [111]. During the initial differentiation of bone progenitor cells, regulatory elements of *Runx2* and *Msx2* genes are bound by Smad1, downstream of BMP signaling, and also by Lef1, activated by Wnt signaling, for cooperative gene activation [112]. Postnatally, Wnt signaling through the Lrp5 receptor is required for bone accrual in mice and humans [80]. In developing bone, osteogenic differentiation and calcification are dependent on sequential activation of BMP, followed by Wnt/β-catenin, signaling [110]. It is possible that a similar regulatory relationship exists in CAVD, but this has not yet been demonstrated.

Notch activation inhibits osteogenesis through suppression of the Wnt/β-catenin pathway and Runx2 transcription factor activity [94, 113, 114]. Loss of Notch1 or Notch2 function promotes osteoblast differentiation and leads to increased bone mass in mice [115]. Notch pathway activation inhibits the progression of osteoblast differentiation through direct binding of the activated Notch1 intracellular domain (N1ICD) to β-catenin, thereby counteracting Wnt-mediated induction of osteogenesis [113, 114]. In addition, the Notch target gene *Hey1* encodes a transcriptional repressor that binds and inhibits Runx2 transcriptional function [115]. Precise levels of Notch signaling are required for cell proliferation and chondrogenic differentiation, with defects in these processes occurring with increased or decreased Notch signaling in mice [116]. In early cartilage precursors, Notch signaling is required for cell proliferation, but increased Notch signaling inhibits terminal differentiation of chondrocytes and endochondral ossification [116]. Loss of Notch signaling has been implicated in CAVD [64], but it is not known if this occurs through inhibition of Wnt/β-catenin signaling, as has been demonstrated for osteoblast differentiation and bone mineralization.

4. Molecular and cellular mechanisms of CAVD

4.1. Overview of CAVD progression

The mature aortic valves are comprised of three ECM layers critical for normal leaflet structure and function [24, 44, 117]. Collagen predominates in the fibrosa layer, which is oriented on the opposite side of blood flow, whereas elastin is enriched in the ventricularis layer on the flow side of the valve. Between the fibrosa and ventricularis layers, is the proteoglycan-rich spongiosa layer [24, 44, 117]. This trilaminar ECM arrangement is preserved among species, and lends both strength and elasticity to the aortic valves [24]. In CAVD, the aortic valve becomes thickened and displays extensive ECM remodeling and mineralization [118-121]. Abnormal thickening (aortic valve sclerosis) and calcification of the aortic valve lead to stiffening of the valve leaflets and can reduce the effective valve opening (aortic valve stenosis), which can impede blood flow and lead to clinical symptoms such as syncope and angina [119, 122, 123]. Histologically, human explanted diseased aortic valves have extensive ECM remodeling and elastic fiber fragmentation with evidence of both macroscopic calcific nodule formation as well as microscopic mineral deposits [119].

Changes in the resident VICs are apparent in CAVD. Under normal conditions, aortic VICs are quiescent and non-proliferative [13, 24, 104, 124]. However, in disease, a subset of aortic VICs exhibits features of myofibroblast activation, which is characterized by expression of α-smooth muscle actin (αSMA), MMP13, non-muscle myosin heavy chain (SMemb), and markers of proliferation [13, 104, 119, 124, 125]. In vivo, the factors responsible for inducing myofibroblast activation are not well defined. However, in culture, TGFβ1 stimulation and mechanical strain are potent inducers of VIC myofibroblast activation [125, 126]. Activated VICs also exhibit characteristics of valve and bone precursor cells as they induce expression of the common mesenchymal markers Sox9, Twist1, and Msx2 [13]. Currently it is unknown where the mesenchymal-like cells come from and what role these proliferative cells play in the progression of CAVD pathogenesis.

Valve calcification, apparent as hydroxyapatite deposits on the surface of or within the leaflets, is a prominent feature of CAVD [119, 127, 128]. Histologically, valve calcific nodules are primarily acellular [13, 129]. Although traditionally thought to be a completely passive deposition of mineral, in some cases, valve calcification is coincident with endochondral bone-like and cartilaginous-like nodules [129, 130]. Aortic valve calcification is observed primarily in the regions of the valves exposed to the greatest physical strain, specifically at the hinge region of the valve and along the line of leaflet coaptation [120]. Furthermore, calcification is predominantly found in the fibrosa layer of the diseased valve, which is similar to early bone matrix as it contains primarily fibrillar collagen [44]. Expression of other bone matrix molecules, such as osteocalcin and osteopontin, are induced during disease [5]. Furthermore, expression of osteogenic factors, such as Runx2, BMP2, and alkaline phosphatase, also is induced in VICs from calcified valves, suggesting that resident VICs may have the potential to undergo osteogenic transdifferentiation and actively contribute to valve calcification (reviewed in [131]).

Extrinsic factors have been implicated in valve calcification. For example, lipid deposition and immune cell infiltration are common histopathological features of CAVD, and it has been proposed that aortic valve calcification occurs by mechanisms similar to arterial calcification in atherosclerosis [119, 132-135]. In addition, altered external physical forces elicit changes in resident VICs, which play an active role in pathological valve calcification [126]. In contrast to VIC response to immune cell infiltration and altered physical forces, cell intrinsic mechanisms may also contribute to valve calcification, as stimulation with factors such as BMP2 or TGFβ1 in cell culture studies can induce VIC calcification in the absence of inflammatory stimulation or altered physical forces [126, 136-138]. Together, these studies suggest that not only is valve calcification an active cell-regulated process, but that many factors likely contribute to progression of calcification during disease. It is also likely that not all CAVD is created equal. Genetic predisposition, the presence of a malformed aortic valve, and other disease comorbidities, such as coronary artery disease, hypertension, and kidney disease, likely affect the pathology and underlying cause of CAVD [64, 139-142].

4.2. Activation of progenitor cell and osteogenesis-related molecular pathways in CAVD

4.2.1. Expression of valve and bone progenitor cell genes in CAVD

The mesenchymal markers Twist1, Msx2, and Sox9 are expressed in adult calcific aortic valves in mesenchymal-like activated VICs [12, 13, 106, 143, 144]. As discussed, these genes are expressed in both valve and bone mesenchymal progenitor cells. A recent study has compared gene expression in pediatric versus adult aortic valve disease and shown that the mesenchymal markers Twist1, Msx2, and Sox9 are increased in both [13]. The observation that both pediatric and adult diseased valves have increased expression of the mesenchymal markers suggests that this expression is related to VIC activation and proliferation, which is common to both, and not related to valve calcification, which is found only in advanced adult disease [13]. In both valve and bone progenitors, Twist1, Msx2, and Sox9 induce proliferation and promote a mesenchymal phenotype, thus reactivation in diseased valves is suggestive of a similar role in valve pathogenesis [38, 40-42, 84, 88, 145]. Although it is presumed that resident VICs re-activate these early mesenchymal markers, other possibilities exist. EMT as a mechanism for VIC activation has not been established in CAVD, however, recent studies report EMT-like events in adult valves. Increased cyclic strain and altered hemodynamics, both recognized features of CAVD, can induce EMT in isolated sheep valve endothelial cells [146, 147]. In addition, cultured valve endothelial cells stimulated with TGFβ adapt a mesenchymal-like phenotype and express markers of both endothelial and mesenchymal cells, suggesting that they can undergo EMT [148, 149]. Likewise, disruption of Notch signaling in adult mice induces aortic valve thickening with evidence of endocardial EMT, as indicated by endocardial cells with more pseudopodial projections, loose endocardial cell-cell junctions, and αSMA expression [150]. Additional sources of mesenchymal-like cells have been suggested. For example, circulating bone marrow-derived hematopoietic stem cells have been shown to integrate into the valve interstitium, adapt fibroblast-like characteristics, and surround regions of prominent valve calcification in human end stage CAVD [33, 130, 151]. It is uncertain what role reactivation of the mesenchymal markers Twist1, Msx2, and Sox9 have in potential valve repair mechanisms or in the progression of CAVD. It is possible that adult VICs maintain a certain "mesenchymal-plasticity" and are able to revert back to an early progenitor-like mesenchymal cell during disease. Alternatively, they may be indicators of newly derived VICs arising from EMT or circulating progenitor cell populations in response to disease conditions.

4.2.2. Osteogenic factors in CAVD

Molecular mechanisms of endochondral ossification and cartilaginous nodule formation are active in CAVD [7, 13]. Studies in human explanted diseased aortic valve tissues have demonstrated increased expression of the osteogenic factors BMP2, TGFβ1, Runx2, osteocalcin (OCN), osteopontin (OPN), osteoprotegerin (OPG), bone sialoprotein (BSP), alkaline phosphatase (ALP), and Osx in disease [5, 13, 106, 118, 137, 152]. At a molecular level, BMP2 signaling is a key inducer of VIC calcification, which is thought to act through p-SMAD1/5/8 and phospho-ERK1/2 signaling to stimulate increases in both Runx2 and OPN expression [138]. Induction of VIC calcification by BMP2 stimulation is highly reminiscent of BMP signaling in bone development, suggesting that some parallels exist between osteogenic bone formation and VIC calcification [9]. Histological studies of explanted human valves further support a role for BMP signaling in valve calcification. Comparison of pediatric diseased valves, which do not acquire calcification, and adult calcified valves demonstrates that increased BMP signaling, evident in p-SMAD1/5/8 activation, is exclusive to adult valves with calcification, indicating that BMP signaling may contribute to valve calcification in human disease [13]. Additionally, TGFβ1 is also a potent inducer of osteogenic-like differentiation of VICs in cell culture, as it stimulates VIC activation and calcification, increases ALP activity, and increases expression of ECM remodeling enzymes [126, 136, 137]. Negative regulators of valve calcification have been demonstrated through in vivo studies. One negative regulator of valve calcification is Notch signaling. Animals haploinsufficient for Notch signaling develop aortic valve calcification with increased BMP signaling and increased expression of Runx2 in the valve leaflets [65, 153]. Studies in isolated aortic VICs further demonstrate that Notch signaling plays an important role in suppressing valve calcification as treatment of VICs with Notch inhibitors induces BMP signaling and subsequent increases in osteogenic gene expression [65, 153]. Another negative regulator of valve calcification is Sox9, which potentially acts through induction of proteoglycan expression, similar to what has been observed in developing cartilage [40, 49]. Conditional heterozygous Sox9 mutant mice develop valve calcification along with increased valve thickness and expression of the osteogenic genes *Runx2, osteonectin, OPN,* and *OPG* [40, 49]. Based on these studies, it is apparent that many factors involved in endochondral bone formation are active in the process of aortic valve calcification.

CAVD has been linked to chronic kidney disease in human patients and animal models [140, 154-157]. A prominent pathological feature of kidney disease is the inability to regulate calcium and phosphate metabolism [158]. Increased blood phosphate levels (hyperphosphatemia) are highly associated with aortic valve sclerosis and valve calcification in humans [140]. Klotho-null mice are a model of accelerated aging that includes development of kidney failure and hyperphosphatemia, along with cardiovascular disease [159-162]. Klotho-null mice exhibit extensive valve annulus calcification with increased expression of osteogenic genes, but minimal CD68 positive macrophage infiltration [73]. Thus, valve calcification in the klotho-null animals parallels bone formation, where increases in crucial osteogenic genes, such as *Col10a1, Runx2, OPN,* and *BSP,* are observed [73]. These observations suggest that increased blood phosphate levels could be one stimulus for inducing advanced aortic valve calcification with osteogenic gene expression, but this has not been definitively demonstrated [73, 140].

Atherogenic lipid deposition and inflammation in the valves also has been linked to induction of osteogenic gene expression and disease [163-165]. Rabbit and mouse models of CAVD, induced with hypercholesterolemic or high fat diets, have increased lipid deposition and macrophage infiltration associated with induction of osteogenic markers such as ALP, OCN, OPN, Runx2, and Osx [165-167]. Although osteogenic gene expression is induced in these models, this type of valve calcification closely mimics vascular calcification observed in atherosclerosis, rather than endochondral bone formation, due to the presence of extensive immune cell infiltration [165, 166]. In support, human aortic VICs stimulated with pro-inflammatory mimetics not only induce the expression of inflammatory cytokines, but also induce the expression of osteogenic factors, such as BMP2 and Runx2, again suggesting that this process may be similar to what is occurring in atherosclerotic disease [164, 168]. Based on this evidence, multiple physiologic factors likely contribute to osteogenic gene induction in calcified diseased aortic valves.

4.2.3. Valvulogenic- and osteogenic-related signaling pathways in CAVD

As in both heart valve and endochondral bone development, BMP, TGFβ, Notch, and Wnt signaling have been implicated in the progression of CAVD (Figure 2; Table 1). Increased BMP ligand expression, particularly BMP2 and BMP4, has been demonstrated histologically in human explanted calcific aortic valves surrounding and throughout regions of valvular calcification [118, 129]. Furthermore, active BMP signaling, as indicated by pSMAD1/5/8 expression, is present in both human explanted diseased aortic valves and animal models of CAVD [13, 169, 170]. Comparison of pediatric diseased valves void of calcification to heavily calcified adult diseased valves demonstrates extensive ECM remodeling and evidence of VIC activation in both; however, increased pSMAD1/5/8 signaling is exclusive to calcified valves [13]. The observation that pSMAD1/5/8 expression is found only in adult calcified valves is suggestive of a critical role for BMP signaling as an initiating osteogenic factor in CAVD [13]. Furthermore, increased pSMAD1/5/8 expression reportedly localizes to the fibrosa layer of human calcific aortic valves, which is the primary sight of aortic valve calcification [169]. Cell culture studies support this and show that BMP2 stimulation promotes osteogenic-like aortic valve calcification in human aortic VICs by inducing the expression of the osteogenic factors Runx2, OPN, and ALP [138, 171]. Based on this evidence, active BMP signaling may be a potential therapeutic target to treat CAVD, however it has not yet been tested.

TGFβ signaling induces α SMA expression and myofibroblast differentiation of porcine aortic VICs, suggesting that TGFβ promotes VIC activation, potentially in response to physical strain [125, 172]. Furthermore, TGFβ signaling may also have a role in aortic valve calcification, as human explanted calcific aortic valves have increased levels of TGFβ1 expression and ovine aortic VICs in culture calcify in response to TGFβ1 induction [136, 137]. TGFβ signaling has also been linked to both Wnt/β-catenin and FGF signaling pathways in CAVD [173, 174]. Specifically, FGF signals have been shown to induce MAPK signaling, which inhibits aortic VIC αSMA expression and myofibroblast response to TGFβ [174]. In addition, TGFβ stimulation of aortic VICs induces nuclear localization and activation of β-catenin, which promotes VIC myofibroblast differentiation [173]. Although the role of TGFβ in CAVD is not well established in vivo, there is accumulating evidence for a role in VIC activation and calcification from studies in cell culture systems.

Whereas both BMP and TGFβ signaling have been found to induce VIC calcification, Notch signaling has been implicated as a negative regulator of valve calcification. Familial studies demonstrated that Notch1 haploinsufficiency is associated with CAVD and aortic stenosis (AS) [64]. During development, Notch1 is expressed in the endothelial cells lining the aortic valve cusps and is also observed at lower levels in the VICs, and this expression pattern is maintained into adulthood [64, 175]. Histological analysis of human explanted aortic valves demonstrates that activated Notch1 intracellular domain (NICD) expression is dramatically reduced in VICs directly adjacent to regions of aortic valve calcification [175]. This observation is consistent with a mechanism whereby Notch signaling inhibits valve calcification and downregulation of Notch expression promotes valve calcification [175]. The idea that Notch signaling functions as a negative regulator of calcification was originally defined in endo-chondral bone formation, where downstream effectors of Notch signaling, Hes1 and Hey1, repress Runx2 transcriptional function, leading to expansion of hypertrophic cartilage and impaired osteoblast differentiation [115]. Notch1 heterozygous or RBPJ heterozygous mice develop CAVD, as evidenced by increased aortic valve calcification, and also display significant increases in BMP/pSMAD1/5/8 signaling and Runx2 expression in the aortic valves [65, 153]. Likewise, deletion of RBPJ in adult mice results in increased aortic valve thickness with evidence of VIC proliferation and potentially, endothelial EMT [150]. Together these in vivo studies support the idea that Notch signaling represses BMP expression, thereby indirectly repressing other osteogenic factors [65, 153]. Cell culture studies indicate that Notch inhibition promotes calcification of VICs by repressing chondrogenic genes, including *Sox9*, and inducing expression of the osteogenic genes *OPN, osteonectin, Runx2, ALP*, and *BMP2* [65, 153, 175]. Specifically, Notch signaling in the aortic valves is thought to induce expression of Sox9, which is a negative regulator of calcification, and to repress the expression of both Runx2 and BMP2, which are known to stimulate osteogenic differentiation [64, 153, 175]. These studies suggest that, in the absence of a negative regulator of calcification, the resident VICs possess an intrinsic calcification mechanism, which becomes activated and subsequently induces valve calcification. Combined, the evidence suggests that Notch signaling is a negative regulator of VIC osteogenic differentiation, and that the absence or dysregulation of Notch signaling can induce valvular calcification.

Wnt/β-catenin signaling is important for osteoblast maturation during embryonic development and contributes to mineralized bone formation (reviewed in [80]). A number of studies have also shown activation of Wnt/β-catenin signaling in aortic valve calcification. Canonical Wnt signaling acts through the frizzled receptors and the Wnt co-receptors Lrp5 and Lrp6, resulting in β-catenin nuclear localization and TCF/LEF1 activation [176]. Human explanted calcific AoVs have increased expression of Lrp5, β-catenin, and Wnt3a ligand as compared to control valves [143]. Increased Wnt signaling in diseased aortic valves also has been observed in multiple animal models of CAVD. Pigs and rabbits maintained on an atherogenic diet develop aortic valve disease and display increased expression levels of β-catenin and Lrp5 receptor [173, 177]. Likewise, in a subset of endothelial nitric oxide synthase (eNOS) deficient mice that develop BAV, expression of Wnt3a ligand and Lrp5 receptor is increased when the animals are fed a high cholesterol diet [178]. Cell culture studies also support the idea that Wnt/β-catenin signaling is important for VIC myofibroblast activation, proliferation, and chondrogenic gene induction. Studies in porcine aortic VICs show that Wnt3a treatment induces significant VIC proliferation and myofibroblast activation [173, 179]. Furthermore, Wnt3a treatment of embryonic chicken aortic VICs results in increased expression of *periostin* and *mgp*, but does not induce the expression of osteogenic-related genes, suggesting that Wnt3a signaling is not sufficient for VIC osteogenic differentiation [60]. However in adult valves, Wnt signaling can promote the VIC calcification response, as loss of Wnt signaling through the Lrp5 receptor in ApoE knockout mice results in decreased aortic valve calcification [180]. Together these studies demonstrate that Wnt signaling likely contributes to VIC activation, proliferation, and calcification in CAVD.

4.3. Matrix remodeling in CAVD

Diseased aortic valves are characterized by changes in the ECM; in particular, disorganized collagen bundles and extensive elastic fiber fragmentation are observed [181, 182]. Insight into the role of elastin fiber disorganization in the pathogenesis of CAVD has been provided through studies of elastin haploinsufficient mice, which display elastin fiber fragmentation, abnormal ECM remodeling, and increased valve stiffness, suggesting that elastin homeostasis is important for maintaining valve function [72, 183]. Collagen synthesis and remodeling are dramatically increased in CAVD, however, overall collagen content in the valve is actually decreased, suggesting that there is extensive collagen proteolysis during disease [184-186]. In contrast to collagens, expression of proteoglycans, including decorin, biglycan, versican, and hyaluronan, is increased particularly in regions of the diseased valve adjacent to calcific nodules [187]. These changes in ECM composition during CAVD can be compared to matrix remodeling events that occur during valve development and also in bone formation. The decreased collagen content and increased proteoglycan matrix found in CAVD is similar to the primitive ECM characteristic of early valve development [188]. Furthermore, parallels can also be drawn between matrix remodeling in CAVD and bone development. Specifically, matrix remodeling in the immature bone is essential for providing a scaffold upon which the calcified matrix is deposited, and subsequent ECM degradation is essential for expansion of the calcified regions of newly forming bone [189]. The parallels between matrix remodeling in bone development and the disease process of CAVD suggest that valve matrix remodeling may contribute to valvular calcification.

Matrix degradation and remodeling in valvulogenesis, osteogenesis, and CAVD occurs concomitant with increased activity of MMPs and cathepsins, along with increased RANKL signaling. A number of studies have shown significant increases in expression of multiple MMPs, including MMP1, MMP3, MMP7, MMP9, and MMP12, with increased cathepsins B, K, and S in human calcific diseased aortic valves, suggesting that extensive ECM remodeling is a key feature of disease [124, 163, 181, 182, 184, 190]. In bone, RANKL signals through the RANK receptor, which can be inhibited via binding to the soluble receptor OPG, and promotes the expression of proteolytic enzymes, such as MMPs and cathepsin K, through activation of NFATc1 [191, 192]. A similar mechanism has been identified in heart valve remodeling [47, 61]. Comparison of sclerotic diseased aortic valves and advanced stenotic aortic valves determined that OPG levels are significantly higher in sclerotic valves without calcification, whereas RANKL expression is higher in stenotic calcified valves [103, 193]. This study concluded that OPG may be protective against valve calcification, whereas elevated RANKL expression may promote valve calcification by promoting upregulation of matrix remodeling enzymes [103, 193]. Furthermore, treatment of human aortic VICs with RANKL results in increased MMP1 and MMP2 activity with increased VIC proliferation, concomitant with increased calcification and osteogenic gene expression [103, 191]. In addition, NFATc1 expression is increased in human explanted aortic valve leaflets with CAVD [106]. Together, these studies are consistent with signaling events during bone development, namely RANKL activation of NFATc1, stimulating matrix remodeling enzymes, and promoting calcification [192].

A number of other signaling pathways are likely involved in ECM changes that occur during CAVD. In particular, TGFβ1 stimulation of cultured VICs stimulates myofibroblast differentiation, leading to increased levels of αSMA stress fibers in the VICs [125, 172]. It has been suggested that these myofibroblasts then exert a contractile force on the surrounding valve ECM and stimulate rearrangement of the matrix, particularly in fibronectin fibers [125]. Furthermore, TGFβ1 stimulation also induces increased type I collagen production and expression of the matrix remodeling enzymes MMP9 and MMP2 in cultured aortic VICs [136, 172]. These studies indicate that TGFβ1 signaling may be a key factor in ECM-related changes during CAVD pathogenesis. Moreover, Wnt signaling may work in concert with TGFβ1 to induce changes in ECM during CAVD [173]. TGFβ1 stimulation promotes nuclear localization and activation of β-catenin in cultured VICs, and, when combined, Wnt and TGFβ1 signaling dramatically increases myofibroblast activation [173]. In contrast to TGFβ1 and Wnt signaling, FGF signaling may work to inhibit ECM remodeling during valve disease. FGF signaling has been shown to block TGFβ1 induced myofibroblast differentiation and αSMA expression in porcine aortic VICs through activation of phospho-ERK1/2 signaling [174]. In addition, FGF signaling inhibits myofibroblast contraction of a collagen matrix, supporting the idea that FGF signaling blocks TGFβ1 stimulation of matrix-related changes [174]. Many parallels exist between signaling factors involved in ECM changes in development and disease. In particular, RANKL, TGFβ1, Wnt, and FGF signaling have demonstrated roles in ECM production and regulation in both heart valve and endochondral bone formation [8, 76]. The shared signaling pathways in these tissues, both in development and disease, suggest that developmental pathways may be reactivated in CAVD to induce matrix changes characteristic of the disease.

5. Therapeutic mechanisms in CAVD

Currently, aortic valve replacement surgery is the only effective treatment option for CAVD [122]. There have been numerous studies, which are summarized below, testing the effectiveness of different pharmacotherapies on preventing the progression of AS. Unfortunately, studies on statin therapies, inhibitors of the renin-angiotensin-aldosterone system, and osteoporosis treatments have not been proven to be effective at preventing the symptoms or the progression of CAVD/AS. Following the summary of these studies, additional treatment options, related to the expression of developmental and osteogenic-related genes in CAVD, are discussed.

5.1. Statins

Lipid deposition and the accumulation of apolipoproteins (Apo) in the aortic valve leaflets have long been associated with CAVD, and many studies have compared the progression of CAVD to atherosclerotic disease [119, 133, 134, 194]. Therefore, it has been hypothesized that cholesterol lowering therapy with statin drugs may be an effective treatment strategy to delay the progression of CAVD. A specialized mouse model called "Reversa" mice develop signs of CAVD when fed a high cholesterol diet, however, when serum cholesterol is lowered via a genetic deletion of the microsomal triglyceride transfer protein (Mttp), reduced levels of aortic valve calcification, as well as decreased expression of the osteogenic markers pSMAD1/5/8, Msx2, Osx, β-catenin, and Runx2, are observed [167, 170]. Thus reducing plasma cholesterol may reduce CAVD pathogenesis, particularly in terms of reducing osteogenic gene expression in the diseased valves. Similarly, statin treatment of human or porcine aortic VICs cultured concomitantly with osteogenic media results in decreased expression of the osteogenic genes ALP, OCN, Lrp5, and OPN, and reduced calcific nodule formation [171, 177, 195]. However, when statin treatment of aortic VICs is initiated after osteogenic transformation or calcific nodule formation, it is ineffective at reducing calcification and expression of osteogenic markers, indicating that statin therapy cannot reverse aortic valve calcification and osteogenic differentiation once it has occurred [195, 196]. Results from animal studies are equally contradictory. Rabbits fed a high cholesterol diet supplemented with atorvastatin have decreased aortic valve thickness, reduced VIC proliferation, and reduced expression of Lrp5, β -catenin, OPN, *Runx2*, and *ALP*, compared to those animals fed only a high cholesterol diet [165, 177]. Similarly, endothelial nitric oxide synthase (eNOS) deficient mice, displaying a BAV phenotype and fed a high cholesterol diet, have reduced *Lrp5* and *Wnt3a* expression as well as reduced aortic valve calcification when treated with statins, compared to animals fed only a high cholesterol diet [178]. In contrast, a long term study in rabbits fed a high cholesterol diet showed that atorvastatin therapy initiated after aortic valve disease is established is not effective at reducing the amount of aortic valve calcification present, although some improvements in other histological parameters were noted [197]. Based on both cell culture and animal studies, statin therapy may improve some measures of aortic valve calcification, specifically in terms of reducing osteogenic gene expression, however, firm conclusions as to potential efficacy as a CAVD treatment cannot be drawn.

Clinicial studies investigating the use of statin therapy in patients with CAVD are also widely contradictory. An early study investigating the use of statin therapy in patients with moderate to severe aortic stenosis (AS) reported that patients treated with statins had less hemodynamic progression of AS over a 2 year time period than patients who were not on statin therapy [198]. In contrast, three larger prospective clinical studies, SALTIRE (Scottish Aortic Stenosis and Lipid Lowering Trial, Impact on Regression), SEAS (Simvastatin and Ezetimibe in Aortic Stenosis), and ASTRONOMER (Aortic Stenosis Progression Observation: Measuring Effects of Rosuvastatin), found that statin therapy was not effective at treating the progression of AS [199-201]. In these trials, three different statin therapies were investigated in patients with mild to moderate AS and it was determined that statin therapy did not alter the progression of CAVD/AS nor prevent outcomes such as the necessity to undergo aortic valve replacement surgery [199-201]. In response to the negative outcomes of these large clinical trials, the use of statin therapy was next investigated in patients with the earliest form of CAVD/AS, aortic valve sclerosis, to determine if statin use could prevent, rather than reverse, AS [202]. In this report, statin therapy was significantly associated with a decreased development of AS and a decreased need for aortic valve replacement surgery, suggesting that statin therapy may be an effective treatment if started at the earliest stages of the disease, prior to any indication of valve calcification [202]. Based on these studies, it can be concluded that in humans, statin therapy is ineffective at preventing the progression of AS and reversing aortic valve calcification. However, statin therapy may be useful at preventing the onset of AS in patients with the earliest stages of aortic valve thickening.

5.2. Angiotensin converting enzyme inhibitors/Angiotensin receptor blockers

Another potential therapy to prevent the progression of CAVD/AS is the use of the anti-hypertensive angiotensin-converting enzyme inhibitors (ACEI) and angiotensin receptor blockers (ARB). Currently, ACEIs and ARBs are prescribed to treat hypertension, and function by acting on the renin-angiotensin-aldosterone system to ultimately inhibit the vasoconstrictor effects of angiotensin II [203]. Previous reports have identified the overlapping expression of angiotensin-converting enzyme (ACE) and angiotensin II in calcified human aortic valves surrounding regions of valvular calcification [133]. It has been hypothesized that ACE inhibition may prevent the progression of CAVD by reducing ACE activity in the diseased valve leaflet [204-206]. A study conducted in ApoE knockout mice with induced chronic renal failure concluded that animals treated with the ACEI enalapril had significantly reduced levels of pathologic aortic valve leaflet thickening and valve fibrosis than untreated animals [206]. Similarly, in a rabbit model of CAVD in which the animals were fed a high vitamin D diet, treatment with the ACEI ramipril significantly reduced the progression to AS, improved valve endothelial cell integrity, and reduced aortic valve calcification [205]. It is uncertain how ACE and angiotensin receptor (AR) inhibition would directly affect molecular changes in the valve leaflets. However, in a study of rabbits fed a high cholesterol diet, treatment with the ARB olmesartan decreased the number of α SMA positive myofibroblasts and reduced expression of the osteogenic markers *Runx2* and OPN, compared to untreated control animals [204]. These animal studies suggest that ACE and/or AR inhibition may reduce pathologic changes in aortic valve disease by limiting valve fibrosis, reducing myofibroblast activation, and decreasing osteogenic gene expression.

Clinical studies testing the therapeutic benefits of ACEIs and ARBs in CAVD progression have had mixed results. In human explanted aortic valve tissues, ARB therapy is associated with reduced aortic valve remodeling and calcification [207]. As in animal studies, this histological analysis suggests that AR inhibition may limit aortic valve calcification [207]. In a small pilot clinical study (Symptomatic Cardiac Obstruction – Pilot Study of Enalapril in

Aortic Stenosis), use of the ACEI Enalapril was associated with improved clinical symptoms in patients with severe symptomatic AS [208]. The majority of studies investigating the use of ACEIs or ARBs in CAVD/AS with positive outcomes have been retrospective. In three different retrospective studies, ACEI or ARB use in patients with mild to moderate AS was associated with decreased mortality, decreased number of adverse cardiovascular events, slower progression of AS, and less accumulation of valvular calcification [209-211]. Additionally, one prospective study followed a small random population of patients over a 4-year period and reported that the use of ACEIs or ARBs was significantly associated with reduced CAVD/AS disease progression [212]. Together, these studies provide evidence that ACEI and ARB may delay CAVD progression. Conversely, there have also been a number of studies that show no association between ACEI and ARB use and improved outcomes in CAVD progression. The JASS study (Japanese Aortic Stenosis Study) reported that ARB therapy in patients with moderate to severe AS had no beneficial outcomes in CAVD progression, although patients with mild asymptomatic AS had some indication of reduced progression to AS [213]. Furthermore, a large study in patients with very mild asymptomatic AS found that patients on ACEI or ARB therapy had no improvement in the progression of AS compared against a control group [202]. Similarly, a small 2-year study observed no difference in the hemodynamic progression of AS with ACEI use versus non-use [198]. Based on both animal and clinical studies, it is unclear whether ACEI or ARB therapy is an effective treatment option to prevent the progression of CAVD/AS, however there are indications that perhaps this therapy may limit valve calcification [204, 207]. A placebo controlled, blinded trial will be necessary to determine the effectiveness of these therapies in treating CAVD.

5.3. Aldosterone-receptor antagonists

Aldosterone is a component of the renin-angiotensin-aldosterone system that plays a key role in the kidney to regulate water and sodium reabsorption and effectively raise blood pressure [203]. Aldosterone-receptor antagonists (ARA) are commonly prescribed for their diuretic effects [203]. Recently, there have been two studies investigating the use of ARAs in the treatment of CAVD/AS. In an animal study, rabbits fed a high cholesterol diet develop aortic valve sclerosis, with thickening of the valve leaflets and microscopic calcific deposits, which was blocked by treatment with the ARA eplerenone [214]. In addition to reducing valve fibrosis and mineralization, evidence of macrophage infiltration was also reduced [214]. Conversely, in a small placebo-controlled human trial of patients with moderate to severe asymptomatic AS, there was no difference in the progression of AS in those patients receiving the ARA eplerenone versus placebo [215]. To our knowledge, no molecular evidence has been reported in studies on ARA therapy in CAVD and it is unknown whether ARA therapy affects myofibroblast activation or osteogenic gene induction. Additional clinical studies will be necessary to determine if ARA use can prevent AS progression if therapy is started in early disease stages.

5.4. Bisphosphonates

Bisphosphonates (BP) are a class of drugs that mimic inorganic pyrophosphate and prevent ectopic soft tissue calcification and inhibit bone resorption [216]. In adults, especially women, BPs are commonly prescribed to treat excessive bone resorption associated with osteoporosis [216]. Human aortic VICs, grown on collagen gels in the presence of a specialized thiol bisphosphonate, have decreased ALP activity and reduced cellular aggregation, a step that precedes calcific nodule formation, as compared to cells grown on collagen alone [217]. This study suggests that bisphosphonates may inhibit VIC calcification in vitro and could serve as a potential therapeutic strategy to prevent aortic valve calcification [217]. Due to the ability of BPs to prevent ectopic calcification in bone and the availability of patient populations currently using BPs, a number of studies have investigated the use of BPs in the inhibition of aortic valve calcification. Three small retrospective human studies compared measurements of AS progression over a 2-year period in patients with AS taking BPs versus those not taking BPs [218-220]. The results of these studies suggest a modest reduction in the progression of AS in those patients taking BPs [218-220]. The large MESA study (Multi-Ethnic Study of Atherosclerosis) followed women taking BPs, compared to those not taking BPs, and their development of CAVD/AS over time [221]. The results of this study were mixed and showed that, in older women, BP therapy was associated with a slight benefit in terms of aortic valve calcification, whereas, younger women taking BPs had significantly more progression of aortic valve calcification compared to women not taking BPs [221]. Most recently, a large retrospective study investigated the progression of AS in women with mild to moderate AS over a 5-year period and compared the outcomes in patients on BP therapy versus those not taking BPs [222]. The evidence from this study shows that there was no change in survival, or in the number of aortic valve replacement surgeries, in women taking BPs compared to those not taking BPs, suggesting that BP therapy does not suppress the progression of CAVD/AS [222]. Thus far, the outcomes of the human studies investigating the use of bisphosphonate therapy in CAVD demonstrate that this therapy is ineffective at preventing or delaying the progression of CAVD/AS. To definitively determine whether or not BP therapy is effective at suppressing the progression of CAVD/AS, placebo-controlled prospective studies will be necessary.

5.5. Nitric oxide bioavailability

Endothelial nitric oxide synthase (eNOS) produces nitric oxide (NO) from L-arginine, and eNOS expression has been identified in the endothelial cells lining the aortic valves [68]. eNOS deficiency has been linked to defective aortic valve development, as approximately 50% of eNOS deficient mice develop a bicuspid, rather than tricuspid, aortic valve [68]. eNOS deficient mice with a BAV phenotype fed a high cholesterol diet develop hemodynamic symptoms of AS and also display microscopic mineralization in the aortic valve leaflets, indicating that eNOS activity may be important for suppressing aortic valve calcification [178]. Nitric Oxide deficiency is also an indicator of endothelial cell dysfunction, and systemic endothelial cell dysfunction is prevalent in patients with aortic valve sclerosis/ stenosis [223-225]. The uncoupling, or dysfunction, of eNOS results in decreased NO production and increased generation of reactive oxygen species (ROS) [223]. ROS activity is present in calcific lesions of human stenotic aortic valves, and it has been suggested that ROS activity may speed aortic valve calcification [144, 226]. In animal studies, rabbits fed a high cholesterol/high vitamin D diet develop aortic valve thickening, small deposits of valve calcification, and increased ROS activity in cells surrounding regions of valve calcification [226]. Furthermore, ROS activity was co-localized to clusters of cells expressing Runx2 and OPN, suggesting that ROS activity is associated with VICs displaying an osteogenic-like phenotype [226]. In VIC culture studies, TGFβ1 stimulation induces increased ROS activity, along with calcific nodule formation and ALP activity [227]. Increasing the availability of NO, via NO donors such as sodium nitroprusside, partially blocks both nodule formation and ALP activity, suggesting that NO levels are important for reducing ROS and inhibiting calcification in VICs [227]. There have been a number of small clinical studies investigating the levels of the NOS inhibitor, asymmetric dimethylarginine (ADMA), an indicator of en-dothelial cell dysfunction, in patients with moderate to severe AS [228-230]. In these studies, plasma levels of ADMA are significantly higher in patients with moderate to severe AS, compared to patients with mild AS or no disease, suggesting that NO production is disrupt-ed in CAVD/AS [228-230]. Combined, these studies suggest that increased ROS production is associated with aortic valve calcification and the induction of osteogenic gene expression. Thus, increasing the bioavailability of NO may be a potential therapeutic avenue to block ROS activity, and thereby disease progression, in CAVD.

5.6. NSAIDs/COX2 inhibitors

Previous reports have demonstrated that immune cell infiltration is common in CAVD [119, 132, 135]. Non-steroidal anti-inflammatory drugs (NSAIDS) are commonly used to treat pain and inflammation, and act by inhibiting the enzymes COX1 and/or COX2 [231-233]. These enzymes function by converting arachidonic acid to prostaglandins (PGs) [233, 234]. There has been one study conducted in human aortic VICs, demonstrating that stimulation of VICs with pro-inflammatory mimetics induces the expression of COX2 and the release of prostaglandins [235]. This study suggests that COX2 inhibition may be one way to treat the immune response associated with CAVD [235]. Interestingly, COX2 and PG signaling are al-so involved in bone formation as well as cellular responses to physical stress and strain, processes that also likely contribute to CAVD (reviewed in [131]). In bone, PG signaling has an anabolic effect, and PG treatment of osteoblast cultures results in increased expression of OCN, BMP2, Runx2, OPN, ALP, and BSP [236-244]. In osteoblast cultures, BMP2 stimulation induces COX2 expression through upregulation of Runx2, which binds to and activates the COX2 promoter [245, 246]. Downstream, PG signaling induces the expression of p38 MAPK through the activation of protein kinase A [243, 247]. Furthermore, fluid shear stress and other physical forces induce COX2 expression in osteoblast-like cells, suggesting that in-creased COX2 and PG signaling is a cellular response to altered mechanical forces [248, 249]. The combined results of these studies suggest that COX2/PG signaling may be an effective therapeutic target to treat CAVD progression, as COX2/PG signaling plays a role in inflam-mation, osteogenesis, and cellular response to physical strain, all of which are thought to be pathological mechanisms involved in CAVD [131, 243, 244, 248-251]. It would be interesting to determine whether COX2 inhibition/NSAID use could reduce CAVD progression. However, one caveat is that COX2 inhibitor therapy can be associated with some rare but significant adverse cardiovascular events such as myocardial infarction and stroke [252, 253]. Perhaps therapeutics designed toward downstream targets of PG signaling, such as p38 MAPK, could improve outcomes of CAVD patients without the cardiovascular side effects of selective coxibs [254].

5.7. Development of new therapeutic approaches based on valvulogenic and osteogenic molecular mechanisms.

As reviewed above, Notch, Wnt, and BMP signaling have been implicated in the progression of CAVD. Pharmacotherapies designed to act as Wnt and BMP inhibitors, or Notch agonists, could be a potential avenue for new therapeutics to treat the progression of CAVD. BMP signaling is thought to be a specific indicator of aortic valve calcification as active BMP signaling is observed in adult diseased valves with prominent calcification and is not found in pediatric diseased valves void of calcification [13]. Furthermore, BMP2 signaling stimulates VIC calcific nodule formation and induces osteogenic gene expression [138, 171]. It is possible that therapies designed to inhibit BMP signaling will block osteogenic-like calcification in diseased aortic valves. Likewise, inhibition of the Wnt/β-catenin signaling pathway may also serve to reduce aortic valve calcification during disease, which is supported by evidence from animal studies in ApoE knockout mice. When fed an atherogenic diet, ApoE knockout mice reportedly develop aortic valve calcification, however, when the Wnt co-receptor Lrp5 is genetically deleted in these mice, the amount of aortic valve calcification is significantly reduced [180]. Therefore, Wnt inhibition may be another potential therapeutic approach for treating CAVD. Lastly, strategies to maintain Notch signaling in the valves may be another potential way to inhibit calcification in CAVD. Notch inhibition of calcification and osteogenic gene expression has been demonstrated in aortic VICs in culture and reduced Notch signaling in vivo leads to CAVD in mice [65, 153, 175]. Furthermore, Notch1 haploinsufficiency in humans is associated with CAVD, indicating that maintaining Notch signaling is important for valve homeostasis [64]. Thus, therapeutic strategies designed to affect one or more of these pathways may serve to prevent valve calcification in CAVD. A potential limitation of this approach is that BMP, Wnt, and Notch signaling pathways are involved in many homeostatic and disease processes. For example, Wnt signaling is increased in many types of cancer, and all three pathways are involved in bone homeostasis. Therefore the development of therapeutics based on these molecular mechanisms must take into account potential effects on multiple organ systems. Nevertheless, targeted approaches based on these pathways could represent a new therapeutic avenue in the development of pharmacologic based approaches to CAVD.

6. Conclusions and future directions

There are numerous examples of shared molecular pathways between valvulogenesis, osteogenesis, and disease pathogenesis of CAVD. In valvulogenesis, signaling factors involved in early cushion formation, such as BMP, Notch, and Wnt/β-catenin pathways are active in osteogenesis and in CAVD [7-9, 14]. Furthermore, transcription factors expressed in the early valve mesenchyme, such as Twist1, Msx2, and Sox9, can also be found in the primitive condensed bone mesenchyme and in the mesenchymal-like cells identified in diseased aortic valve tissues [8, 13, 80, 255]. In addition to signaling and transcription factors, molecular pathways governing ECM production and remodeling, such as the RANKL – NFATc1 – CtsK pathway are shared amongst valve progenitor, developing bone, and diseased valve tissues [11, 47, 103, 106, 193]. This commonality suggests that the mesenchymal cells found within these tissues are governed by common molecular pathways and that these developmental pathways are reactivated during disease. Additional parallels can be drawn between calcification of the embryonic bone tissues and calcification observed in diseased aortic valves. For example, the endochondral bone factors Runx2, OCN, and BSP are reactivated during aortic valve disease, suggesting that osteogenic molecular pathways are activated during CAVD and may contribute to pathogenic calcification [5, 13, 76, 80, 106, 152]. Effective pharmacological therapies to treat CAVD remain elusive and identifying potential targets for new pharmacotherapies is a priority, as the only effective treatment for CAVD with AS is valve replacement surgery [256]. Studies testing the effectiveness of statin therapy, inhibitors of the renin-angiotensin-aldosterone, and bisphosphonates in slowing the progression of CAVD have been disappointing (see therapeutic section). New therapeutic strategies are needed and, perhaps, targeted inhibition of BMP and Wnt signaling or maintenance of Notch signaling may provide new avenues for potential CAVD treatments.

Author details

Elaine E. Wirrig and Katherine E. Yutzey[*]

*Address all correspondence to: Katherine.yutzey@cchmc.org

The Heart Institute, Cincinnati Children's Hospital Medical Center, Cincinnati, Ohio, USA

References

[1] Roger VL, Go AS, Lloyd-Jones DM, Adams RJ, Berry JD, Brown TM, et al. Heart disease and stroke statistics--2011 update: A report from the American Heart Association Circulation. 2011;123:e18-e209.

[2] Otto CM. Valvular aortic stenosis: disease severity and timing of intervention. J Am Coll Cardiol. 2006;47:2141-2151.

[3] Bonow RO, Carabello BA, Kanu C, de Leon AC, Jr., Faxon DP, Freed MD, et al. ACC/AHA 2006 guidelines for the management of patients with valvular heart disease: a report of the American College of Cardiology/American Heart Association

Task Force on Practice Guidelines (writing committee to revise the 1998 Guidelines for the Management of Patients With Valvular Heart Disease). Circulation. 2006;114:e84-231.

[4] Roberts WC, Ko JM. Frequency by decades of unicuspid, bicuspid and tricuspid aortic valves in adults having isolated aortic valve replacement for aortic stenosis, with or without associated aortic regurgitation. Circulation. 2005;111:920-925.

[5] Rajamannan NM, Subramaniam M, Rickard DJ, Stock SR, Donovan J, Springett M, et al. Human aortic valve calcification is associated with an osteoblast phenotype. Circulation. 2003;107:2181-2184.

[6] O'Brien KD. Pathogenesis of calcific aortic valve disease: a disease process comes of age (and a good deal more). Arterioscler Thromb Vasc Biol. 2006;26:1721-1728.

[7] Bostrom K, Rajamannan NM, Towler DA. The regulation of valvular and vascular sclerosis by osteogenic morphogens. Circ Res. 2011;109:564-577.

[8] Combs MD, Yutzey KE. Heart valve development: Regulatory networks in development and disease. Circ Res. 2009;105:408-421.

[9] Karsenty G, Kronenberg HM, Settembre C. Genetic control of bone formation. Annu Rev Cell Dev Biol. 2009;25:629-648.

[10] Hinton RB, Yutzey KE. Heart valve structure and function in development and disease. Annu Rev Physiol. 2011;73:29-46.

[11] Lincoln J, Lange AW, Yutzey KE. Hearts and bones: Shared regulatory mechanisms in heart valve, cartilage, tendon, and bone development. Dev Biol. 2006;294:292-302.

[12] Chakraborty S, Wirrig EE, Hinton RB, Merrill WH, Spicer DB, Yutzey KE. Twist1 promotes heart valve cell proliferation and extracellular matrix gene expression during development in vivo and is expressed in human diseased aortic valves. Dev Biol. 2010;347:167-179.

[13] Wirrig EE, Hinton RB, Yutzey KE. Differential expression of cartilage and bone-related proteins in pediatric and adult diseased aortic valves. J Mol Cell Cardiol. 2011;50:561-569.

[14] Miller JD, Weiss RM, Heistad DD. Calcific aortic valve stenosis: Methods, models, and mechanisms. Circ Res. 2011;108:1392-1412.

[15] Schroeder JA, Jackson LF, Lee DC, Camenisch TD. Form and function of developing heart valves: coordination by extracellular matrix growth and signaling. J Mol Med. 2003;81:392-403.

[16] Person AD, Klewer SE, Runyan RB. Cell biology of cardiac cushion development. Int Rev Cytol. 2005;243:287-335.

[17] Camenisch TD, Molin DG, Person A, Runyan RB, Gittenberger-de Groot AC, McDonald JA, et al. Temporal and distinct TGFbeta ligand requirements during mouse and avian endocardial cushion morphogenesis. Dev Biol. 2002;248:170-181.

[18] Ma L, Lu MF, Schwartz RJ, Martin JF. Bmp2 is essential for cardiac cushion epithelial-mesenchymal transition and myocardial patterning. Development. 2005;132:5601-5611.

[19] Rivera-Feliciano J, Tabin CJ. Bmp2 instructs cardiac progenitors to form the heart-valve-inducing field. Dev Biol. 2006;295:580-588.

[20] McCulley DJ, Kang JO, Martin JF, Black BL. BMP4 is required in the anterior heart field and its derivatives for endocardial cushion remodeling, outflow tract septation, and semilunar valve development. Dev Dyn. 2008;237:3200-3209.

[21] Snarr BS, Kern CB, Wessels A. Origin and fate of cardiac mesenchyme. Dev Dyn. 2008;237:2804-2819.

[22] Lin C-J, Lin C-Y, Chen C-H, Zhou B, Chang C-P. Partitioning the heart: mechanisms of cardiac septation and valve development. Development. 2012;139:3277-3299.

[23] Lincoln J, Alfieri CM, Yutzey KE. Development of heart valve leaflets and supporting apparatus in chicken and mouse embryos. Dev Dyn. 2004;230:239-250.

[24] Hinton RB, Lincoln J, Deutsch GH, Osinska H, Manning PB, Benson DW, et al. Extracellular matrix remodeling and organization in developing and diseased aortic valves. Circ Res. 2006;98:1431-1438.

[25] deLange FJ, Moorman AFM, Anderson RH, Manner J, Soufan AT, deGier-deVries C, et al. Lineage and morphogenetic analysis of the cardiac valves. Circ Res. 2004;95:645-654.

[26] Rochais F, Mesbah K, Kelly RG. Signaling pathways controlling second heart field development. Circ Res. 2009;104:933-942.

[27] Nakamura T, Colbert MC, Robbins J. Neural crest cells retain multipotential characteristics in the developing valves and label the cardiac conduction system. Circ Res. 2006;98:1547-1554.

[28] Jiang X, Rowitch DH, Soriano P, McMahon AP, Sucov HM. Fate of the mammalian cardiac neural crest. Development. 2000;127:1607-1616.

[29] Jain R, Engleka KA, Rentschler SL, Manderfield LJ, Li L, Yuan L, et al. Cardiac neural crest orchestrates remodeling and functional maturation of mouse semilunar valves. J Clin Invest. 2011;121:422-430.

[30] Zhang J, Chang JY, Huang Y, Lin X, Schwartz RJ, Martin JF, et al. The FGF-BMP signaling axis regulates outflow tract valve primordium formation by promoting cushion neural crest cell differentiation. Circ Res. 2010;107:1209-1219.

[31] Wessels A, van den Hoff MJ, Adamo RF, Phelps AL, Lockhart MM, Sauls K, et al. Epicardially derived fibroblasts preferentially contribute to the parietal leaflets of the atrioventricular valves in the murine heart. Dev Biol. 2012;366:111-124.

[32] Zhou B, Ma Q, Rajagopal S, Wu SM, Domian I, Rivera-Feliciano J, et al. Epicardial progenitors contribute to the cardiomyocyte lineage in the developing heart. Nature. 2008;454:109-113.

[33] Visconti RP, Ebihara Y, LaRue AC, Fleming PA, McQuinn TC, Masuya M, et al. An in vivo analysis of hematopoietic stem cell potential: hematopoietic origin of cardiac valve interstitial cells. Circ Res. 2006;98:690-696.

[34] Hajdu Z, Romeo SJ, Fleming PA, Markwald RR, Visconti RP, Drake CJ. Recruitment of bone marrow-derived valve interstitial cells is a normal homeostatic process. J Mol Cell Cardiol. 2011;51:955-965.

[35] Chakraborty S, Combs MD, Yutzey KE. Transcriptional regulation of heart valve progenitor cells. Pediatr Cardiol. 2010;31:414-421.

[36] Timmerman LA, Grego-Bessa J, Raya A, Bertran E, Perez-Pomares JM, Diez J, et al. Notch promotes epithelial-mesenchymal transition during cardiac development and oncogenic transformation. Genes Dev. 2004;18:99-115.

[37] Tao G, Levay AK, Gridley T, Lincoln J. Mmp15 is a direct target of Snail1 during endothelial to mesenchymal transformation and endocardial cushion development. Dev Biol. 2011;359:209-221.

[38] Shelton EL, Yutzey KE. Twist1 function in endocardial cell proliferation, migration, and differentiation during heart valve development. Dev Biol. 2008;317:282-295.

[39] Shelton EL, Yutzey KE. Tbx20 regulation of endocardial cushion cell proliferation and extracellular matrix gene expression. Dev Biol. 2007;302:376-388.

[40] Lincoln J, Kist R, Scherer G, Yutzey KE. Sox9 is required for precursor cell expansion and extracellular matrix gene expression. Dev Biol. 2007;302:376-388.

[41] Chen YH, Ishii M, Sukov HM, Maxson RE. Msx1 and Msx2 are required for endothelial-mesenchymal transformation of the atrioventricular cushions and patterning of the atrioventricular myocardium. BMC Dev Biol. 2008;8:75.

[42] Lee MP, Yutzey KE. Twist1 directly regulates genes that promote cell proliferation and migration in developing heart valves. PLoS One. 2011;6:e29758.

[43] Chakraborty S, Cheek J, Sakthivel B, Aronow BJ, Yutzey KE. Shared gene expression profiles in developing heart valves and osteoblasts. Physiol Genomics. 2008;35:75-85.

[44] Aikawa E, Whittaker P, Farber M, Mendelson K, Padera RF, Aikawa M, et al. Human semilunar cardiac valve remodeling by activated cells from fetus to adult. Circulation. 2006;113:1344-1352.

[45] de la Pompa JL, Timmerman LA, Takimoto H, Yoshida H, Elia AJ, Samper E, et al. Role of NF-ATc transcription factor in morphogenesis of cardiac valves and septum. Nature. 1998;392:182-186.

[46] Ranger AM, Grusby MJ, Gravallese EM, de la Brousse FC, Hoey T, Mickanin C, et al. The transcription factor NF-ATc is essential for cardiac valve formation. Nature. 1998;392:186-190.

[47] Combs MD, Yutzey KE. VEGF and RANKL regulation of NFATc1 in heart valve development. Circ Res. 2009;105:565-574.

[48] Lincoln J, Alfieri CM, Yutzey KE. BMP and FGF regulatory pathways control cell lineage diversification of heart valve precursor cells. Dev Biol. 2006;292:290-302.

[49] Peacock JD, Levay AK, Gillaspie DB, Tao G, Lincoln J. Reduced Sox9 function promotes heart valve calcification phenotypes in vivo. Circ Res. 2010;106:712-719.

[50] Levay AK, Peacock JD, Lu Y, Koch M, Hinton RB, Kadler KE, et al. Scleraxis is required for cell lineage differentiation and extracellular matrix remodeling during murine heart formation in vivo. Circ Res. 2008;103:948-956.

[51] Luna-Zurita L, Prados B, Grego-Bessa J, Luxan G, del Monte G, Benguria A, et al. Integration of a Notch-dependent mesenchymal gene program and BMP2-driven cell invasiveness regulates murine cardiac valve formation. J Clin Invest. 2010;120:3493-3507.

[52] Dor Y, Camenisch TD, Itin A, Fishman GI, McDonald JA, Carmeliet P, et al. A novel role for VEGF in endocardial cushion formation and its potential contribution to congenital heart defects. Development. 2001;128:1531-1538.

[53] Liebner S, Cattelino A, Gallini R, Rudini N, Iurlaro M, Piccolo S, et al. β-catenin is required for endothelial-mesenchymal transformation during heart cushion development in the mouse. J Cell Biol. 2004;166:359-367.

[54] Person AD, Garriock RJ, Krieg PA, Runyan RB, Klewer SE. Frzb modulates Wnt-9a-mediated β-catenin signaling during avian atrioventricular cardiac cushion development. Dev Biol. 2005;278:35-48.

[55] Jackson LF, Qiu TH, Sunnarborg SW, Chang A, Zhang C, Patterson C, et al. Defective valvulogenesis in HB-EGF and TACE-null mice is associated with aberrant BMP signaling. EMBO J. 2003;22:2704-2716.

[56] Delot EC, Bahamonde ME, Zhao M, Lyons KM. BMP signaling is required for septation of the outflow tract of the mammalian heart. Development. 2003;130:209-220.

[57] Beppu H, Malhotra RR, Beppu Y, Lepore JJ, Parmacek MS, Bloch KD. BMP type II receptor regulates positioning of the outflow tract and remodeling of the atrioventricular cushion during cardiogenesis. Dev Biol. 2009;331:167-175.

[58] Galvin KM, Donovan MJ, Lynch CA, Meyer RI, Paul RJ, Lorenz JN, et al. A role for smad6 in development and homeostasis of the cardiovascular system. Nat Genet. 2000;24:171-174.

[59] Zhao B, Etter L, Hinton RB, Benson DW. BMP and FGF regulatory pathways in semilunar valve precursor cells. Dev Dyn. 2007;236:971-980.

[60] Alfieri CM, Cheek J, Chakraborty S, Yutzey KE. Wnt signaling in heart valve development and osteogenic gene induction. Dev Biol. 2010;338:127-135.

[61] Lange AW, Yutzey KE. NFATc1 expression in the developing heart valves is responsive to the RANKL pathway and is required for endocardial expression of cathepsin K. Dev Biol. 2006;292:407-417.

[62] del Monte G, Grego-Bessa J, Gozalez-Rajal A, Bolos V, delaPompa JL. Monitoring Notch1 activity in development: evidence for a feedback regulatory loop. Dev Dyn. 2007;236:2594-2614.

[63] Cripe L, Andelfinger G, Martin LJ, Shooner K, Benson DW. Bicuspid aortic valve is heritable. J Am Coll Cardiol. 2004;44:138-143.

[64] Garg V, Muth AN, Ransom JF, Schluterman MK, Barnes R, King IN, et al. Mutations in NOTCH1 cause aortic valve disease. Nature. 2005;437:270-274.

[65] Nus M, MacGrogan D, Martinez-Poveda B, Benito Y, Casanova JC, Fernandez-Aviles F, et al. Diet-induced aortic valve disease in mice haploinsufficient for the Notch pathway effector RBPJK/CSL. Arterioscler Thromb Vasc Biol. 2011;31:1580-1588.

[66] Laforest B, Andelfinger G, Nemer M. Loss of Gata5 in mice leads to bicuspid aortic valve. J Clin Invest. 2011;121:2876-2887.

[67] Padang R, Bagnall RD, Richmond DR, Bannon PG, Semsarian C. Rare non-synonymous variations in the transcriptional activation domains of GATA5 in bicupid aortic valve disease. J Mol Cell Cardiol. 2012;53:277-291.

[68] Lee TC, Zhao YD, Courtman DW, Stewart DJ. Abnormal aortic valve development in mice lacking endothelial nitric oxide synthase. Circulation. 2000;101:2345-2348.

[69] Schoen FJ. Evolving concepts of cardiac valve dynamics. Circulation. 2008;118:1864-1880.

[70] Snider P, Hinton RB, Moreno-Rodriguez R, Wang J, Rogers R, Lindsley A, et al. Periostin is required for maturation and extracellular matrix stabilization of noncardiomyocyte lineages of the heart. Circ Res. 2008;102:752-760.

[71] Norris RA, Moreno-Rodriguez RA, Sugi Y, Hoffman S, Amos J, Hart MM, et al. Periostin regulates atrioventricular valve maturation. Dev Biol. 2008;316:200-213.

[72] Hinton RB, Adelman-Brown J, Witt S, Krishnamurthy VK, Osinska H, Sakthivel B, et al. Elastin haploinsufficiency results in progressive aortic valve malformation and latent valve disease in a mouse model. Circ Res. 2010;107:549-557.

[73] Cheek JD, Wirrig EE, Alfieri CM, James JF, Yutzey KE. Differential activation of val-
      vulogenic, chondrogenic, and osteogenic pathways in mouse models of myxomatous
      and calcific aortic valve disease. J Mol Cell Cardiol. 2012;52:689-700.

[74] Kern CB, Wessels A, McGarity J, Dixon LJ, Alston E, Argraves WS, et al. Reduced
      versican cleavage due to Adamts9 haploinsufficiency is associated with cardiac and
      aortic anomalies. Matrix Biol. 2010;29:304-316.

[75] Dupuis LE, McCulloch DR, McGarity JD, Bahan A, Wessels A, Weber D, et al. Al-
      tered versican cleavage in ADAMTS5 deficient mice; a novel etiology of myxomatous
      valve disease. Dev Biol. 2011;357:152-164.

[76] Karsenty G, Wagner EF. Reaching a genetic and molecular understanding of skeletal
      development. Dev Cell. 2002;2:389-406.

[77] Lefebvre V, Bhattaram P. Vertebrate skeletogenesis. Curr Top Dev Biol.
      2010;90:291-317.

[78] Chai Y, Jiang X, Ito Y, Bringas P, Jr., Han J, Rowitch DH, et al. Fate of the mammalian
      cranial neural crest during tooth and mandibular morphogenesis. Development.
      2000;127:1671-1679.

[79] Karsenty G. Transcriptional control of skeletogenesis. Annu Rev Genomics Hum
      Genet. 2008;9:183-196.

[80] Long F. Building strong bones: molecular regulation of the osteoblast lineage. Nat
      Rev Mol Cell Biol. 2012;13:27-38.

[81] Goldring MB, Tsuchimochi K, Ijiri K. The control of chondrogenesis. J Cell Biochem.
      2006;97:33-44.

[82] Yoshioka M, Yuasa S, Matsumura K, Kimura K, Shiomi T, Kimura N, et al. Chondro-
      modulin-I maintains cardiac valvular function by preventing angiogenesis. Nat Med.
      2006;12:1151-1159.

[83] Nakashima K, Zhou X, Kunkel G, Zhang Z, Deng JM, Behringer RR, et al. The novel
      zinc finger-containing transcription factor osterix is required for osteoblast differen-
      tiation and bone formation. Cell. 2002;108:17-29.

[84] Bialek P, Kern B, Yang X, Schrock M, Sosoc D, Hong N, et al. A Twist code deter-
      mines the onset of osteoblast differentiation. Dev Cell. 2004;6:423-435.

[85] Gu S, Boyer TG, Naski M. Basic helix-loop-helix transcription factor Twist1 inhibits
      transactivator function of master chondrogenic regulator Sox9. J Biol Chem.
      2012;287:21082-21092.

[86] Yousfi M, Lasmoles F, Lomri A, Delannoy P, Marie PJ. Increased bone formation and
      decreased osteocalcin expression induced by reduced Twist dosage in Saethre-Chot-
      zen syndrome. J Clin Invest. 2001;107:1153-1161.

[87] Dodig M, Tadic T, Kronenberg MS, Dacic S, Liu YH, Maxson RE, et al. Ectopic Msx2 overexpression inhibits and Msx2 antisense stimulates calvarial osteoblast differentiation. Dev Biol. 1999;209:298-307.

[88] Akiyama H, Chaboissier M-C, Martin JF, Schedl A, de Crombrugghe B. The transcription factor Sox9 has essential roles in successive steps of the chondrocyte differentiation pathway and is required for expression of Sox5 and Sox6. Genes Dev. 2002;16:2813-2828.

[89] Chimal-Monroy J, Rodriguez-Leon J, Montero JA, Ganan Y, Macias D, Merino R, et al. Analysis of the molecular cascade responsible for mesodermal limb chondrogenesis: Sox genes and BMP signaling. Dev Biol. 2003;257:292-301.

[90] Lefebvre V, Huang W, Harley VR, Goodfellow PN, de Crombrugghe B. SOX9 is a potent activator of the chondrocyte-specific enhancer of the pro alpha1(II) collagen gene. Mol Cell Biol. 1997;17:2336-2346.

[91] Sekiya I, Tsuji K, Koopman P, Watanabe T, Yamada Y, Shinomiya K, et al. SOX9 enhances aggrecan gene promoter/enhancer activity and is up-regulated by retinoic acids in a cartilage-derived cell line, TC6. J Biol Chem. 2000;275:10738-10744.

[92] Dy P, Wang W, Bhattaram P, Wang Q, Wang L, Ballock RT, et al. Sox9 directs hypertrophic maturation and blocks osteoblast differentiation of growth plate chondrocytes. Dev Cell. 2012;22:597-609.

[93] Ducy P, Zhang R, Geoffroy V, Ridall AL, Karsenty G. Osf/Cbfa1: a transcriptional activator of osteoblast differentiation. Cell. 1997;89:747-754.

[94] Zamurovic N, Cappellen D, Rohner D, Susa M. Coordinated activation of Notch, Wnt, and transforming growth factor-beta signaling pathways in bone morphogenetic 2-induced osteogenesis. J Biol Chem. 2004;279:37704-37715.

[95] Ducy P, Starbuck M, Priemel M, Shen J, Pinero G, Geoffroy V, et al. A Cbfa1-dependent genetic pathway controls bone formation beyond embryonic development. Genes Dev. 1999;13:1025-1036.

[96] Boyle WJ, Simonet WS, Lacey DL. Osteoclast differentiation and activation. Nature. 2003;423:337-342.

[97] Takayanagi H, Kim S, Koga T, Nishina H, Isshiki M, Yoshida H, et al. Induction and activation of the transcription factor NFATc1 (NFAT2) integrate RANKL signaling and terminal differentiation of osteoclasts. Dev Cell. 2002;8:889-901.

[98] Ishida N, Hayashi K, Hoshijima M, Ogawa T, Koga S, Miyatake Y, et al. Large scale gene expression analysis of osteoclastogenesis in vitro and elucidation of NFAT2 as a key regulator. J Biol Chem. 2002;277:41147-41156.

[99] Simonet WS, Lacey DL, Dunstan CR, Kelley M, Chang MS, Luthy R, et al. Osteoprotegerin: a novel secreted protein involved in the regulation of bone density. Cell. 1997;89:309-319.

[100] Yasuda H, Shima N, Nakagawa N, Mochizuki SA, Yano K, Fujise N, et al. Identity of osteoclastogenesis inhibitor factor (OCIF) and osteoprotegerin (OPG): a mechanism by which OPG/OCIF inhibits osteoclastogenesis in vitro. Endocrinology. 1998;139:1329-1337.

[101] Koga T, Matsui Y, Asagiri M, Kodama T, de Crombrugge B, Nakashima K, et al. NFAT and Osterix cooperatively regulate bone formation. Nat Med. 2005;11:880-885.

[102] Winslow MM, Pan M, Starbuck M, Gallo EM, Deng L, Karsenty G, et al. Calcineurin/NFAT signaling in osteoblasts regulates bone mass. Dev Cell. 2006;10:771-782.

[103] Kaden JJ, Bickelhaupt S, Grobholz R, Haase KK, Sarikoc A, Kilic R, et al. Receptor activator of nuclear factor kB ligand and osteoprotegerin regulate aortic valve calcification. J Mol Cell Cardiol. 2004;36:57-66.

[104] Rabkin-Aikawa E, Farber M, Aikawa M, Schoen FJ. Dynamic and reversible changes in interstitial cell phenotype during remodeling of cardiac valves. J Heart Valve Disease. 2004;13:841-847.

[105] Nishimura R, Wakabayashi M, Hata K, Matsubara T, Honma S, Wakisaka S, et al. Osterix regulates calcification and degradation of chondrogenic matrices through matrix metalloproteinase (MMP13) expression in association with transcription factor Runx2 during endochondral ossification. J Biol Chem. 2012;287:33179-33190.

[106] Alexopoulos A, Bravou V, Peroukides S, Kaklamanis L, Varakis J, Alexopoulos D, et al. Bone regulatory factors NFATc1 and Osterix in human calcific aortic valves. Int J Cardiol. 2010;139:142-149.

[107] Kobayashi T, Kronenberg H. Trascriptional regulation in development of bone. Endocrinology. 2005;146:1012-1017.

[108] Wozney JM, Rosen V, A.J. C, Mitsock LM, Whitters MJ, Kriz RW, et al. Novel regulators of bone formation: molecular clones and activities. Science. 1988;242:1528-1534.

[109] Nishimura R, Hata K, Matsubara T, Wakabayashi M, Yoneda T. Regulation of bone and cartilage development by network between BMP signaling and transcription factors. J Biochem. 2012;151:247-254.

[110] Lin GL, Hakenson KD. Integration of BMP, Wnt, and Notch signaling pathways in osteoblast differentiation. J Cell Biochem. 2011;112:3491-3501.

[111] Rawadi G, Vayssiere B, Dunn F, Baron R, Roman-Roman S. BMP-2 controls alkaline phosphatase expression and osteoblast mineralization by a Wnt auotcrine loop. J Bone Min Res. 2003;18:1842-1853.

[112] Rodriguez-Carballo E, Ulsamer A, Susperregui AR, Manzanares-Cespedes C, Sanchez-Garcia E, Bartrons R, et al. Conserved regulatory motifs in osteogenic gene promoters integrate cooperative effects of canonical Wnt and BMP pathways. J Bone Miner Res. 2011;26:718-729.

[113] Sciaudone M, Gazzerro E, Priest L, Delanty AM, Canalis E. Notch1 impairs osteoblastic cell differentiation. Endocrinology. 2003;144:5631-5639.

[114] Deregowski V, Gazzerro E, Priest L, Rydziel S, Canalis E. Notch 1 overexpression inhibits osteoblastogenesis by suppressing Wnt/β-catenin but not bone morphogenetic protein signaling. J Biol Chem. 2006;218:6203-6210.

[115] Hilton MJ, Tu X, Wu X, Bai S, Zhao H, Kobayashi T, et al. Notch signaling maintains bone marrow mesenchyme progenitors by suppressing osteoblast differentiation. Nat Med. 2008;14:306-314.

[116] Mead TJ, Yutzey KE. Notch pathway regulation of chondrocyte differentiation and proliferation during appendicular and axial skeleton development. Proc Natl Acad Sci USA. 2009;106:14420-14425.

[117] Gross L, Kugel MA. Topographic Anatomy and Histology of the Valves in the Human Heart. Am J Pathol. 1931;7:445-474.

[118] Kaden JJ, Bickelhaupt S, Grobholz R, Vahl CF, Hagl S, Brueckmann M, et al. Expression of bone sialoprotein and bone morphogenetic protein-2 in calcific aortic stenosis. J Heart Valve Dis. 2004;13:560-566.

[119] Otto CM, Kuusisto J, Reichenbach DD, Gown AM, O'Brien KD. Characterization of the early lesion of 'degenerative' valvular aortic stenosis. Histological and immunohistochemical studies. Circulation. 1994;90:844-853.

[120] Thubrikar MJ, Jaffar A, Nolan SP. Patterns of calcific deposits in operatively excised stenotic or purely regurgitant aortic valves and their relation to mechanical stress. Am J Cardiol. 1986;58:304-308.

[121] Turri M, Thiene G, Bortolotti U, Milano A, Mazzucco A, Gallucci V. Surgical pathology of aortic valve disease. A study based on 602 specimens. Eur J Cardiothorac Surg. 1990;4:556-560.

[122] Bonow RO, Carabello BA, Chatterjee K, de Leon AC, Jr., Faxon DP, Freed MD, et al. 2008 Focused update incorporated into the ACC/AHA 2006 guidelines for the management of patients with valvular heart disease: a report of the American College of Cardiology/American Heart Association Task Force on Practice Guidelines (Writing Committee to Revise the 1998 Guidelines for the Management of Patients With Valvular Heart Disease). Circulation. 2008;118:e523-661.

[123] Cosmi JE, Kort S, Tunick PA, Rosenzweig BP, Freedberg RS, Katz ES, et al. The risk of the development of aortic stenosis in patients with "benign" aortic valve thickening. Arch Intern Med. 2002;162:2345-2347.

[124] Rabkin E, Aikawa M, Stone JR, Fukumoto Y, Libby P, Schoen FJ. Activated interstitial myofibroblasts express catabolic enzymes and mediate matrix remodeling in myxomatous heart valves. Circulation. 2001;104:2525-2532.

[125] Walker GA, Masters KS, Shah DN, Anseth KS, Leinwand LA. Valvular myofibroblast activation by transforming growth factor β. Circ Res. 2004;95:253-260.

[126] Fisher CI, Chen J, Merryman WD. Calcific nodule morphogenesis by heart valve interstitial cells is strain dependent. Biomech Model Mechanobiol. 2012; In Press.

[127] Ortlepp JR, Schmitz F, Mevissen V, Weiss S, Huster J, Dronskowski R, et al. The amount of calcium-deficient hexagonal hydroxyapatite in aortic valves is influenced by gender and associated with genetic polymorphisms in patients with severe calcific aortic stenosis. Eur Heart J. 2004;25:514-522.

[128] Weska RF, Aimoli CG, Nogueira GM, Leirner AA, Maizato MJ, Higa OZ, et al. Natural and prosthetic heart valve calcification: morphology and chemical composition characterization. Artif Organs. 2010;34:311-318.

[129] Mohler ER, Gannon F, Reynolds C, Zimmerman R, Keane MG, Kaplan FS. Bone formation and inflammation in cardiac valves. Circulation. 2001;103:1522-1528.

[130] Egan KP, Kim JH, Mohler ER, 3rd, Pignolo RJ. Role for circulating osteogenic precursor cells in aortic valvular disease. Arterioscler Thromb Vasc Biol. 2011;31:2965-2971.

[131] Li C, Xu S, Gotlieb AI. The progression of calcific aortic valve disease through injury, cell dysfunction, and disruptive biologic and physical force feedback loops. Cardiovasc Pathol. 2012; In Press.

[132] Mazzone A, Epistolato MC, De Caterina R, Storti S, Vittorini S, Sbrana S, et al. Neoangiogenesis, T-lymphocyte infiltration, and heat shock protein-60 are biological hallmarks of an immunomediated inflammatory process in end-stage calcified aortic valve stenosis. J Am Coll Cardiol. 2004;43:1670-1676.

[133] O'Brien KD, Shavelle DM, Caulfield MT, McDonald TO, Olin-Lewis K, Otto CM, et al. Association of angiotensin-converting enzyme with low-density lipoprotein in aortic valvular lesions and in human plasma. Circulation. 2002;106:2224-2230.

[134] Olsson M, Thyberg J, Nilsson J. Presence of oxidized low density lipoprotein in non-rheumatic stenotic aortic valves. Arterioscler Thromb Vasc Biol. 1999;19:1218-1222.

[135] Steiner I, Krbal L, Rozkos T, Harrer J, Laco J. Calcific aortic valve stenosis: Immunohistochemical analysis of inflammatory infiltrate. Pathol Res Pract. 2012;208:231-234.

[136] Clark-Greuel JN, Connolly JM, Sorichillo E, Narula NR, Rapoport HS, Mohler ER, et al. Transforming growth factor-β1 mechanisms in aortic valve calcification: increased alkaline phosphatase and related events. Ann Thorac Surg. 2007;83:946-953.

[137] ian B, Narula N, Li QY, Mohler ER, 3rd, Levy RJ. Progression of aortic valve stenosis: TGF-beta1 is present in calcified aortic valve cusps and promotes aortic valve interstitial cell calcification via apoptosis. Ann Thorac Surg. 2003;75:457-465.

[138] Yang X, Meng X, Su X, Mauchley DC, Ao L, Cleveland JC, et al. Bone morphogenetic protein 2 induces Runx2 and osteopontin expression in human aortic valve intersti-

tial cells: Role of Smad1 and extracellular signal-regulated kinase 1/2. J Thorac Cardiovasc Surg. 2009;138:1008-1015.

[139] Beppu S, Suzuki S, Matsuda H, Ohmori F, Nagata S, Miyatake K. Rapidity of progression of aortic stenosis in patients with congenital bicuspid aortic valves. Am J Cardiol. 1993;71:322-327.

[140] Linefsky JP, O'Brien KD, Katz R, de Boer IH, Barasch E, Jenny NS, et al. Association of serum phosphate levels with aortic valve sclerosis and annular calcification: the cardiovascular health study. J Am Coll Cardiol. 2011;58:291-297.

[141] Rosenhek R, Klaar U, Schemper M, Scholten C, Heger M, Gabriel H, et al. Mild and moderate aortic stenosis. Natural history and risk stratification by echocardiography. Eur Heart J. 2004;25:199-205.

[142] Varadarajan P, Kapoor N, Bansal RC, Pai RG. Clinical profile and natural history of 453 nonsurgically managed patients with severe aortic stenosis. Ann Thorac Surg. 2006;82:2111-2115.

[143] Caira FC, Stock SR, Gleason TG, McGee EC, Huang J, Bonow RO, et al. Human degenerative valve disease is associated with up-regulation of low-density lipoprotein-related protein 5 receptor-mediated bone formation J Am Coll Cardiol. 2006;47:1707-1712.

[144] Miller JD, Chu Y, Brooks RM, Richenbacher WE, Pena-Silva R, Heistad DD. Dysregulation of antioxidant mechanisms contributes to increased oxidative stress in calcific aortic valvular stenosis in humans. J Am Coll Cardiol. 2008;52:843-850.

[145] Satokata I, Ma L, Ohshima H, Bei M, Woo I, Nishizawa K, et al. Msx2 deficiency in mice causes pleiotropic defects in bone growth and ectodermal organ formation. Nat Genet. 2000;24:391-395.

[146] Balachandran K, Alford PW, Wylie-Sears J, Goss JA, Bischoff J, Aikawa E, et al. Cyclic strain induces dual-mode endothelial-mesenchymal transformation of the cardiac valve. Proc Natl Acad Sci USA. 2011;108:19943-19948.

[147] Dal-Bianco JP, Aikawa E, Bischoff J, Guerrero JL, Handschumacher MD, Sullivan S, et al. Active adaptation of the tethered mitral valve: Insights into a compensatory mechanism for functional mitral regurgitation. Circulation. 2009;120:334-342.

[148] Paranya G, Vineberg S, Dvorin E, Kaushal S, Roth SJ, Rabkin E, et al. Aortic valve endothelial cells undergo transforming growth factor-beta-mediated and non-transforming growth factor-beta-mediated transdifferentiation in vitro. Am J Pathol. 2001;159:1335-1343.

[149] Paruchuri S, Yang JH, Aikawa E, Melero-Martin JM, Khan ZA, Loukogeorgakis S, et al. Human pulmonary valve progenitor cells exhibit endothelial/mesenchymal plasticity in response to vascular endothelial growth factor-A and transforming growth factor-beta2. Circ Res. 2006;99:861-869.

[150] Li Z, Feng L, Wang CM, Zheng QJ, Zhao BJ, Yi W, et al. Deletion of RBP-J in adult mice leads to the onset of aortic valve degenerative diseases. Mol Biol Rep. 2012;39:3837-3845.

[151] Hajdu Z, Romeo SJ, Fleming PA, Markwald RR, Visconti RP, Drake CJ. Recruitment of bone marrow-derived valve interstitial cells is a normal homeostatic process. J Mol Cell Cardiol. 2011;51:955-965.

[152] Pohjolainen V, Taskinen P, Soini Y, Rysa J, Ilves M, Juvonen T, et al. Noncollagenous bone matrix proteins as a part of calcific aortic valve disease regulation. Hum Pathol. 2008;39:1695-1701.

[153] Nigam V, Srivastava D. Notch1 represses osteogenic pathways in aortic valve cells. J Mol Cell Cardiol. 2009;47:828-834.

[154] Aikawa E, Aikawa M, Libby P, Figueiredo J-L, Rusanescu G, Iwamoto Y, et al. Arterial and aortic valve calcification abolished by elastolytic cathepsin S deficiency in chronic renal disease. Circulation. 2009;119:1785-1794.

[155] Hjortnaes J, Butcher J, Figueiredo J-L, Riccio M, Kohler RH, Kozloff KM, et al. Arterial and aortic valve calcification inversely correlates with osteoporotic bone remodeling: a role for inflammation. Eur Heart J. 2010;31:1975-1984.

[156] Ix JH, Shlipak MG, Katz R, Budoff MJ, Shavelle DM, Probstfield JL, et al. Kidney function and aortic valve and mitral annular calcification in the Multi-Ethnic Study of Atherosclerosis (MESA). Am J Kidney Dis. 2007;50:412-420.

[157] Shuvy M, Abedat S, Beeri R, Danenberg HD, Planer D, Ben-Dov IZ, et al. Uraemic hyperparathyroidism causes a reversible inflammatory process of aortic valve calcification in rats. Cardiovasc Res. 2008;79:492-499.

[158] Shanahan CM, Crouthamel MH, Kapustin A, Giachelli C. Arterial calcification in chronic kidney disease: key roles for calcium and phosphate. Circ Res. 2011;109:697-711.

[159] Hu MC, Kuro-o M, Moe OW. Klotho and kidney disease. J Nephrol. 2010;23 Suppl 16:S136-144.

[160] Kuro-o M, Matsumura Y, Aizawa H, Kawaguchi H, Suga T, Utsugi T, et al. Mutation of the mouse klotho gene leads to a syndrome resembling ageing. Nature. 1997;390:45-51.

[161] Segawa H, Yamanaka S, Ohno Y, Onitsuka A, Shiozawa K, Aranami F, et al. Correlation between hyperphosphatemia and type II Na-Pi cotransporter activity in klotho mice. Am J Physiol Renal Physiol. 2007;292:F769-779.

[162] Takeshita K, Fujimori T, Kurotaki Y, Honjo T, Tsujikawa H, Yasui K, et al. Sinoatrial node dysfunction and early unexpected death of mice with a defect of klotho gene expression. Circulation. 2004;109:1776-1782.

[163] Aikawa E, Nahrendorf M, Sosnovik D, Lok VM, Jaffer FA, Aikawa M, et al. Multimodality molecular imaging identifies proteolytic and osteogenic activities in early aortic valve disease. Circulation. 2007;115:377-386.

[164] Meng X, Ao L, Song Y, Babu A, Yang X, Wang M, et al. Expression of functional Toll-like receptors 2 and 4 in human aortic valve interstitial cells: potential roles in aortic valve inflammation and stenosis. Am J Physiol Cell Physiol. 2008;294:C29-35.

[165] Rajamannan NM, Subramaniam M, Springett M, Sebo TC, Niekrasz M, McConnell JP, et al. Atorvastatin inhibits hypercholesterolemia-induced cellular proliferation and bone matrix production in the rabbit aortic valve. Circulation. 2002;105:2660-2665.

[166] Aikawa E, Nahrendorf M, Figueiredo JL, Swirski FK, Shtatland T, Kohler RH, et al. Osteogenesis associates with inflammation in early-stage atherosclerosis evaluated by molecular imaging in vivo. Circulation. 2007;116:2841-2850.

[167] Miller JD, Weiss RM, Serrano KM, Brooks RM, Berry CJ, Zimmerman K, et al. Lowering plasma cholesterol levels halts progression of aortic valve disease in mice. Circulation. 2009;119:2693-2701.

[168] Babu AN, Meng X, Zou N, Yang X, Wang M, Song Y, et al. Lipopolysaccharide stimulation of human aortic valve interstitial cells activates inflammation and osteogenesis. Ann Thorac Surg. 2008;86:71-76.

[169] Ankeny RF, Thourani VH, Weiss D, Vega JD, Taylor WR, Nerem RM, et al. Preferential activation of SMAD1/5/8 on the fibrosa endothelium in calcificed human aortic valves - Association with low BMP antagonists and SMAD6. PLoS One. 2011;6:e20969.

[170] Miller JD, Weiss RM, Serrano KM, Casteneda LE, Brooks RM, Zimmerman K, et al. Evidence for active regulation of pro-osteogenic signaling in advanced aortic valve disease. Arterioscler Thromb Vasc Biol. 2010;30:2482-2486.

[171] Osman L, Yacoub MH, Latif N, Amrani M, Chester AH. Role of human valve interstitial cells in valve calcification and their response to atorvastatin. Circulation. 2006;114:I-547-I-552.

[172] Merryman WD, Lukoff HD, Long RA, Engelmayr GC, Jr., Hopkins RA, Sacks MS. Synergistic effects of cyclic tension and transforming growth factor-beta1 on the aortic valve myofibroblast. Cardiovasc Pathol. 2007;16:268-276.

[173] Chen JH, Chen WLK, Sider KL, Yip CYY, Simmons CA. beta-catenin mediated mechanically regulated, transforming growth factor-beta1-induced myofibroblast differentiation of aortic valve interstitial cells. Arterioscler Thromb Vasc Biol. 2011;31:590-597.

[174] Cushing MC, Mariner PD, Liao JT, Sims EA, Anseth KS. Fibroblast growth factor represses Smad-mediated myofibroblast activation in aortic valvular interstitial cells. FASEB J. 2008;22:1769-1777.

[175] Acharya A, Hans CP, Keonig SN, Nichols HA, Galindo CL, Garner HR, et al. Inhibitory role for Notch1 in calcific aortic valve disease. PLoS One. 2011;6:e27743.

[176] Tamai K, Zeng X, Liu C, Zhang X, Harada Y, Chang Z, et al. A mechanism for Wnt coreceptor activation. Mol Cell. 2004;13:149-156.

[177] Rajamannan NM, Subramaniam M, Caira F, Stock SR, Spelsberg TC. Atorvastatin inhibits hypercholesterolemia-induced calcification in the aortic valves via the Lrp5 receptor pathway. Circulation. 2005;112:I229-I234.

[178] Rajamannan NM. Oxidative-mechanical stress signals stem cell niche mediated Lrp5 osteogenesis in eNOS(-/-) null mice. J Cell Biochem. 2012;113:1623-1634.

[179] Xu S, Gotlieb AI. Wnt3a/beta-catenin increases proliferation in heart valve interstitial cells. Cardiovasc Pathol. 2012; In Press.

[180] Rajamannan NM. The role of Lrp5/6 in cardiac valve disease: experimental hypercholesterolemia in the ApoE-/- /Lrp5-/- mice. J Cell Biochem. 2011;112:2987-2991.

[181] Fondard O, Detaint D, Iung B, Choqueux C, Adle-Biassette H, Jarraya M, et al. Extracellular matrix remodelling in human aortic valve disease: the role of matrix metalloproteinases and their tissue inhibitors. Eur Heart J. 2005;26:1333-1341.

[182] Perrotta I, Russo E, Camastra C, Filice G, Di Mizio G, Colosimo F, et al. New evidence for a critical role of elastin in calcification of native heart valves: immunohistochemical and ultrastructural study with literature review. Histopathology. 2011;59:504-513.

[183] Krishnamurthy VK, Opoka AM, Kern CB, Guilak F, Narmoneva DA, Hinton RB. Maladaptive matrix remodeling and regional biomechanical dysfunction in a mouse model of aortic valve disease. Matrix Biol. 2012;31:197-205.

[184] Bosse Y, Miqdad A, Fournier D, Pepin A, Pibarot P, Mathieu P. Refining molecular pathways leading to calcific aortic valve stenosis by studying gene expression profile of normal and calcified stenotic human aortic valves. Circ Cardiovasc Genet. 2009;2:489-498.

[185] Eriksen HA, Satta J, Risteli J, Veijola M, Vare P, Soini Y. Type I and type III collagen synthesis and composition in the valve matrix in aortic valve stenosis. Atherosclerosis. 2006;189:91-98.

[186] Matsumoto KI, Satoh K, Maniwa T, Araki A, Maruyama R, Oda T. Noticeable Decreased Expression of Tenascin-X in Calcific Aortic Valves. Connect Tissue Res. 2012; In Press.

[187] Stephens EH, Shangkuan J, Kuo JJ, Carroll JL, Kearney DL, Carberry KE, et al. Extracellular matrix remodeling and cell phenotypic changes in dysplastic and hemodynamically altered semilunar human cardiac valves. Cardiovasc Pathol. 2011;20:e157-167.

[188] Lockhart M, Wirrig E, Phelps A, Wessels A. Extracellular matrix and heart development. Birth Defects Res A Clin Mol Teratol. 2011;91:535-550.

[189] Mackie EJ, Tatarczuch L, Mirams M. The skeleton: a multi-functional complex organ: the growth plate chondrocyte and endochondral ossification. J Endocrinol. 2011;211:109-121.

[190] Balachandran K, Sucosky P, Jo H, Yoganathan AP. Elevated cyclic stretch alters matrix remodeling in aortic valve cusps: implications for degenerative aortic valve disease. Am J Physiol Heart Circ Physiol. 2009;296:H756-764.

[191] Kaden JJ, Dempfle CE, Kilic R, Sarikoc A, Hagl S, Lang S, et al. Influence of receptor activator of nuclear factor kappa B on human aortic valve myofibroblasts. Exp Mol Pathol. 2005;78:36-40.

[192] Takayanagi H. Mechanistic insight into osteoclast differentiation in osteoimmunology. J Mol Med (Berl). 2005;83:170-179.

[193] Steinmetz M, Skowasch D, Wernert N, Welsch U, Preusse CJ, Welz A, et al. Differential profile of the OPG/RANKL/RANK-system in degenerative aortic native and bioprosthetic valves. J Heart Valve Dis. 2008;17:187-193.

[194] O'Brien KD, Reichenbach DD, Marcovina SM, Kuusisto J, Alpers CE, Otto CM. Apolipoproteins B, (a), and E accumulate in the morphologically early lesion of 'degenerative' valvular aortic stenosis. Arterioscler Thromb Vasc Biol. 1996;16:523-532.

[195] Benton JA, Kern HB, Leinwand LA, Mariner PD, Anseth KS. Statins block calcific nodule formation of valvular interstitial cells by inhibiting alpha-smooth muscle actin expression. Arterioscler Thromb Vasc Biol. 2009;29:1950-1957.

[196] Monzack EL, Masters KS. A time-course investigation of the statin paradox among valvular interstitial cell phenotypes. Am J Physiol Heart Circ Physiol. 2012; 303:H903-9.

[197] Hamilton AM, Boughner DR, Drangova M, Rogers KA. Statin treatment of hypercholesterolemic-induced aortic valve sclerosis. Cardiovasc Pathol. 2011;20:84-92.

[198] Rosenhek R, Rader F, Loho N, Gabriel H, Heger M, Klaar U, et al. Statins but not angiotensin-converting enzyme inhibitors delay progression of aortic stenosis. Circulation. 2004;110:1291-1295.

[199] Chan KL, Teo K, Dumesnil JG, Ni A, Tam J. Effect of Lipid lowering with rosuvastatin on progression of aortic stenosis: results of the aortic stenosis progression observation: measuring effects of rosuvastatin (ASTRONOMER) trial. Circulation. 2010;121:306-314.

[200] Cowell SJ, Newby DE, Prescott RJ, Bloomfield P, Reid J, Northridge DB, et al. A randomized trial of intensive lipid-lowering therapy in calcific aortic stenosis. N Engl J Med. 2005;352:2389-2397.

[201] Rossebo AB, Pedersen TR, Boman K, Brudi P, Chambers JB, Egstrup K, et al. Intensive lipid lowering with simvastatin and ezetimibe in aortic stenosis. N Engl J Med. 2008;359:1343-1356.

[202] Ardehali R, Leeper NJ, Wilson AM, Heidenreich PA. The effect of angiotensin-converting enzyme inhibitors and statins on the progression of aortic sclerosis and mortality. J Heart Valve Dis. 2012;21:337-343.

[203] Powers B, Greene L, Balfe LM. Updates on the treatment of essential hypertension: a summary of AHRQ's comparative effectiveness review of angiotensin-converting enzyme inhibitors, angiotensin II receptor blockers, and direct renin inhibitors. J Manag Care Pharm. 2011;17(8 Suppl):S1-14.

[204] Arishiro K, Hoshiga M, Negoro N, Jin D, Takai S, Miyazaki M, et al. Angiotensin receptor-1 blocker inhibits atherosclerotic changes and endothelial disruption of the aortic valve in hypercholesterolemic rabbits. J Am Coll Cardiol. 2007;49:1482-1489.

[205] Ngo DT, Stafford I, Sverdlov AL, Qi W, Wuttke RD, Zhang Y, et al. Ramipril retards development of aortic valve stenosis in a rabbit model: mechanistic considerations. Br J Pharmacol. 2011;162:722-732.

[206] Simolin MA, Pedersen TX, Bro S, Mayranpaa MI, Helske S, Nielsen LB, et al. ACE inhibition attenuates uremia-induced aortic valve thickening in a novel mouse model. BMC Cardiovasc Disord. 2009;9:10.

[207] Cote N, Couture C, Pibarot P, Despres JP, Mathieu P. Angiotensin receptor blockers are associated with a lower remodelling score of stenotic aortic valves. Eur J Clin Invest. 2011;41:1172-1179.

[208] Chockalingam A, Venkatesan S, Subramaniam T, Jagannathan V, Elangovan S, Alagesan R, et al. Safety and efficacy of angiotensin-converting enzyme inhibitors in symptomatic severe aortic stenosis: Symptomatic Cardiac Obstruction-Pilot Study of Enalapril in Aortic Stenosis (SCOPE-AS). Am Heart J. 2004;147:E19.

[209] Nadir MA, Wei L, Elder DH, Libianto R, Lim TK, Pauriah M, et al. Impact of renin-angiotensin system blockade therapy on outcome in aortic stenosis. J Am Coll Cardiol. 2011;58:570-576.

[210] O'Brien KD, Probstfield JL, Caulfield MT, Nasir K, Takasu J, Shavelle DM, et al. Angiotensin-converting enzyme inhibitors and change in aortic valve calcium. Arch Intern Med. 2005;165:858-862.

[211] Wakabayashi K, Tsujino T, Naito Y, Ezumi A, Lee-Kawabata M, Nakao S, et al. Administration of angiotensin-converting enzyme inhibitors is associated with slow progression of mild aortic stenosis in Japanese patients. Heart Vessels. 2011;26:252-257.

[212] Sverdlov AL, Ngo DT, Chan WP, Chirkov YY, Gersh BJ, McNeil JJ, et al. Determinants of aortic sclerosis progression: implications regarding impairment of nitric oxide signaling and potential therapeutics. Eur Heart J. 2012; 33:2419-2425.

[213] Yamamoto K, Yamamoto H, Yoshida K, Kisanuki A, Hirano Y, Ohte N, et al. Prognostic factors for progression of early- and late-stage calcific aortic valve disease in Japanese: the Japanese Aortic Stenosis Study (JASS) Retrospective Analysis. Hypertens Res. 2010;33:269-274.

[214] Gkizas S, Koumoundourou D, Sirinian X, Rokidi S, Mavrilas D, Koutsoukos P, et al. Aldosterone receptor blockade inhibits degenerative processes in the early stage of calcific aortic stenosis. Eur J Pharmacol. 2010;642:107-112.

[215] Stewart RA, Kerr AJ, Cowan BR, Young AA, Occleshaw C, Richards AM, et al. A randomized trial of the aldosterone-receptor antagonist eplerenone in asymptomatic moderate-severe aortic stenosis. Am Heart J. 2008;156:348-355.

[216] Russell RG. Bisphosphonates: mode of action and pharmacology. Pediatrics. 2007;119 Suppl 2:S150-162.

[217] Rapoport HS, Connolly JM, Fulmer J, Dai N, Murti BH, Gorman RC, et al. Mechanisms of the in vivo inhibition of calcification of bioprosthetic porcine aortic valve cusps and aortic wall with triglycidylamine/mercapto bisphosphonate. Biomaterials. 2007;28:690-699.

[218] Innasimuthu AL, Katz WE. Effect of bisphosphonates on the progression of degenerative aortic stenosis. Echocardiography. 2011;28:1-7.

[219] Skolnick AH, Osranek M, Formica P, Kronzon I. Osteoporosis treatment and progression of aortic stenosis. Am J Cardiol. 2009;104:122-124.

[220] Sterbakova G, Vyskocil V, Linhartova K. Bisphosphonates in calcific aortic stenosis: association with slower progression in mild disease--a pilot retrospective study. Cardiology. 2010;117:184-189.

[221] Elmariah S, Delaney JA, O'Brien KD, Budoff MJ, Vogel-Claussen J, Fuster V, et al. Bisphosphonate Use and Prevalence of Valvular and Vascular Calcification in Women MESA (The Multi-Ethnic Study of Atherosclerosis). J Am Coll Cardiol. 2010;56:1752-1759.

[222] Aksoy O, Cam A, Goel SS, Houghtaling PL, Williams S, Ruiz-Rodriguez E, et al. Do bisphosphonates slow the progression of aortic stenosis? J Am Coll Cardiol. 2012;59:1452-1459.

[223] Kietadisorn R, Juni RP, Moens AL. Tackling endothelial dysfunction by modulating NOS uncoupling: new insights into its pathogenesis and therapeutic possibilities. Am J Physiol Endocrinol Metab. 2012;302:E481-495.

[224] Matsumoto Y, Adams V, Walther C, Kleinecke C, Brugger P, Linke A, et al. Reduced number and function of endothelial progenitor cells in patients with aortic valve stenosis: a novel concept for valvular endothelial cell repair. Eur Heart J. 2009;30:346-355.

[225] Poggianti E, Venneri L, Chubuchny V, Jambrik Z, Baroncini LA, Picano E. Aortic valve sclerosis is associated with systemic endothelial dysfunction. J Am Coll Cardiol. 2003;41:136-141.

[226] Liberman M, Bassi E, Martinatti MK, Lario FC, Wosniak J, Jr., Pomerantzeff PM, et al. Oxidant generation predominates around calcifying foci and enhances progression of aortic valve calcification. Arterioscler Thromb Vasc Biol. 2008;28:463-470.

[227] Kennedy JA, Hua X, Mishra K, Murphy GA, Rosenkranz AC, Horowitz JD. Inhibition of calcifying nodule formation in cultured porcine aortic valve cells by nitric oxide donors. Eur J Pharmacol. 2009;602:28-35.

[228] Cagirci G, Cay S, Canga A, Karakurt O, Yazihan N, Kilic H, et al. Association between plasma asymmetrical dimethylarginine activity and severity of aortic valve stenosis. J Cardiovasc Med. 2011;12:96-101.

[229] Ngo DT, Heresztyn T, Mishra K, Marwick TH, Horowitz JD. Aortic stenosis is associated with elevated plasma levels of asymmetric dimethylarginine (ADMA). Nitric Oxide. 2007;16:197-201.

[230] Schumm J, Luetzkendorf S, Rademacher W, Franz M, Schmidt-Winter C, Kiehntopf M, et al. In patients with aortic stenosis increased flow-mediated dilation is independently associated with higher peak jet velocity and lower asymmetric dimethylarginine levels. Am Heart J. 2011;161:893-899.

[231] Boursinos LA, Karachalios T, Poultsides L, Malizos KN. Do steroids, conventional non-steroidal anti-inflammatory drugs and selective Cox-2 inhibitors adversely affect fracture healing? J Musculoskelet Neuronal Interact. 2009;9:44-52.

[232] Grosser T. Variability in the response to cyclooxygenase inhibitors: toward the individualization of nonsteroidal anti-inflammatory drug therapy. J Investig Med. 2009;57:709-716.

[233] Smith WL, DeWitt DL, Garavito RM. Cyclooxygenases: structural, cellular, and molecular biology. Annu Rev Biochem. 2000;69:145-182.

[234] Narumiya S, Sugimoto Y, Ushikubi F. Prostanoid receptors: structures, properties, and functions. Physiol Rev. 1999;79:1193-1226.

[235] Lopez J, Fernandez-Pisonero I, Duenas AI, Maeso P, Roman JA, Crespo MS, et al. Viral and bacterial patterns induce TLR-mediated sustained inflammation and calcification in aortic valve interstitial cells. Int J Cardiol. 2012;158:18-25.

[236] Alander CB, Raisz LG. Effects of selective prostaglandins E2 receptor agonists on cultured calvarial murine osteoblastic cells. Prostaglandins Other Lipid Mediat. 2006;81:178-183.

[237] Choudhary S, Alander C, Zhan P, Gao Q, Pilbeam C, Raisz L. Effect of deletion of the prostaglandin EP2 receptor on the anabolic response to prostaglandin E2 and a selective EP2 receptor agonist. Prostaglandins Other Lipid Mediat. 2008;86:35-40.

[238] Chyun YS, Raisz LG. Stimulation of bone formation by prostaglandin E2. Prostaglandins. 1984;27:97-103.

[239] Gao Q, Xu M, Alander CB, Choudhary S, Pilbeam CC, Raisz LG. Effects of prostaglandin E2 on bone in mice in vivo. Prostaglandins Other Lipid Mediat. 2009;89:20-25.

[240] Jee WS, Ueno K, Kimmel DB, Woodbury DM, Price P, Woodbury LA. The role of bone cells in increasing metaphyseal hard tissue in rapidly growing rats treated with prostaglandin E2. Bone. 1987;8:171-178.

[241] Kaneki H, Takasugi I, Fujieda M, Kiriu M, Mizuochi S, Ide H. Prostaglandin E2 stimulates the formation of mineralized bone nodules by a cAMP-independent mechanism in the culture of adult rat calvarial osteoblasts. J Cell Biochem. 1999;73:36-48.

[242] Li M, Healy DR, Li Y, Simmons HA, Crawford DT, Ke HZ, et al. Osteopenia and impaired fracture healing in aged EP4 receptor knockout mice. Bone. 2005;37:46-54.

[243] Minamizaki T, Yoshiko Y, Kozai K, Aubin JE, Maeda N. EP2 and EP4 receptors differentially mediate MAPK pathways underlying anabolic actions of prostaglandin E2 on bone formation in rat calvaria cell cultures. Bone. 2009;44:1177-1185.

[244] Zhang X, Schwarz EM, Young DA, Puzas JE, Rosier RN, O'Keefe RJ. Cyclooxygenase-2 regulates mesenchymal cell differentiation into the osteoblast lineage and is critically involved in bone repair. J Clin Invest. 2002;109:1405-1415.

[245] Chikazu D, Li X, Kawaguchi H, Sakuma Y, Voznesensky OS, Adams DJ, et al. Bone morphogenetic protein 2 induces cyclo-oxygenase 2 in osteoblasts via a Cbfa1 binding site: role in effects of bone morphogenetic protein 2 in vitro and in vivo. J Bone Miner Res. 2002;17:1430-1440.

[246] Susperregui AR, Gamell C, Rodriguez-Carballo E, Ortuno MJ, Bartrons R, Rosa JL, et al. Noncanonical BMP signaling regulates cyclooxygenase-2 transcription. Mol Endocrinol. 2011;25:1006-1017.

[247] Kakita A, Suzuki A, Ono Y, Miura Y, Itoh M, Oiso Y. Possible involvement of p38 MAP kinase in prostaglandin E1-induced ALP activity in osteoblast-like cells. Prostaglandins Leukot Essent Fatty Acids. 2004;70:469-474.

[248] Celil Aydemir AB, Minematsu H, Gardner TR, Kim KO, Ahn JM, Lee FY. Nuclear factor of activated T cells mediates fluid shear stress- and tensile strain-induced Cox2 in human and murine bone cells. Bone. 2010;46:167-175.

[249] Mehrotra M, Saegusa M, Voznesensky O, Pilbeam C. Role of Cbfa1/Runx2 in the fluid shear stress induction of COX-2 in osteoblasts. Biochem Biophys Res Commun. 2006;341:1225-1230.

[250] Boniface K, Bak-Jensen KS, Li Y, Blumenschein WM, McGeachy MJ, McClanahan TK, et al. Prostaglandin E2 regulates Th17 cell differentiation and function through cyclic AMP and EP2/EP4 receptor signaling. J Exp Med. 2009;206:535-548.

[251] Yao C, Sakata D, Esaki Y, Li Y, Matsuoka T, Kuroiwa K, et al. Prostaglandin E2-EP4 signaling promotes immune inflammation through Th1 cell differentiation and Th17 cell expansion. Nat Med. 2009;15:633-640.

[252] Garcia Rodriguez LA, Gonzalez-Perez A, Bueno H, Hwa J. NSAID use selectively increases the risk of non-fatal myocardial infarction: a systematic review of randomised trials and observational studies. PLoS One. 2011;6:e16780.

[253] Salvo F, Fourrier-Reglat A, Bazin F, Robinson P, Riera-Guardia N, Haag M, et al. Cardiovascular and gastrointestinal safety of NSAIDs: a systematic review of meta-analyses of randomized clinical trials. Clin Pharmacol Ther. 2011;89:855-866.

[254] Willette RN, Eybye ME, Olzinski AR, Behm DJ, Aiyar N, Maniscalco K, et al. Differential effects of p38 mitogen-activated protein kinase and cyclooxygenase 2 inhibitors in a model of cardiovascular disease. J Pharmacol Exp Ther. 2009;330:964-970.

[255] Wirrig EE, Yutzey KE. Transcriptional regulation of heart valve development and disease. Cardiovasc Pathol. 2011;20:162-167.

[256] Rajamannan NM, Evans FJ, Aikawa E, Grande-Allen KJ, Demer LL, Heistad DD, et al. Calcific aortic valve disease: not simply a degenerative process: A review and agenda for research from the National Heart and Lung and Blood Institute Aortic Stenosis Working Group. Executive summary: Calcific aortic valve disease-2011 update. Circulation. 2011;124:1783-1791.

Chapter 4

Notch Signaling in Congenital and Acquired Aortic Valve Disease

Erik Fung and Masanori Aikawa

Additional information is available at the end of the chapter

1. Introduction

Calcific aortic valve disease represents the predominant pathology of tricuspid (trileaflet) and bicuspid aortic valves in developed countries (Ladich et al., 2011). Accounting for approximately half of anatomically isolated aortic stenosis and 25 percent of patients with aortic regurgitation (Roberts, 1970), calcific bicuspid aortic valves requiring surgical intervention present at least two decades earlier than the tricuspid counterpart (Ward, 2000). Mechanisms important in cardiac and organ development — notably, the Notch pathway — have emerged as central players recapitulated and reused during the pathogenesis of calcific aortic valve disease, and support also a common etiology for bicuspid aortic valve and aortic valve calcification (Garg et al., 2005) (Table 1). Active engagement of inflammatory, remodeling, neovascularization and osteogenic (Aikawa et al., 2007a; Aikawa et al., 2007b; Miller et al., 2010; Rajamannan et al., 2003) pathways has conceptually replaced 'degeneration' in calcific aortic valve disease pathogenesis and progression (Dweck et al., 2012). Moreover, these pathways invoke similar mechanisms during cardiac morphogenesis. Dysregulated Notch activity has also been reported in vascular inflammation, macrophage activation (Fung et al., 2007), cardiometabolic disorder, and vascular and aortic valve calcification (Fukuda et al., 2012). Preclinical studies suggest that specific blockade of Notch ligand–receptor signaling potently suppresses vascular calcification and calcific aortic valve disease (Fukuda et al., 2012). In this chapter, we review the mechanisms of Notch signaling, aortic valve dysmorphology pertinent to accelerated valve calcification, and discuss the pathways involving Notch that lead to aortic valve calcification and disease.

	Role in cardiac and aortic valve development	Role in aortic valve calcification
NOTCH1	cardiac morphogenesis	inhibits calcification
Hey1/2	downstream effector of Notch inhibits action of BMP2	inhibits calcification, decreases ostepontin
BMP2	coordination of cardiac patterning and EMT required for valve formation	promotes calcification
Sox9	increased by Hey2 and mediates chondrogenesis	suppresses osteogenesis
Runx2	repressed by NOTCH1 and Hey1/2	promotes calcification
JAG1	boundary definition in myocardium; vasculogenesis	inhibits calcification
DLL4	formation of heart fields and boundary definition in endocardium; vasculogenesis	neovascularization (angioneogenesis) & hemorrhage leading to calcific aortic valve disease

Table 1. Major components of the Notch1-Hey-BMP2 axis and their actions in cardiac and aortic valve development, and in aortic valve calcification. BMP, bone morphogenetic protein. DLL4, Delta-like 4. JAG1, Jagged1.

2. Notch signaling

The human Notch receptor family comprises four members, Notch1 through Notch4, expressed as transmembrane molecules on the cell surface of neighboring cells that enable canonical signaling in a contact-dependent manner (Bray, 2006; Kopan and Ilagan, 2009). Canonical Notch signaling describes the 'classic' interaction between membrane-bound receptors and ligands expressed on the surface of neighboring (signaling and receiving) cells, whereas non-canonical signaling encompasses a diverse group of structurally unrelated ligands that contribute to the pleiotropic effect of Notch signaling (Kopan and Ilagan, 2009). In mammals, five members of the Delta-Serrate-LAG-2 (DSL) family have the capacity to activate or modify canonical Notch signaling — Delta-like 1 (Dll1), Dll3, Dll4, Jagged1, and Jagged2. Interaction between Notch receptor and ligand is tightly controlled, and the signaling outcome is determined by the receptor:ligand ratio (Artavanis-Tsakonas and Muskavitch, 2010; Gibert and Simpson, 2003; Heitzler and Simpson, 1991; Wilkinson et al., 1994) that critically determines asymmetry in cell fate and development of neighboring cells. This interaction between receptor and ligand can be modified posttranslationally through Notch glycosylation by lunatic, manic and radical glycosyltransferases (Bray, 2006). The receptor:ligand ratio is dependent on the differential expression of competing ligands on neighboring cells in *trans*, as opposed to *cis* interaction through which receptor and ligand expressed on the same cell can also modulate Notch signaling. The complexity of receptor–ligand interaction is further increased by the requirement of heterodimerization of the receptor (Kopan and Ilagan, 2009). Canonical interaction between Notch receptor and ligand leads to two sequential cleavage events at site 2 (S2) and S3. S2 is a 'permissive' extracellular juxtamembrane cleavage by a disintegrin and metalloprotease 17 (ADAM17, known also as tumor necrosis factor-α converting enzyme/TACE) and/or ADAM10 (Artavanis-Tsakonas and Muskavitch, 2010;

Bray, 2006), whereas S3 is executed by γ-secretase, a protease with many substrates (McCarthy et al., 2009; Wakabayashi and De Strooper, 2008). S1 cleavage is carried out by a furin-like convertase occurring posttranslationally in the trans-Golgi apparatus before translocation of the nascent Notch receptor to the cell surface (Bray, 2006; Kopan and Ilagan, 2009). Following S3 cleavage, the Notch intracellular domain is liberated and enters the nucleus to form a transcription activational complex with the transcriptional factor RBP-Jκ, and the transcriptional coactivator Mastermind to promote target gene transcription (Bray, 2006; Kopan and Ilagan, 2009). Targets indicative of Notch activity include the basic-helix-loop-helix genes of the hairy and enhancer of split (HES) and the hairy-related (HRT or Hey) family (Bray, 2006; Kopan and Ilagan, 2009).

Functionality of Notch signaling components is highly context-dependent and conventionally requires cell-to-cell contact to specify cell fate, differentiation, growth, proliferation, survival and apoptosis (Bray, 2006; Fiuza and Arias, 2007; Guruharsha et al., 2012). Interaction between Notch receptor and ligand on adjacent cells results in asymmetric signal transduction, leading to potentially divergent cell fate decision, phenotypic development and growth (Bray, 2006; Kopan and Ilagan, 2009).

3. Congenital aortic valve disease

3.1. Notch dysfunction in aortic valve anomalies and other congenital heart diseases

Congenital aortic valve anomalies frequently associate with other abnormalities in neighboring structures, including the aortic root (e.g. dilatation, aneurysm), aorta (e.g. coarctation of aorta), ventricular outflow tract (e.g. septal defect, transposition of great vessels), and/or coronary arteries (e.g. coronary anomalies) (Perloff, 2003; Ward, 2000). The association of anomalies is due in part to the complexity and critical function of the endocardial cushion, and its formation during cardiac valve and septum development (Camenisch et al., 2010).

The tight regulation of Notch signaling during murine cardiac morphogenesis, particularly of the cardiac outflow tract and semilunar (aortic and pulmonary) valves, have been recently reviewed in detail by de la Pompa and Epstein (de la Pompa and Epstein, 2012). The evolutionarily conserved nature of Notch across mammalian species is generally recognized to be applicable to human. The highly coordinated action of Notch in progenitor cell proliferation and differentiation is instrumental during development. Earliest signs of cardiac morphogenesis occur with formation of the cardiac crescent by midline fusion of first and second heart fields that feature expression of Notch1, Dll4 and Jagged1 in the primitive endocardium (de la Pompa and Epstein, 2012; del Monte et al., 2007; Duarte et al., 2004). Continuing cell proliferation and development leads to the generation of the heart tube, consisting of an outer myocardial layer, middle cardiac jelly of extracellular matrix, and an inner endocardial endothelium (Camenisch et al., 2010; de la Pompa and Epstein, 2012). Demarcation of boundary and tissue layers is marked by expression of Jagged1 limited to the myocardial layer, and Dll4, Notch1, Notch2 and Notch4 in the endocardium. The heart tube gradually undergoes a complex morphologic change with a rightward bend, converting the anterior-posterior polarity of the heart tube into a right-left (R-) loop. As the looped heart further develops, the valve territories of the atrioventricular canal (AVC) and outflow tract (OFT) are demarcated. The AVC and OFT cushions become the sites for formation of the mitral and aortic valves, respectively, in the left ventricle and the tricuspid and pulmonary valves in the right ventricule (Person et al., 2005). Contribution of endocardium-derived mesenchyme to the development of AVC and OFT valve primordia diverge as the neural crest contribute additionally to the development of the OFT valve primordium (de la Pompa and Epstein, 2012; Zhang et al., 2010). At this stage of development, Jagged1 expression is present in the endocardium and chamber myocardium, whereas expression of Dll4 and Notch1 localizes to the valve and atrial endo-cardium. Here, Notch coordinates cardiac patterning through regulation of the Notch-Hey-Bmp2 axis (MacGrogan et al., 2011). Bmp2, or bone morphogenetic protein 2, is responsible for AVC specification together with Tbx2/3, members of the T-box transcription factor family with crucial roles in cardiac development (de la Pompa and Epstein, 2012; Ma et al., 2005). Tbx2 is repressible by Tbx20, which has regulatory function in ion channel expression (Shen et al., 2011). Importantly, *TBX20* nonsense and missense germline mutations result in complex septal, chamber and valvular anomalies in human (Kirk et al., 2007). Tbx transcription factors carry strong activation and repression domains and, especially Tbx20, interact with other important cardiac developmental factors including Nkx2.5, Gata4, Gata5 and Tbx5 (Brown et al., 2005; Combs and Yutzey, 2009; Kirk et al., 2007; Plageman and Yutzey, 2005; Stennard et al., 2003). Targeted disruption of *Gata5* has been demonstrated to associate with the develop-ment of bicuspid aortic valve in the mouse (Laforest et al., 2011), and one study on patients with bicuspid aortic valve found that approximately 4% had rare non-synonymous mutations within the *GATA5* transcriptional activation domains (Padang et al., 2012). A functional connection between *gata5* and *notch1* was reported in a zebrafish study of endoderm formation (Kikuchi et al., 2004), and those findings may potentially be generalized to human, given the evolutionarily conserved nature of the Notch pathway (Artavanis-Tsakonas and Muskavitch, 2010).

Cardiac valve formation begins with myocardial cells signaling to endocardial cells in the AVC and OFT cushions to undergo epithelial-mesenchymal transformation (transition) (EMT) (de la Pompa and Epstein, 2012). Coordinated by Notch and RBP-Jκ (del Monte et al., 2007; Timmerman et al., 2004), Bmp2 instructs cushion endocardial cells to invade the extracellular matrix and become the cushion mesenchyme (Hinton and Yutzey, 2011), and acting via Snail1/2, the Notch–Hey–Bmp2/4 axis promotes EMT and subsequent completion of valve tissue development (MacGrogan et al., 2011) (Figure 1). Interference with Notch signaling results in abnormal development of the aortic valve and cardiac outflow tract as demonstrated in animal studies (de la Pompa and Epstein, 2012; Garg et al., 2005; Mohamed et al., 2006; van den Akker et al., 2012). As discussed below, BMP2 also mediates aortic valve calcification.

Bicuspid aortic valve represents one of the most common anomalies of the heart or vessels (Roberts, 1970; Roberts et al., 2012; Ward, 2000), and its association with other anomalies is well recognized. For instance, ~10% of relatives of patients with hypoplastic left heart syn-drome have bicuspid aortic valve (Loffredo et al., 2004), and aortic abnormalities such as coarctation of aorta and interrupted aortic arch are present in 20–85% (Presbitero et al., 1987;

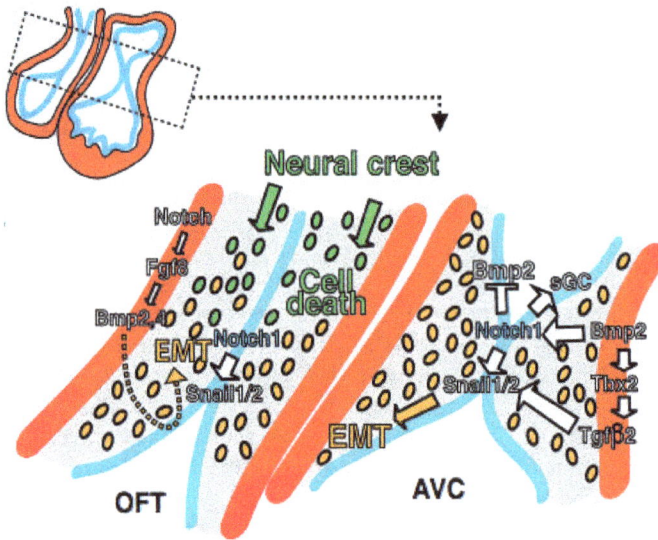

Figure 1. Diagram of a looped heart expanded to show the outflow tract (OFT) and the atrioventricular canal (AVC) endocardial cushions where epithelial-mesenchymal transition (EMT) occurs and precedes the development of semilunar and atrioventricular valves, respectively. Factors important during cardiac EMT and valve morphogenesis are shown. Myocardium, red; endocardium, blue; extracellular matrix, gray. Bmp, bone morphogenetic protein. Fgf, fibroblast growth factor. sGC, soluble guanylyl cyclase. Tbx, T-box transcription factor. Tgf, transforming growth factor. Adapted with permission from Elsevier.

Stewart et al., 1993) and ~27% (Roberts et al., 2012) of cases, respectively. Individuals with bicuspid aortic valve consistently have dilatation of the ascending aorta (Hahn et al., 1992). As a common variation noted by several investigators (Higgins and Wexler, 1975; Hutchins et al., 1978), a higher incidence of left coronary arterial system dominance (defined by the presence of the posterior descending artery arising from the left circumflex artery, as opposed to the right coronary artery) is observed in patients with bicuspid aortic valve. The phenotypic heterogeneity and overlap suggest common developmental mechanisms and gene networks that closely interact; the extent of the interactions may vary depending on the penetrance of the mutation(s), effect size of the variants, and the interaction between genes and signaling pathway.

In a study of two unrelated families, one of which included five generations, Garg and colleagues observed mutations in *NOTCH1* that segregated with aortic valve disease, particularly with bicuspid aortic valve and aortic valve calcification; but also, to a lesser extent, with tetralogy of Fallot, ventricular septal defect, mitral atresia, double-outlet right ventricle, or hypoplastic left ventricle (Garg et al., 2005). *NOTCH1* is located on chromosome 9q34.3 and encodes the 2,556-amino acid transmembrane Notch1 receptor. Affected members of one of the families analyzed had autosomal dominant inheritance of a point mutation (R1108X) resulting from a C-to-T transition of nucleotide 3322. Another unrelated family analyzed had a single base pair deletion leading to a frameshift mutation (H1505del) at position 4515. These mutations produced truncated transcripts that are believed to undergo nonsense-mediated decay, supporting haploinsufficiency of *NOTCH1* in the pathogenesis of congenital heart disease (Garg et al., 2005). Of note, despite the high propensity to development of bicuspid aortic valve and other cardiac anomalies in individuals with the *NOTCH1* mutation (R1108X) (Garg et al., 2005), aortic valve calcification was present even in a minority of family members with the mutation who did not have bicuspid or dysmorphic aortic valves, suggesting that the penetrance of the *NOTCH1* mutation is variable (or the effects compensated for by another Notch receptor or other mechanisms), and that maldistribution of mechanical stress alone can not explain accelerated valve calcification in these individuals.

Mutations or abnormal copy number variants in the gene (*JAG1*) encoding Jagged1, a Notch ligand, on chromosome 20p12 can cause a range of cardiovascular anomalies (McElhinney et al., 2002; Oda et al., 1997). However, the distribution and manifestations of cardiovascular anomalies, including the frequency of bicuspid aortic valve and calcific aortic valve disease, differ considerably between the *JAG1* and *NOTCH1* mutations (Garg et al., 2005; McElhinney et al., 2002). Although *JAG1* mutation is well recognized as a primary cause of Alagille syndome, familial as well as 'sporadic' tetralogy of Fallot, among other anomalies, has been reported (Eldadah et al., 2001; Greenway et al., 2009). Tetralogy of Fallot is a syndrome that comprises ventricular septal defect, pulmonary stenosis, right ventricular hypertrophy and an overriding aorta, in association with aortic regurgitation in ~6% of patients (Abraham et al., 1979). Mutations in *JAG1* have been identified in 60–75% of individuals with Alagille syndrome (Colliton et al., 2001; Li et al., 1997; Oda et al., 1997; Spinner et al., 2001), a condition charac-terized by cholestatic jaundice due to biliary tree anomalies, skeletal deformities, systemic vascular malformations and aneurysms (Kamath et al., 2004), and a high frequency of right-sided cardiovascular anomalies (62% of 200 patients) (McElhinney et al., 2002). In patients with left-sided anomalies (22 of 200 individuals (McElhinney et al., 2002)), a comparison of those with (n = 17) and without (n = 5) *JAG1* mutation did not reveal an obvious trend favoring the distribution nor preponderance of valvular aortic stenosis, supravalvular aortic stenosis, aortic coarctation, or bicuspid aortic stenosis without stenosis (McElhinney et al., 2002). Those findings suggest that aortic valve disease, such as bicuspid aortic valve and at least moderate-severe aortic stenosis, is relatively uncommon (<5%) in patients with Alagille syndrome (McElhinney et al., 2002), and implies that *JAG1* mutation *per se* does not predispose to aortic valve calcification in human, as evidenced by the paucity of left-sided abnormalities. Interest-ingly, although previous mouse studies have reported high lethality associated with endo-thelial-specific deletion of *Jag1* (Benedito et al., 2009; High et al., 2008), one recent study demonstrated a high frequency of cardiac, great vessel, coronary, and valve defects resembling features of tetralogy of Fallot in human; and in animals, chondrogenic nodules and calcification were observed in the aortic valve (5 of 10 transgenic animals versus 0 of 10 controls) (Hofmann et al., 2012). The authors of the study postulated that murine *Jag1* was essential to morpho-genesis of the interventricular septum and cardiac valves, and particularly, in valve remodel-ing postnatally through modulation of extracellular matrix (Hofmann et al., 2012).

The complexity of gene-phenotype effects in human is highlighted by variable penetrance of *JAG1* mutation (e.g. G274D missense mutation) and phenotypic expression, as demonstrated by differences in the degree of glycosylation, protein trafficking and cell-surface protein expression given the same mutation (Lu et al., 2003). This heterogeneity is reminiscent of the variable effects of *NOTCH1* in the pathogenesis of bicuspid aortic valve and other cardiovascular anomalies (Garg et al., 2005), and epigenetic factors such as intracardiac fluid forces may be important contributors that couple with transcription factors to affect cardiogenesis and valve development (Hove et al., 2003; Lee et al., 2006; Vermot et al., 2009).

3.2. Aortic valve dysmorphology, bicuspid aortic valve and calcification

Anomalies of the aortic valve can be classified based on size, shape, the number of valve leaflets, cuspal inequality, nature of commissures (e.g. unicomissural, acquired fusion), and location of a false raphé if present (Perloff, 2003; Ward, 2000). Unicuspid, quadricuspid and six-cuspid aortic valves occur rarely (Perloff, 2003), and associated mutations have not been reported, unlike bicuspid aortic valves resulting from impaired Notch1 signaling (Garg et al., 2005). Unicuspid and bicuspid aortic valves often prematurely develop valve calcification at least two decades earlier than their normal trileaflet counterpart (Pachulski and Chan, 1993). Although maldistribution of mechanical stress contributes to the fibrocalcific process, additional factors apart from biomechanical forces including inflammatory and profibrotic processes direct the differentiation of valve fibroblasts into myofibroblasts and osteoblasts that promote osteogenesis (Dweck et al., 2012; Rajamannan et al., 2003).

Maldistribution of shear stress on valve cusps is thought to promote calcification of the aortic valve seen in unicuspid, bicuspid, and tricuspid aortic valve with cuspal inequality (Perloff, 2003). Bicuspid aortic valve is found in 1–2% of the general population in the United States, with a slight male predominance reported in some studies (Roberts et al., 2012; Ward, 2000). Maldistribution of diastolic force among valve cusps and sinus attachment is thought also to promote ascending aortic dilatation or aneurysm (Burks et al., 1998; Perloff, 2003; Roberts, 1970). However, it remains unclear whether these aortic manifestations are genetically determined or represent a byproduct of mechanical stress, given that aortic dilatation is indistinct among regurgitant, stenotic and functionally normal bicuspid aortic valves (Hahn et al., 1992). Emerging evidence supports increased proteolytic activity in the aortic valve and adjacent areas including the aorta that may enhance the remodeling processes (Aikawa et al., 2007b).

Valvular calcification in the early stages causes aortic sclerosis, which predicts increased risks for cardiovascular morbidity and mortality (Otto et al., 1999). As the process progresses, the aortic valve orifice narrows while the valve anatomy and function become gradually distorted to produce valvular aortic stenosis with or without regurgitation, myocardial hypertrophic response, myocardial fibrosis, heart failure, and hemodynamic instability (Dweck et al., 2012). In recent years, the concept of degeneration in the pathogenesis of calcific aortic valve disease has been superseded by that of phenotypic modulation recapitulating embryonic development, angiogenesis, acquired and innate immune activation, wound healing and bone formation (Hakuno et al., 2009).

4. Acquired aortic valve disease

4.1. Aortic valve calcification and systemic inflammation

Aortic valve sclerosis has been estimated to affect at least 20% of adults over 65 years of age in the general population (Lindroos et al., 1993; Stewart et al., 1997). Calcific aortic valve disease represents a continuum of maladapted calcification in the aortic valve arising from active inflammatory and oxidative processes (Kaden et al., 2004; New and Aikawa, 2011; Towler, 2008), as well as a shift in the valve interstitial phenotype from chondrogenic to osteogenic. Early calcification of the aortic valve leads to increased valve leaflet thickness and stiffness in a condition termed aortic valve sclerosis (Otto et al., 1999). Continuation of the inflammatory process propagates angioneogenesis and biomineralization, leading to formation of calcium nodules that distort valve geometry and function, culminating in outflow-limiting aortic stenosis with or without regurgitation (Dweck et al., 2012; Rajamannan et al., 2011). Conditions that promote systemic inflammation, such as atherosclerosis, dyslipidemia and diabetes mellitus, have been shown to exacerbate the development of calcific aortic valve disease (Rajamannan et al., 2011). While statins may stabilize atheromatous plaques, reduce vascular calcification and clinical adverse outcomes, they have unfortunately not been shown to benefit calcific aortic valve disease in disease progression or patient outcomes (Chan et al., 2010; Cowell et al., 2005; Rossebo et al., 2008).

Studies exploring Notch signaling beyond congenital disorders and developmental biology identified Dll4 in macrophage-mediated inflammation (Fung et al., 2007). Recently, Fukuda and colleagues demonstrated that blockade of Dll4-Notch signaling using anti-Dll4 monoclonal antibody decreased BMP2, a central regulator of osteogenesis and bone mineralization (Fukuda et al., 2012), in line with other studies showing reduced aortic valve calcification with BMP2 knockdown by siRNA (Nigam and Srivastava, 2009), and the proinflammatory cytokine, TNF-α, accelerated BMP2-mediated calcification of human aortic valve interstitial cells from patients with calcific aortic valve stenosis (Yu et al., 2011). BMP2 mediates aortic valve calcification via Runx2 (Osf2/Cbfa1), a transcriptional activator of osteoblast development or gene expression (Ducy et al., 1997; Kaden et al., 2004; Mohler et al., 2001), and is suppressible by activation of Notch1 via Hey (HRT) (Acharya et al., 2011; Nigam and Srivastava, 2009). Moreover, the marked attenuation of aortic valvular calcification and stenosis through the blockade of angiogenesis-promoting Dll4 in a mouse model of hypercholesterolemia (Figure 2) also supports the current theory that angioneogenesis is a crucial stage in the natural history of calcific aortic valve disease (Dweck et al., 2012), recapitulating cardiogenesis and valve development (de la Pompa and Epstein, 2012; van den Akker et al., 2012). Thus, Dll4 critically bridges inflammation and angioneogenesis to osteogenesis in calcific aortic valve disease (Fukuda et al., 2012). These effects are probably independent of Notch 1 (Nus et al., 2011), since activation of the receptor presumably leads to inhibition of valve calcification (Acharya et al., 2011), whereas evidence on the benefits of Dll4 blockade (i.e. interruption of Dll4–Notch signaling) suggests that a Notch receptor other than Notch1, when activated, potentiates the development and progression of valve calcification. A shift in the Notch receptor:ligand ratio and/or the DLL:Jagged (Notch ligands) ratio may plausibly alter the cell-to-cell signalling strength and modality *in cis* and/or *in trans*, thus, modifying the final functional outcome. Much work remains to be done to fully delineate the mechanisms through which anti-Dll4 antibody exert inhibitory effects on inflammation and calcification.

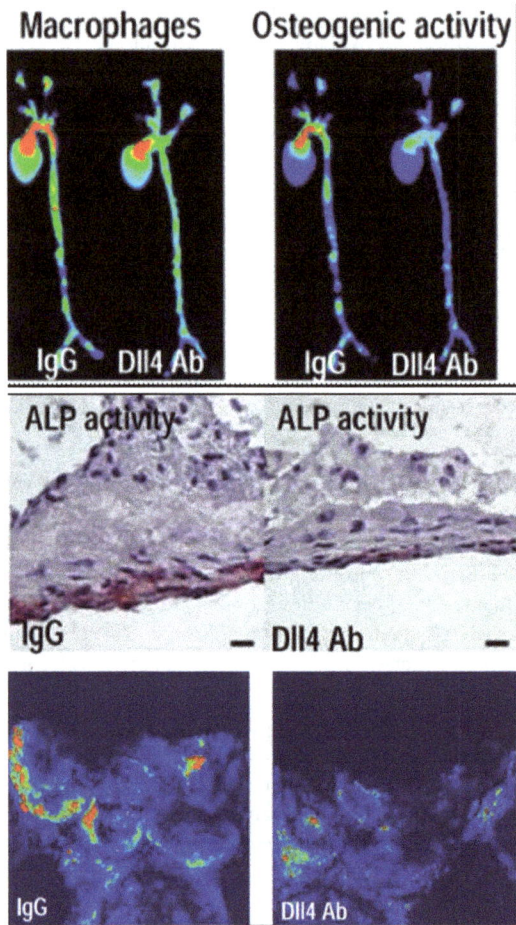

Figure 2. *Ex vivo* mapping using fluorescence reflectance imaging to grossly visualize the biomineralization of the hearts and vessels of atherosclerosis-prone (low-density lipoprotein receptor-deficient, *Ldlr*-/-) animals fed a hypercholesterolemic diet, and independently treated with IgG isotype control or anti-Dll4 monoclonal antibody (Dll4 Ab). 750-nm CLIO750 nanoparticles were used to image macrophages, and 680-nm VisEn OsteoSense680 was used for the detection of osteogenic activity (top and bottom rows). Decreased osteogenic activity in the anti-Dll4 monoclonal antibody treated specimen is visualized using alkaline phosphatase (ALP) staining (middle row). Adapted from Fukuda and colleagues (Fukuda et al., 2012).

5. Clinical implications

Calcific aortic valve disease in individuals with severe aortic stenosis can progress quickly after presentation with symptoms, usually portending limited short-term survival (Turina et al., 1987). Clinical trials on medical therapy including statins have found little benefit and utility in forestalling disease progression, with no demonstrated impact on survival. Since the evidence suggests that inflammatory cells, particularly macrophages, play a crucial role in calcification, anti-inflammatory therapies may prevent development of arterial and valvular calcification. We and others have demonstrated that lipid lowering reduces inflammation (Aikawa et al., 1998; Aikawa et al., 2001; Chu et al., 2012; Libby and Aikawa, 2002; Libby et al., 2011). However, clinical trials (e.g. SALTIRE, SEAS, etc.) have failed to demonstrate that lipid lowering attenuates development of aortic stenosis. Preclinical findings suggest that macrophage accumulation precedes calcific changes in arteries and valves while lesions with advanced calcification are often unassociated with macrophages (Aikawa et al., 2007a; Aikawa et al., 2007b). This may suggest that anti-inflammatory therapies need to be initiated early (Aikawa and Otto, 2012), and thus clinical trials involving patients who had been diagnosed with aortic stenosis due to advanced calcification did not show substantial benefits of lipid lowering therapy. To establish more effective therapies, it is crucial to better understand the complex mechanisms for aortic valve calcification. To identify individuals with subclinical aortic valve calcification and those with high probability or propensity of developing severe aortic valvular stenosis, methods for early detection of calcific changes (e.g., molecular imaging, biomarkers) need to be developed. National Institutes of Health of the United States of America has formed the Working Group of Calcific Aortic Valve Disease to facilitate basic research on this devastating global health threat and initiated federal funding (Rajamannan et al., 2011).

Author details

Erik Fung[1,2] and Masanori Aikawa[3]

1 Section of Cardiology, Heart & Vascular Center, Dartmouth-Hitchcock Medical Center, Lebanon, New Hampshire, USA

2 Geisel School of Medicine at Dartmouth, Dartmouth College, Hanover, New Hampshire, USA

3 Center for Excellence in Vascular Biology, Cardiovascular Division, Brigham and Women's Hospital and Harvard Medical School, Boston, Massachusetts, USA

References

[1] Abraham, K.A., Cherian, G., Rao, V.D., Sukumar, I.P., Krishnaswami, S., and John, S. (1979). Tetralogy of Fallot in adults. A report on 147 patients. Am J Med 66, 811-816.

[2] Acharya, A., Hans, C.P., Koenig, S.N., Nichols, H.A., Galindo, C.L., Garner, H.R., Merrill, W.H., Hinton, R.B., and Garg, V. (2011). Inhibitory role of Notch1 in calcific aortic valve disease. PLoS One 6, e27743.

[3] Aikawa, E., Nahrendorf, M., Figueiredo, J.L., Swirski, F.K., Shtatland, T., Kohler, R.H., Jaffer, F.A., Aikawa, M., and Weissleder, R. (2007a). Osteogenesis associates with inflammation in early-stage atherosclerosis evaluated by molecular imaging in vivo. Circulation 116, 2841-2850.

[4] Aikawa, E., Nahrendorf, M., Sosnovik, D., Lok, V.M., Jaffer, F.A., Aikawa, M., and Weissleder, R. (2007b). Multimodality molecular imaging identifies proteolytic and osteogenic activities in early aortic valve disease. Circulation 115, 377-386.

[5] Aikawa, E., and Otto, C.M. (2012). Look more closely at the valve: imaging calcific aortic valve disease. Circulation 125, 9-11.

[6] Aikawa, M., Rabkin, E., Okada, Y., Voglic, S.J., Clinton, S.K., Brinckerhoff, C.E., Su-khova, G.K., and Libby, P. (1998). Lipid lowering by diet reduces matrix metallopro-teinase activity and increases collagen content of rabbit atheroma: a potential mechanism of lesion stabilization. Circulation 97, 2433-2444.

[7] Aikawa, M., Rabkin, E., Sugiyama, S., Voglic, S.J., Fukumoto, Y., Furukawa, Y., Shio-mi, M., Schoen, F.J., and Libby, P. (2001). An HMG-CoA reductase inhibitor, cerivas-tatin, suppresses growth of macrophages expressing matrix metalloproteinases and tissue factor in vivo and in vitro. Circulation 103, 276-283.

[8] Artavanis-Tsakonas, S., and Muskavitch, M.A. (2010). Notch: the past, the present, and the future. Curr Top Dev Biol 92, 1-29.

[9] Benedito, R., Roca, C., Sorensen, I., Adams, S., Gossler, A., Fruttiger, M., and Adams, R.H. (2009). The notch ligands Dll4 and Jagged1 have opposing effects on angiogene-sis. Cell 137, 1124-1135.

[10] Bray, S.J. (2006). Notch signalling: a simple pathway becomes complex. Nat Rev Mol Cell Biol 7, 678-689.

[11] Brown, D.D., Martz, S.N., Binder, O., Goetz, S.C., Price, B.M., Smith, J.C., and Con-lon, F.L. (2005). Tbx5 and Tbx20 act synergistically to control vertebrate heart mor-phogenesis. Development 132, 553-563.

[12] Burks, J.M., Illes, R.W., Keating, E.C., and Lubbe, W.J. (1998). Ascending aortic aneurysm and dissection in young adults with bicuspid aortic valve: implications for echocardiographic surveillance. Clin Cardiol 21, 439-443.

[13] Camenisch, T.D., Runyan, R.B., and Markwald, R.R., eds.Molecular regulation of cushion morphogenesis, In: Heart Development and Regeneration, 363-413, 1st edn (London, UK, Academic Press).

[14] Chan, K.L., Teo, K., Dumesnil, J.G., Ni, A., and Tam, J. (2010). Effect of Lipid lowering with rosuvastatin on progression of aortic stenosis: results of the aortic stenosis progression observation: measuring effects of rosuvastatin (ASTRONOMER) trial. Circulation 121, 306-314.

[15] Chu, A.Y., Guilianini, F., Barratt, B.J., Nyberg, F., Chasman, D.I., and Ridker, P.M. (2012). Pharmacogenetic determinants of statin-induced reductions in C-reactive protein. Circ Cardiovasc Genet 5, 58-65.

[16] Colliton, R.P., Bason, L., Lu, F.M., Piccoli, D.A., Krantz, I.D., and Spinner, N.B. (2001). Mutation analysis of Jagged1 (JAG1) in Alagille syndrome patients. Hum Mutat 17, 151-152.

[17] Combs, M.D., and Yutzey, K.E. (2009). Heart valve development: regulatory networks in development and disease. Circ Res 105, 408-421.

[18] Cowell, S.J., Newby, D.E., Prescott, R.J., Bloomfield, P., Reid, J., Northridge, D.B., and Boon, N.A. (2005). A randomized trial of intensive lipid-lowering therapy in calcific aortic stenosis. N Engl J Med 352, 2389-2397.

[19] de la Pompa, J.L., and Epstein, J.A. (2012). Coordinating tissue interactions: Notch signaling in cardiac development and disease. Dev Cell 22, 244-254.

[20] Del Monte, G., Grego-Bessa, J., Gonzalez-Rajal, A., Bolos, V., and De La Pompa, J.L. (2007). Monitoring Notch1 activity in development: evidence for a feedback regulatory loop. Dev Dyn 236, 2594-2614.

[21] Duarte, A., Hirashima, M., Benedito, R., Trindade, A., Diniz, P., Bekman, E., Costa, L., Henrique, D., and Rossant, J. (2004). Dosage-sensitive requirement for mouse Dll4 in artery development. Genes Dev 18, 2474-2478.

[22] Ducy, P., Zhang, R., Geoffroy, V., Ridall, A.L., and Karsenty, G. (1997). Osf2/Cbfa1: a transcriptional activator of osteoblast differentiation. Cell 89, 747-754.

[23] Dweck, M.R., Boon, N.A., and Newby, D.E. (2012). Calcific aortic stenosis: a disease of the valve and the myocardium. J Am Coll Cardiol 60, 1854-1863.

[24] Eldadah, Z.A., Hamosh, A., Biery, N.J., Montgomery, R.A., Duke, M., Elkins, R., and Dietz, H.C. (2001). Familial Tetralogy of Fallot caused by mutation in the jagged1 gene. Hum Mol Genet 10, 163-169.

[25] Fiuza, U.M., and Arias, A.M. (2007). Cell and molecular biology of Notch. J Endocrinol 194, 459-474.

[26] Fukuda, D., Aikawa, E., Swirski, F.K., Novobrantseva, T.I., Kotelianski, V., Gorgun, C.Z., Chudnovskiy, A., Yamazaki, H., Croce, K., Weissleder, R., et al. (2012). Notch

ligand Delta-like 4 blockade attenuates atherosclerosis and metabolic disorders. Proc Natl Acad Sci U S A 109, E1868-1877.

[27] Fung, E., Tang, S.M., Canner, J.P., Morishige, K., Arboleda-Velasquez, J.F., Cardoso, A.A., Carlesso, N., Aster, J.C., and Aikawa, M. (2007). Delta-like 4 induces notch signaling in macrophages: implications for inflammation. Circulation 115, 2948-2956.

[28] Garg, V., Muth, A.N., Ransom, J.F., Schluterman, M.K., Barnes, R., King, I.N., Grossfeld, P.D., and Srivastava, D. (2005). Mutations in NOTCH1 cause aortic valve disease. Nature 437, 270-274.

[29] Gibert, J.M., and Simpson, P. (2003). Evolution of cis-regulation of the proneural genes. Int J Dev Biol 47, 643-651.

[30] Greenway, S.C., Pereira, A.C., Lin, J.C., DePalma, S.R., Israel, S.J., Mesquita, S.M., Ergul, E., Conta, J.H., Korn, J.M., McCarroll, S.A., et al. (2009). De novo copy number variants identify new genes and loci in isolated sporadic tetralogy of Fallot. Nat Genet 41, 931-935.

[31] Guruharsha, K.G., Kankel, M.W., and Artavanis-Tsakonas, S. (2012). The Notch signalling system: recent insights into the complexity of a conserved pathway. Nat Rev Genet 13, 654-666.

[32] Hahn, R.T., Roman, M.J., Mogtader, A.H., and Devereux, R.B. (1992). Association of aortic dilation with regurgitant, stenotic and functionally normal bicuspid aortic valves. J Am Coll Cardiol 19, 283-288.

[33] Hakuno, D., Kimura, N., Yoshioka, M., and Fukuda, K. (2009). Molecular mechanisms underlying the onset of degenerative aortic valve disease. J Mol Med (Berl) 87, 17-24.

[34] Heitzler, P., and Simpson, P. (1991). The choice of cell fate in the epidermis of Drosophila. Cell 64, 1083-1092.

[35] Higgins, C.B., and Wexler, L. (1975). Reversal of dominance of the coronary arterial system in isolated aortic stenosis and bicuspid aortic valve. Circulation 52, 292-296.

[36] High, F.A., Lu, M.M., Pear, W.S., Loomes, K.M., Kaestner, K.H., and Epstein, J.A. (2008). Endothelial expression of the Notch ligand Jagged1 is required for vascular smooth muscle development. Proc Natl Acad Sci U S A 105, 1955-1959.

[37] Hinton, R.B., and Yutzey, K.E. (2011). Heart valve structure and function in development and disease. Annu Rev Physiol 73, 29-46.

[38] Hofmann, J.J., Briot, A., Enciso, J., Zovein, A.C., Ren, S., Zhang, Z.W., Radtke, F., Simons, M., Wang, Y., and Iruela-Arispe, M.L. (2012). Endothelial deletion of murine Jag1 leads to valve calcification and congenital heart defects associated with Alagille syndrome. Development 139, 4449-4460.

[39] Hove, J.R., Koster, R.W., Forouhar, A.S., Acevedo-Bolton, G., Fraser, S.E., and Gharib, M. (2003). Intracardiac fluid forces are an essential epigenetic factor for embryonic cardiogenesis. Nature 421, 172-177.

[40] Hutchins, G.M., Nazarian, I.H., and Bulkley, B.H. (1978). Association of left dominant coronary arterial system with congenital bicuspid aortic valve. Am J Cardiol 42, 57-59.

[41] Kaden, J.J., Bickelhaupt, S., Grobholz, R., Vahl, C.F., Hagl, S., Brueckmann, M., Haase, K.K., Dempfle, C.E., and Borggrefe, M. (2004). Expression of bone sialoprotein and bone morphogenetic protein-2 in calcific aortic stenosis. J Heart Valve Dis 13, 560-566.

[42] Kamath, B.M., Spinner, N.B., Emerick, K.M., Chudley, A.E., Booth, C., Piccoli, D.A., and Krantz, I.D. (2004). Vascular anomalies in Alagille syndrome: a significant cause of morbidity and mortality. Circulation 109, 1354-1358.

[43] Kikuchi, Y., Verkade, H., Reiter, J.F., Kim, C.H., Chitnis, A.B., Kuroiwa, A., and Stainier, D.Y. (2004). Notch signaling can regulate endoderm formation in zebrafish. Dev Dyn 229, 756-762.

[44] Kirk, E.P., Sunde, M., Costa, M.W., Rankin, S.A., Wolstein, O., Castro, M.L., Butler, T.L., Hyun, C., Guo, G., Otway, R., et al. (2007). Mutations in cardiac T-box factor gene TBX20 are associated with diverse cardiac pathologies, including defects of septation and valvulogenesis and cardiomyopathy. Am J Hum Genet 81, 280-291.

[45] Kopan, R., and Ilagan, M.X. (2009). The canonical Notch signaling pathway: unfolding the activation mechanism. Cell 137, 216-233.

[46] Ladich, E., Nakano, M., Carter-Monroe, N., and Virmani, R. (2011). Pathology of calcific aortic stenosis. Future Cardiol 7, 629-642.

[47] Laforest, B., Andelfinger, G., and Nemer, M. (2011). Loss of Gata5 in mice leads to bicuspid aortic valve. J Clin Invest 121, 2876-2887.

[48] Lee, J.S., Yu, Q., Shin, J.T., Sebzda, E., Bertozzi, C., Chen, M., Mericko, P., Stadtfeld, M., Zhou, D., Cheng, L., et al. (2006). Klf2 is an essential regulator of vascular hemodynamic forces in vivo. Dev Cell 11, 845-857.

[49] Li, L., Krantz, I.D., Deng, Y., Genin, A., Banta, A.B., Collins, C.C., Qi, M., Trask, B.J., Kuo, W.L., Cochran, J., et al. (1997). Alagille syndrome is caused by mutations in human Jagged1, which encodes a ligand for Notch1. Nat Genet 16, 243-251.

[50] Libby, P., and Aikawa, M. (2002). Stabilization of atherosclerotic plaques: new mechanisms and clinical targets. Nat Med 8, 1257-1262.

[51] Libby, P., Ridker, P.M., and Hansson, G.K. (2011). Progress and challenges in translating the biology of atherosclerosis. Nature 473, 317-325.

[52] Lindroos, M., Kupari, M., Heikkila, J., and Tilvis, R. (1993). Prevalence of aortic valve abnormalities in the elderly: an echocardiographic study of a random population sample. J Am Coll Cardiol 21, 1220-1225.

[53] Loffredo, C.A., Chokkalingam, A., Sill, A.M., Boughman, J.A., Clark, E.B., Scheel, J., and Brenner, J.I. (2004). Prevalence of congenital cardiovascular malformations among relatives of infants with hypoplastic left heart, coarctation of the aorta, and d-transposition of the great arteries. Am J Med Genet A 124A, 225-230.

[54] Lu, F., Morrissette, J.J., and Spinner, N.B. (2003). Conditional JAG1 mutation shows the developing heart is more sensitive than developing liver to JAG1 dosage. Am J Hum Genet 72, 1065-1070.

[55] Ma, L., Lu, M.F., Schwartz, R.J., and Martin, J.F. (2005). Bmp2 is essential for cardiac cushion epithelial-mesenchymal transition and myocardial patterning. Development 132, 5601-5611.

[56] MacGrogan, D., Luna-Zurita, L., and de la Pompa, J.L. (2011). Notch signaling in cardiac valve development and disease. Birth Defects Res A Clin Mol Teratol 91, 449-459.

[57] McCarthy, J.V., Twomey, C., and Wujek, P. (2009). Presenilin-dependent regulated intramembrane proteolysis and gamma-secretase activity. Cell Mol Life Sci 66, 1534-1555.

[58] McElhinney, D.B., Krantz, I.D., Bason, L., Piccoli, D.A., Emerick, K.M., Spinner, N.B., and Goldmuntz, E. (2002). Analysis of cardiovascular phenotype and genotype-phenotype correlation in individuals with a JAG1 mutation and/or Alagille syndrome. Circulation 106, 2567-2574.

[59] Miller, J.D., Weiss, R.M., Serrano, K.M., Castaneda, L.E., Brooks, R.M., Zimmerman, K., and Heistad, D.D. (2010). Evidence for active regulation of pro-osteogenic signaling in advanced aortic valve disease. Arterioscler Thromb Vasc Biol 30, 2482-2486.

[60] Mohamed, S.A., Aherrahrou, Z., Liptau, H., Erasmi, A.W., Hagemann, C., Wrobel, S., Borzym, K., Schunkert, H., Sievers, H.H., and Erdmann, J. (2006). Novel missense mutations (p.T596M and p.P1797H) in NOTCH1 in patients with bicuspid aortic valve. Biochem Biophys Res Commun 345, 1460-1465.

[61] Mohler, E.R., 3rd, Gannon, F., Reynolds, C., Zimmerman, R., Keane, M.G., and Kaplan, F.S. (2001). Bone formation and inflammation in cardiac valves. Circulation 103, 1522-1528.

[62] New, S.E., and Aikawa, E. (2011). Molecular imaging insights into early inflammatory stages of arterial and aortic valve calcification. Circ Res 108, 1381-1391.

[63] Nigam, V., and Srivastava, D. (2009). Notch1 represses osteogenic pathways in aortic valve cells. J Mol Cell Cardiol 47, 828-834.

[64] Nus, M, MacGrogan, D, Martínez-Poveda, B, Benito, Y, Casanova, J. C, Fernández-Avilés, F, Bermejo, J, de la Pompa J. L. (2011). Diet-induced aortic valve disease in mice haploinsufficient for the Notch pathway effector RBPJK/CSL. Arterioscler Thromb Vasc Biol, 31, 1580-1588.

[65] Oda, T., Elkahloun, A.G., Pike, B.L., Okajima, K., Krantz, I.D., Genin, A., Piccoli, D.A., Meltzer, P.S., Spinner, N.B., Collins, F.S., et al. (1997). Mutations in the human Jagged1 gene are responsible for Alagille syndrome. Nat Genet 16, 235-242.

[66] Otto, C.M., Lind, B.K., Kitzman, D.W., Gersh, B.J., and Siscovick, D.S. (1999). Association of aortic-valve sclerosis with cardiovascular mortality and morbidity in the elderly. N Engl J Med 341, 142-147.

[67] Pachulski, R.T., and Chan, K.L. (1993). Progression of aortic valve dysfunction in 51 adult patients with congenital bicuspid aortic valve: assessment and follow up by Doppler echocardiography. Br Heart J 69, 237-240.

[68] Padang, R., Bagnall, R.D., Richmond, D.R., Bannon, P.G., and Semsarian, C. (2012). Rare non-synonymous variations in the transcriptional activation domains of GATA5 in bicuspid aortic valve disease. J Mol Cell Cardiol 53, 277-281.

[69] Perloff, J.K. (2003). Congenital aortic stenosis, In: The Clinical Recognition of Congenital Heart Disease, 81-112, 3rd edn (Philadelphia, PA, Saunders).

[70] Person, A.D., Klewer, S.E., and Runyan, R.B. (2005). Cell biology of cardiac cushion development. Int Rev Cytol 243, 287-335.

[71] Plageman, T.F., Jr., and Yutzey, K.E. (2005). T-box genes and heart development: putting the "T" in heart. Dev Dyn 232, 11-20.

[72] Presbitero, P., Demarie, D., Villani, M., Perinetto, E.A., Riva, G., Orzan, F., Bobbio, M., Morea, M., and Brusca, A. (1987). Long term results (15-30 years) of surgical repair of aortic coarctation. Br Heart J 57, 462-467.

[73] Rajamannan, N.M., Evans, F.J., Aikawa, E., Grande-Allen, K.J., Demer, L.L., Heistad, D.D., Simmons, C.A., Masters, K.S., Mathieu, P., O'Brien, K.D., et al. (2011). Calcific aortic valve disease: not simply a degenerative process: A review and agenda for research from the National Heart and Lung and Blood Institute Aortic Stenosis Working Group. Executive summary: Calcific aortic valve disease-2011 update. Circulation 124, 1783-1791.

[74] Rajamannan, N.M., Subramaniam, M., Rickard, D., Stock, S.R., Donovan, J., Springett, M., Orszulak, T., Fullerton, D.A., Tajik, A.J., Bonow, R.O., et al. (2003). Human aortic valve calcification is associated with an osteoblast phenotype. Circulation 107, 2181-2184.

[75] Roberts, W.C. (1970). The structure of the aortic valve in clinically isolated aortic stenosis: an autopsy study of 162 patients over 15 years of age. Circulation 42, 91-97.

[76] Roberts, W.C., Vowels, T.J., and Ko, J.M. (2012). Natural history of adults with con-
      genitally malformed aortic valves (unicuspid or bicuspid). Medicine (Baltimore) 91,
      287-308.

[77] Rossebo, A.B., Pedersen, T.R., Boman, K., Brudi, P., Chambers, J.B., Egstrup, K.,
      Gerdts, E., Gohlke-Barwolf, C., Holme, I., Kesaniemi, Y.A., et al. (2008). Intensive lip-
      id lowering with simvastatin and ezetimibe in aortic stenosis. N Engl J Med 359,
      1343-1356.

[78] Shen, T., Aneas, I., Sakabe, N., Dirschinger, R.J., Wang, G., Smemo, S., Westlund,
      J.M., Cheng, H., Dalton, N., Gu, Y., et al. (2011). Tbx20 regulates a genetic program
      essential to adult mouse cardiomyocyte function. J Clin Invest 121, 4640-4654.

[79] Spinner, N.B., Colliton, R.P., Crosnier, C., Krantz, I.D., Hadchouel, M., and Meunier-
      Rotival, M. (2001). Jagged1 mutations in alagille syndrome. Hum Mutat 17, 18-33.

[80] Stennard, F.A., Costa, M.W., Elliott, D.A., Rankin, S., Haast, S.J., Lai, D., McDonald,
      L.P., Niederreither, K., Dolle, P., Bruneau, B.G., et al. (2003). Cardiac T-box factor
      Tbx20 directly interacts with Nkx2-5, GATA4, and GATA5 in regulation of gene ex-
      pression in the developing heart. Dev Biol 262, 206-224.

[81] Stewart, A.B., Ahmed, R., Travill, C.M., and Newman, C.G. (1993). Coarctation of the
      aorta life and health 20-44 years after surgical repair. Br Heart J 69, 65-70.

[82] Stewart, B.F., Siscovick, D., Lind, B.K., Gardin, J.M., Gottdiener, J.S., Smith, V.E.,
      Kitzman, D.W., and Otto, C.M. (1997). Clinical factors associated with calcific aortic
      valve disease. Cardiovascular Health Study. J Am Coll Cardiol 29, 630-634.

[83] Timmerman, L.A., Grego-Bessa, J., Raya, A., Bertran, E., Perez-Pomares, J.M., Diez, J.,
      Aranda, S., Palomo, S., McCormick, F., Izpisua-Belmonte, J.C., et al. (2004). Notch
      promotes epithelial-mesenchymal transition during cardiac development and onco-
      genic transformation. Genes Dev 18, 99-115.

[84] Towler, D.A. (2008). Oxidation, inflammation, and aortic valve calcification peroxide
      paves an osteogenic path. J Am Coll Cardiol 52, 851-854.

[85] Turina, J., Hess, O., Sepulcri, F., and Krayenbuehl, H.P. (1987). Spontaneous course of
      aortic valve disease. Eur Heart J 8, 471-483.

[86] van den Akker, N.M., Caolo, V., and Molin, D.G. (2012). Cellular decisions in cardiac
      outflow tract and coronary development: an act by VEGF and NOTCH. Differentia-
      tion 84, 62-78.

[87] Vermot, J., Forouhar, A.S., Liebling, M., Wu, D., Plummer, D., Gharib, M., and Fraser,
      S.E. (2009). Reversing blood flows act through klf2a to ensure normal valvulogenesis
      in the developing heart. PLoS Biol 7, e1000246.

[88] Wakabayashi, T., and De Strooper, B. (2008). Presenilins: members of the gamma-sec-
      retase quartets, but part-time soloists too. Physiology (Bethesda) 23, 194-204.

[89] Ward, C. (2000). Clinical significance of the bicuspid aortic valve. Heart 83, 81-85.

[90] Wilkinson, H.A., Fitzgerald, K., and Greenwald, I. (1994). Reciprocal changes in expression of the receptor lin-12 and its ligand lag-2 prior to commitment in a C. elegans cell fate decision. Cell 79, 1187-1198.

[91] Yu, Z., Seya, K., Daitoku, K., Motomura, S., Fukuda, I., and Furukawa, K. (2011). Tumor necrosis factor-alpha accelerates the calcification of human aortic valve interstitial cells obtained from patients with calcific aortic valve stenosis via the BMP2-Dlx5 pathway. J Pharmacol Exp Ther 337, 16-23.

[92] Zhang, J., Chang, J.Y., Huang, Y., Lin, X., Luo, Y., Schwartz, R.J., Martin, J.F., and Wang, F. (2010). The FGF-BMP signaling axis regulates outflow tract valve primordium formation by promoting cushion neural crest cell differentiation. Circ Res 107, 1209-1219.

Chapter 5

Role of MicroRNAs in Cardiovascular Calcification

Claudia Goettsch and Elena Aikawa

Additional information is available at the end of the chapter

1. Introduction

With a growing older population, cardiovascular diseases are becoming an increasing economic and social burden in Western societies. Cardiovascular calcification is a major characteristic of chronic inflammatory disorders — such as chronic renal disease (CRD), type 2 diabetes (T2D), atherosclerosis and calcific aortic valve disease (CAVD) — that associate with significant morbidity and mortality. Cardiovascular calcification also associates with osteoporosis in humans and animal models [1, 2] — the so-called "calcification paradox" [3]. The concept that similar pathways control both bone remodeling and vascular calcification is currently widely accepted, but the precise mechanisms of calcification remain largely unknown. Osteogenic transition of vascular smooth muscle cells (SMCs), valvular interstitial cells (VIC) or stem cells is induced by bone morphogenetic proteins, inflammation, oxidative stress, or high phosphate levels, and leads to a unique molecular pattern marked by osteogenic transcription factors [4]. Loss of mineralization inhibitors, such as matrix γ-carboxyglutamic acid Gla protein (MGP) and fetuin-A also contribute to cardiovascular calcification. The physiological balance between induction and inhibition of calcification becomes dysregulated in CRD, T2D, atherosclerosis, and CAVD. Consequently, calcification may occur at several sites in the cardiovascular system, including the intima and media of vessels and cardiac valves [3].

The central role of miRNAs as fine-tune regulators in the cardiovascular system and bone biology has gained acceptance and has raised the possibility for novel therapeutic targets. Circulating miRNAs have been proposed as biomarkers for a wide range of cardiovascular diseases, but knowledge of miRNA biology in cardiovascular calcification is very limited.

2. Micro-RNA biology: Biosynthesis and function

Micro-RNAs (miRNAs) are a large class of evolutionarily conserved, small, endogenous, non-coding RNAs serving as essential post-transcriptional modulators of gene expression [5]. miRNAs regulate biological processes by binding to mRNA 3'-untranslated region (UTR) sequences to attenuate protein synthesis or messenger RNA (mRNA) stability [6]. Acting as genetic switches or fine-tuners, miRNAs are key regulators of diverse biological and pathological processes, including development, organogenesis, apoptosis, and cell proliferation and differentiation. miRNA dysregulation often results in impaired cellular function and disease progression. It has been estimated that the whole human genome encodes for about 1000 miRNAs which may be located within introns of coding or non-coding genes, within host exons or within intergenic regions [7].

miRNA biogenesis is shown in Figure 1. The transcription process is mediated by the RNA-polymerase II that produces long precursor RNAs known as "primary miRNA" (pri-miRNA) with a typical hairpin morphology [8]. A nuclear endonuclease, called DROSHA, then crops the distal stem portion of pri-RNA obtaining shorter chains (pre-miRNA) [9]. Pre-miRNA is transported to the cytoplasm by the nuclear receptor Exportin-5 [10] and processed by DICER, an RNase III, to short double-stranded RNA sequence containing the miRNA and the 'star strand' (miRNA*). miRNA* is degraded after stripping the miRNA strand to obtain mature miRNA [11]. Mature miRNA interact with proteins like Argonaute endonuclease (Arg 2), in order to form the RNA-induced silencing complex (RICS), which directs mature miRNA towards the targeted mRNA and bind on their 3' untranslated region (UTR) [6].

A single miRNA may modulate hundreds of miRNAs, and one mRNA has multiple predicted binding sites for miRNAs in their 3'UTR. Furthermore, after cleavage of a target mRNA, miRNAs are not Destroyed; so they may recognise and modulate other mRNAs [5, 12].

3. miRNAs and cardiovascular disease

Cardiovascular calcification is an independent risk factor for cardiovascular morbidity and mortality. Several risk factors can accelerate atherosclerosis and cardiovascular calcification, including age, hypercholesterolemia, metabolic syndrome, CRD, and T2D. Cardiovascular calcification can be distinguished by location — as intimal (atherosclerotic) , medial (CRD, T2D), or valvular [3]. Atherosclerotic calcification occurs as a part of atherogenic progress in the vessel intima. Small hydroxyapatite mineral crystals (microcalcification) can be visualized in early lesions [13]. Medial calcification occurs primarily in association with CRD and T2D, independently of hypercholesterolemia. Aortic valve calcification leads to impaired movement of aortic valve leaflets, and causes valve dysfunction [2]. All three processes shared risk factors and etiological factors, including inflammation and oxidative stress.

The identification of circulating miRNA as a novel biomarker in various diseases is a growing area of research investigation. Many pioneering studies describe specific miRNA patterns in

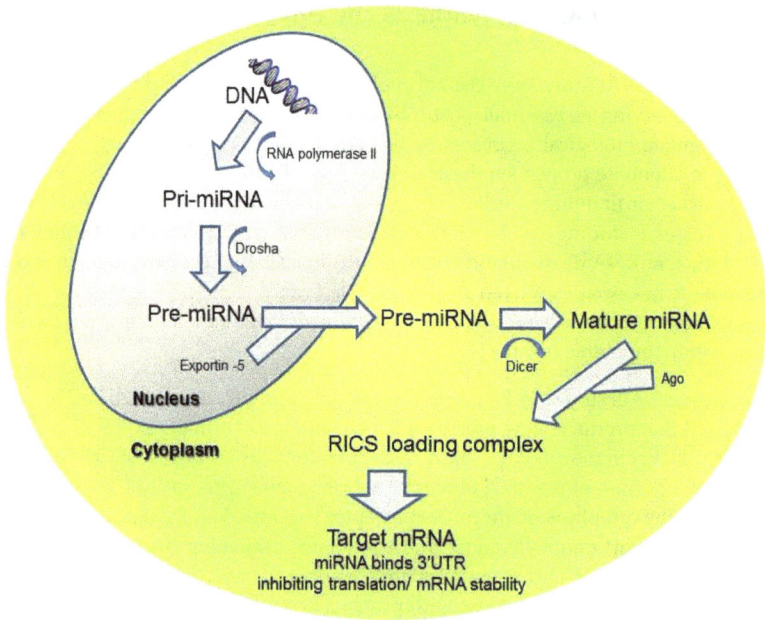

Figure 1. Schematic overview of miRNA biogenesis.

cardiovascular diseases. The first study reporting circulating miRNAs in patients with atherosclerosis was published in 2010, demonstrating a reduction of circulating vascular- and inflammation-associated miRNAs (miR-126, miR-17, miR-92a, miR-155) in patients with coronary artery disease (CAD) [14]. In addition, tissue levels of miRNAs were investigated.

Here we summarize and discuss the current knowledge on circulating and tissue miRNAs in diseases associated with cardiovascular calcification (Tables 1 and 2).

3.1. miRNAs in coronary artery disease

Studies about miRNA expression in calcified vessels are rare. Li *et al.* analyzed the expression of miRNAs in patients with peripheral artery disease (arteriosclerosis obliterans), characterized by fibrosis of the tunica intima and calcification of the tunica media [15]. miR-21, miR-130a, miR-27b, let-7f, and miR-210 were significantly increased, while miR-221 and miR-222 were decreased in the sclerotic intima, compared to normal vessels [15]. Higher levels of miR-21 and miR-210 were confirmed in a study that compared atherosclerotic with non-atherosclerotic left internal thoracic arteries [16]. In addition, the expression of miR-34a, miR-146a, miR146b-5p, and miR-210 increased more than 4-fold in atherosclerotic arteries. Several predicted targets were downregulated [16]. Another study found a different miRNA pattern using plaque material from the carotid artery, compared with the arteria mammaria interna as control tissue [17]. The healthy vessel expressed higher levels of miR-520b and miR-105, whereas miR-10b, miR-218, miR-30e, miR-26b, and miR-125a were predominantly expressed in atherosclerotic plaque [17]. The investigators in both studies, however, did not examine miRNAs in calcified lesions. Microcalcification is thought to cause plaque rupture [18, 19]. Destabilized human plaques are characterized by a specific miRNA expression profile (high levels of miR-100, miR-127, miR-145, miR-133a, miR-133b). Target genes of these miRNAs (Nox1, MMP9, CD40) may play a role in vascular calcification [7]. Thus, miRNAs could participate in the formation of hydroxyapatite crystals, and thereby have an important role in regulating atherosclerotic plaque toward unstable phenotypes and rupture [20].

Fichtlscherer *et al.* authored the first study investigating circulating miRNA in CAD [14]. Plasma levels of miR-17, miR-92a, miR-126, miR-145, and miR-155 were reduced in CAD compared to healthy controls, whereas miR-133a and miR-208a were increased [14]. Another study demonstrated a positive correlation of plasma miR-122 and miR-370 levels with the presence and severity of CAD [21]. Both miRNAs were significantly increased in hyperlipidemia patients, compared to controls [21]. Increased levels of miR-27b, miR-130a, and miR-210 were observed in the serum of arteriosclerosis obliterans patients [15].

Comparison of published studies is challenging mainly because of the different sources of circulating miRNAs, which include serum, whole blood, PBMCs, EPCs, and platelets (Table 1). The miRNA profiles obtained from the different studies, therefore, are often not the same. In this context, a recent report suggested the necessity of careful selection for reference miRNAs by showing that hemolysis may significantly affect the levels of plasma miRNAs previously used as controls [22].

Polymorphisms in the 3'UTR may alter miRNA binding, leading to post-transcriptional dysregulation of the target gene and aberrant protein level. Functional single-nucleotide polymorphisms (SNPs) of miRNA-binding sites associate with the risk of cardiovascular disease. Wu *et al.* discovered a SNP in the miR-149 binding site of the 5,10-methylenetetrahydrofolate reductase (MTHFR) gene that associated with increased risk for CAD [23]. Furthermore, a larger study in a Chinese population of 956 CAD patients and 620 controls revealed that a SNP in the binding sites for miR-196a2 and miR-499 associated with the occurrence and prognosis of CAD [24].

3.2. miRNAs in diabetes and chronic renal disease (CRD)

T2D is a major risk factor for cardiovascular disease. Zampetaki *et al.* identified a plasma miRNA signature for T2D that includes reduced levels of miR-223, miR-15, miR-20b, miR-21, miR-24, miR-29b, miR-126, miR-150, miR-191, miR-197, miR-320, and miR-486, and elevated levels of miR-28-3p [33]. Reduced miR-126 levels antedated diabetes manifestation, and might explain the impaired peripheral angiogenic signaling in patients with T2D. Reduction of circulating miR-21 and miR-126 was confirmed by Meng *et al.*, who also found a decrease of miR-27a,b and miR-130a in T2D patients [35]. Another study demonstrated mostly elevated miRNA levels (miR-9, miR-29a, miR-30d, miR-34a, miR-124a, miR-146a, and miR-375) in serum from T2D patients, compared with pre-diabetic and/or normal glucose tolerance

miRNA	Disease	Source	Finding	Reference number
miR-17, -21, -20a, -22a, -27a, -92a, -126, -145, -155, -221, -130a, -208b, let-7d	CAD	Serum	Decreased	[14]
miR-133a, -208a			Increased	
miR-146a/b	CAD	PBMC	Increased	[25]
miR-34a	CAD	EPC	Increased	[26]
miR-221, -222	CAD	EPC	Increased	[27]
miR-135a, -147	CAD	PBMC	Decreased	[28]
miR-140, -182	CAD	Whole blood	Decreased	[29]
miR-122, -370	CAD	Plasma	Increased	[21]
miR-181a	CAD	Monocytes	Decreased	[30]
Let-7i	CAD	Monocytes	Decreased	[31]
miR-340, -624	CAD	Platelets	Increased	[32]
miR-20b, -21, -24, -29b, -15a, -126, -150, -191, -197, -223, -320, -486	T2D	Plasma	Decreased	[33]
miR-28-3p			Increased	
miR-146a	T2D	PBMC	Decreased	[34]
miR-21, -27a, b, -126, -130a	T2D	EPC	Decreased	[35]
miR-9, -29a, -30d, -34a, -124a, -146a, -375	T2D	Serum	Increased	[36]
miR-16, -21, -155, -210, -638	CRD	Plasma	Decreased	[37]
miR-188-5p, -135*, -323-3p, -509-3p, -520-3p, -572, -573, 629*, -632	HC	HDL	Decreased	[38]
miR-24, -106a, -191, -218, -222, -223, -342-3p, -412, let-7p			Increased	
miR-21, -27b, -130a, -210	AO	Serum	Increased	[15]

CRD, chronic renal disease; T2D, type 2 diabetes; CAD, coronary artery disease; AS, aortic stenosis; HC, familial hyper-cholesterolemia; AO, arteriosclerosis obliterans; PBMC, peripheral blood mononuclear cell; EPC, endothelial progenitor cell; HDL, high-density lipoprotein.

Table 1. Circulating miRNA in diseases associated with vascular calcification.

conditions [36]. In contrast, reduced miR-146a levels in PMBCs from Asian Indian T2D patients associated with insulin resistance, poor glycemic control, and several proinflammatory cytokine genes [34]. miR-146a participates in the transcriptional circuitry regulating fibronectin in T2D animals.[39].

The high incidence of cardiovascular complications in patients with CRD is partly explained by more aggressive development of atherosclerotic lesions and accelerated calcification [40]. To our knowledge, only one study reports circulating miRNA in patients with CRD. Neal *et al.* found that plasma levels of total and specific miRNAs (miR-16, miR-21, miR-155, miR-210, and miR-638) are reduced in CRD patients, compared to patients with normal renal function [37]. A strong correlation exists between detected circulating miRNAs and estimated glomerular filtration rate [37]. Interestingly, miR-638 was the only miRNA that showed a differential urine excretion in CRD patients [37]. Transforming growth factor beta (TGF-β), a pro-fibrotic key mediator of CRD, reduces levels of miR-192 [41] and miR-29a [42] and increases miR-377 levels [43] *in vitro* and *in vivo*, thereby promoting the expression of extracellular matrix components.

3.3. miRNAs and aortic valve disease

Aortic stenosis (AS) is typically caused by calcific aortic valve disease. To our knowledge, no study to date describes a specific miRNA signature in the circulation of patients with AS. Nigam *et al.* identified a miRNA pattern specific to AS using tissue from whole bicuspid valves and linking them to calcification-related genes, such as Smad1/3, Runx2, and BMP2 [44]. miR-26a, miR-30b, and miR-195 were decreased in the aortic valves of patients requiring replacement due to AS, compared to those requiring replacement due to aortic insufficiency [44]. Another group compared bicuspid with tricuspid aortic valve leaflets by miRNA microarray, and found a number of modulated miRNAs [45]. Particularly, miR-141 had the most dramatic change, showing a 14.5-fold decrease in the bicuspid versus tricuspid valve tissue, while the levels of calcification were comparable between the two groups.

3.4. Similar miRNA profiles may represent common miRNAs in diseases associated with cardiovascular calcification

Our detailed investigation using currently published literature revealed common circulating miRNAs in diseases associated with vascular calcification. Seven miRNAs (miR-21, miR-27, miR-34a, miR-126, miR-146a, miR-155, and miR210) were useful biomarkers in atherosclerosis, T2D, and/or CRD, and only miR-21 was common among all three diseases [14, 33, 37] (Table 3).

Atherosclerotic arteries [16] and sclerotic intima from lower-extremity vessels [15] expressed higher miR-21 levels than did healthy vessels. Circulating levels of miR-21 in atherosclerosis, T2D, and/or CRD were reduced [14, 33, 37]. The reason for this discrepancy is unknown, and requires further investigation.

miR-146a is an inflammation-related miRNA, implicated in atherosclerosis and osteoclastogenesis [46]. Circulating miR-146a is increased in CAD patients [25] and T2D [36]. In addition, miR-146a was more highly expressed in atherosclerotic arteries in an animal model [16], and associated with CRD *in vivo* [47]. miR-155, another inflammation-associated miRNA, is decreased in CAD [14] and CRD [37]. Deficiency of miR155 enhanced atherosclerotic plaque development and decreased plaque stability [48], suggesting that it acts as an anti-inflammatory and atheroprotective miRNA. miR-155 is also highly expressed in endothelial cells (ECs) and SMCs, where it targets angiotensin-II receptor [49]. The renin–angiotensin system participates in cardiovascular calcification [50, 51]. Angiotensin-receptor blockade can inhibit

miRNA	Disease	Tissue type	Finding	Reference number
miR-21, -34a, -146a, -146b-5p, -210	CAD	Atherosclerotic arteries	Increased	[16]
miR-105, -520b	CAD	Atherosclerotic carotid artery	Decreased	[17]
miR-10b, -26b, -30e, -125a, -218,			Increased	
miR-100, -127, -133a,b -145	CAD	Destabilized plaque	Increased	[20]
miR-221, -222	AO	Sclerotic intima from lower extremities vessels	Decreased	[15]
miR-21, -27b, -210, -130a, let-7f			Increased	
miR-22, -27a, -141, -124, -125b, -185, -187, -194, -211, -330, -370, -449, -486, -551, -564, -575, -585, -622, -637, -648, -1202, -1282, -1469, -1908, -1972	AS	Bicuspid aortic valve	Decreased	[45]
miR-30e, -32, -145, -151, -152, -190, -373, -768			Increased	
miR-26a, -30b, -195	AS	Whole bicuspid valves	Decreased	[44]

CAD, coronary artery disease; AS, aortic stenosis; AO, arteriosclerosis obliterans.

Table 2. miRNAs expressed in human calcified tissue.

CAD	T2D	CRD
miR-21 ↓	miR-21 ↓	miR-21 ↓
miR-27 ↓	miR-27 ↓	
miR-34a ↑	miR-34a ↑	
miR-126 ↓	miR-126 ↓	
miR-155 ↓		miR-155 ↓

CRD, chronic renal disease; T2D, type 2 diabetes; CAD, coronary artery disease

Table 3. Common circulating miRNA in diseases associated with vascular calcification.

arterial calcification by disrupting vascular osteogenesis *in vivo* [52]. In addition, an observational study showed reduced progression of AV disease in patients taking angiotensin-converting enzyme inhibitors [53]. Furthermore, miR-155 represses osteoblastogenesis by targeting Smad proteins [54]. Thus, high expression of miR-155 may prevent cardiovascular calcification by inhibiting the BMP signalling pathway or the renin–angiotensin system, making it a promising anti-calcification therapeutic target.

In summary, a set of circulating miRNAs (consisting of miR-21, miR-27, miR-34a, miR-126, miR-146a, miR-155, and miR-210) is dysregulated in various pro-inflammatory diseases and may represent a miRNA signature for cardiovascular calcification. Of note, systemic and local inflammation paradoxically affects cardiovascular calcification and bone loss, which supports the concept of inflammation-dependent cardiovascular calcification previously proposed by our group and others [13, 40, 55-57].

4. miRNA and osteogenesis in the vascular wall

Cardiovascular calcification is an active, cell-regulated process. Various studies provide evidence of phenotypic transition or transition/dedifferentiation of mature SMCs or VICs into an osteogenic phenotype — a key feature in cardiovascular calcification. In medial calcification, SMCs undergo dedifferentiation from a contractile to a pro-atherogenic synthestic phenotype, lose the expression of their marker genes, acquire osteogenic markers, and deposit a mineralized bone-like matrix. In valvular calcification, VICs can undergo the transition to osteoblast-like bone-forming cells [58]. Recently, a novel concept emerged of circulating cells harboring osteogenic potential that can home to atherosclerotic lesions and contribute to intimal calcification [59, 60]. Comparing the sources of cells that contribute to atherosclerotic intimal calcification revealed that SMCs are the major contributors that reprogram its lineage towards osteochondrogenesis/blastogenesis; circulating bone marrow-derived cells, however, also contribute to early osteochondrogenic differentiation in atherosclerotic vessels [61]. The master transcription factors, including Runx2/Cbfa1, Msx2, and Osterix, designate cells for osteoblast lineages through the induction of downstream genes such as alkaline phosphatase, osteopontin, and osteocalcin. Here we summarize miRNAs involved in SMC differentiation, as well as in osteogenesis, with targets involved in cardiovascular calcification.

The SMC phenotype is dependent on the miR-143/145 cluster [62-64]. Circulating miR-145 levels are reduced in CAD patients [14]. miR-145 is one of the most recognized arterial miRNAs [65]. Inhibition of miR-143/145 promotes a phenotypic switch to the synthetic, pro-atherogenic SMC state [62], including the inhibition of SMC marker-like alpha-smooth muscle actin and smooth muscle myosin heavy chain [66] — both diminished in osteogenic SMCs [67]. miR-145 modulates SMC differentiation by targeting Krüppel-like factor 4 (KLF4) [63]. KLF4 mediates high phosphate-induced conversion of SMCs into osteogenic cells [68]. Conversely, miR-145-deficient mice [69] and overexpression of miR-145 [66] both reduce neointima formation in vascular injury.

Similar to miR-145, miR-133 has a potent inhibitory role on the vascular SMC phenotypic switch [70]. Runx2, a cell-fate determining osteoblastic transcription factor, is a target of miR-133 [71]. Runx2 acts as a critical regulator of osteogenic lineage and a modulator of bone-related genes [72]. Runx2 is essential and sufficient for regulating osteogenesis in SMC and VIC [73, 74, 75, 76]. Discovered in the bone biology field, a program of miRNAs controls Runx2 expression to prevent skeletal disorders [77]. Three of these miRNAs (miR-133a, miR-135a, and miR-218) are altered in cardiovascular diseases associated with vascular calcification [14, 17, 20, 28]. Klotho mutant mice, which display vascular calcification due to hyperphosphatemia and through a Runx2-dependent mechanism [78], show overexpression of miR-135a (together with miR-762, miR-714, and miR-712) in the aortic media, which causes SMC calcification by disruption of Ca^{2+} transporters and increasing intracellular Ca^{2+} concentrations [79]. More recently, miR-204, another candidate of the Runx2-cluster, was found to contribute to SMC calcification *in vitro* and *in vivo* [80]. Downstream targets of Runx2 are bone-specific genes like osteopontin, osterix and osteocalcin, all present in the cardiovascular osteogenic cell phenotype [2, 81]. We recently demonstrated that miR-125b, which inhibits osteoblast differentiation [82] regulates the transition of SMCs into osteoblast-like cells partially by targeting the transcription factor osterix, providing the first miR-dependent mechanism in the progression of vascular calcification [83]. Additionally, miRNA-processing enzymes — essential for SMC function [84] — were reduced in calcified SMCs [83].

Another potent regulator of vascular and valvular calcification is the BMP signaling pathway (reviewed in detail elsewhere [85]). BMP2 and BMP4 are potent osteogenic differentiation factors detected in calcified valve and atherosclerotic lesions [86-88]. BMPs elicit their effects through activation of receptor complex composed of type I and type II receptors and activate receptor-type–dependent and ligand-dependent Smad transcription factors, which modulate the expression of Runx2 [85]. MiR-26a, miR-135, and miR-155 were previously reported as Smad-regulating miRNAs related to osteoblastogenesis; they functionally repress osteoblast differentiation by targeting Smad1 and Smad5, respectively [54]. miR-155 is one of the circulating miRNAs that is decreased in CAD [14] and CRD [37] (discussed earlier). miR-26a was repressed in aortic valve leaflets of patients with aortic stenosis, and human aortic valvular interstitial cells showed decreased mRNA levels of BMP2 and Smad1 when treated with miR-26a mimic [44]. The same group found lower expression of miR-30b, which targets Smad1 and Smad3. Another group reported deceased miR-141 levels together with increased BMP2 levels in bicuspid versus tricuspid aortic valve leaflets, and showed *in vitro* that miR-141 represses the VIC response to calcification, in part through BMP2-dependent calcification [45]. Itoh *et al.* identified miR-141 as a pre-osteoblast differentiation-related miRNA, which modulated the BMP2-induced pre-osteoblast differentiation by direct translational repression of Dlx5, a transcription factor for osterix [89].

Activation of canonical wingless-type (WNT) signaling is crucial for osteoblast function [90] and for the programming of valvular and vascular cells during cardiovascular calcification [85]. Activation of the Wnt/β-catenin signaling pathway occurs in human calcified aortic valve stenosis [91], in LDL receptor (LDLR)-deficient mice [92, 93], and in osteogenic SMCs *in vitro* [94]. Dickkopf (Dkk)1 is an extracellular antagonist of the canonical Wnt signaling that plays a crucial role in bone remodeling by binding to and inactivating signaling from LDLR-related protein 5/6 [95, 96]. Dkk-1 may also play a role in vascular calcification. In CRD patients, Dkk1 serum levels correlated negatively with arterial stiffness [97]. Dkk-1 prevents warfarin-induced activation of β-catenin, and osteogenic transdifferentiation of SMCs [98] and TNF α-induced induction of alkaline phosphatase activity [92]. Remarkably, two miRNAs targeting bone Dkk-1 (miR-335-5p, miR-29a) increase with age [99, 100] — a risk for cardiovascular calcification. miR-335-5p directly targets and represses Wnt inhibitor Dkk-1, thereby enhancing Wnt signaling and promoting osteoblast differentiation [101]. To date, no publications exist regarding the role of miR-335-5p in the cardiovascular system. Yet, the age-dependent increase of miR-335 in rat renal tissue inhibited the expression and function of the enzymes implicated in oxidative stress defense [99]. Likewise, miR-29a potentiates osteoblastogenesis by modulating Wnt signaling. Canonical Wnt signaling induces miR-29a expression, which negatively targets regulators of Wnt signaling, including Dkk-1, sFRP2, Kremen, and osteonectin [102, 103]. miR-29 increased age-dependently in mouse aortic tissue and associated with reduced extracellular matrix components, such as collagen and elastin [100]. Elastolysis accelerates arterial and aortic valve calcification [40]. Furthermore, MMP-2, another target of miR-29 [104], was shown to promote arterial calcification in CRD [105] and valvular calcification [106].

The contribution of osteoclasts to cardiovascular calcification is still controversial [59]. The observation of osteoclast-like cells in calcified atherosclerotic lesions suggested this bone-related cell is active in the vessel wall. The evidence was strengthened recently by Sun et al., who demonstrated the functional role of SMC-derived Runx2 promoting infiltration of macrophages into the calcified lesion to form osteoclast-like cells — suggesting that the development of vascular calcification is coupled with the formation of osteoclast-like cells, paralleling the bone remodeling process [74]. The receptor activator of the nuclear factor-kappa B (NF-kappa B) ligand (RANKL)/osteoprotegerin (OPG) system controls proper osteoclastogenesis, and actes as a biomarker for CAD [107, 108]. In silico analysis revealed RANKL as a target of miR-126 [109], which is decreased in the plasma of CAD [14] and T2D [33] patients. miR-146a, highly expressed in atherosclerotic arteries [16], inhibits osteoclastogenesis [46]. The number of tartrate-resistant acid phosphatase-positive multinucleated cells was significantly reduced by miR-146a in a dose-dependent manner [46]. Furthermore, miR-155, which is decreased in plasma of CRD [37] and CAD [14] patients, was shown to inhibit osteoclast function [110].

Taken together, osteogenic processes in both bone and the cardiovascular system are tightly controlled by miRNAs (Figure 2). Further studies are needed to elucidate whether interplay of miRNAs could explain the bone-vascular axis "calcification paradox," or whether they act independently in the calcifying vessel and bone.

5. Circulating miRNAs as biomarkers and extracellular communicators

miRNAs are present in blood (plasma, platelets, erythrocytes, nucleated blood cells) with high stability. miRNAs can circulate in extracellular vesicles [111], in a protein complex (Ago2), or in a lipoprotein complex (HDL) [38], which prevents their degradation. Depending on the size and type, extracellular vesicles are broadly classified as ectosomes (also called shedding microvesicles), exosomes, matrix vesicles (MVs), and apoptotic bodies. Ectosomes are large extracellular vesicles 50-1000 nm in diameter; exosomes are small membranous vesicles of endocytic origin, 40-100 nm in diameter; MVs are 30-300 nm in diameter, are produced by

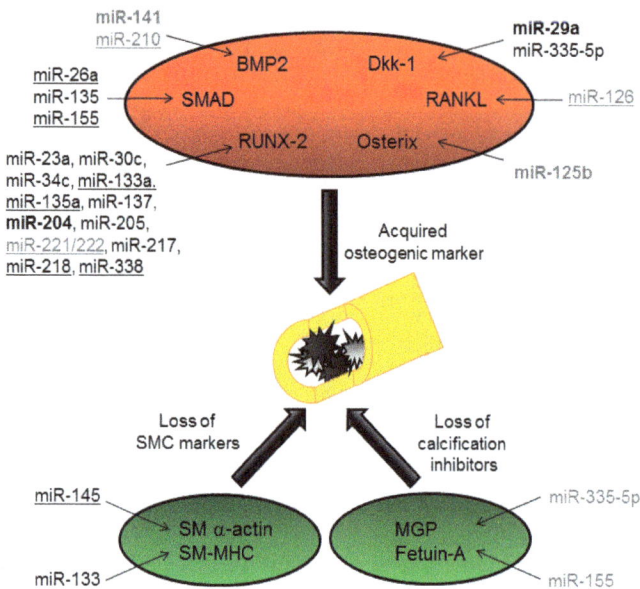

Figure 2. Potential and established miRNAs contributing to osteogenic regulation of vascular calcification. Bold, established miRNAs in vascular calcification; underlined, dysregulated in cardiovascular disease (circulating or tissue); gray, predicted miRNA binding sites.

blebbing of the plasma membrane, and can calcify; and apoptotic bodies, 50-5000 nm in diameter, are released from fragmented apoptotic cells.

The majority of miRNAs are independent of vesicles [111] and co-purify with the Ago2 complex [112, 113]. But in CAD patients, most plasma miRNAs associate with extracellular vesicles, and only a small amount are found in extracellular vesicle-free plasma [114]. A cell-type-specific miRNA release and different export systems are implicated, as the miRNA release pattern within vesicles is different from that associated with Ago2 complexes [112]. Thus, cells can select miRNA and pre-miRNA for controlled cellular release [115, 116]. miRNA profiles of extracellular vesicles are different from their maternal cell profiles, indicating an active mechanism of selective miRNA packing from cells into vesicles [114]. We have limited knowledge about miRNA secretion. Blockade of sphingomyelinase inhibits exosome generation and miRNA secretion, and intercellular miRNA transfer implicates a ceramide-dependent mechanism [117, 118]. Ago2–miRNA complexes may be passively produced by dead cells, released by live cells, or actively transported though cell-membrane–associated channels or receptors [119].

Extracellular vesicles use miRNA to mediate intercellular communication over long distances or on a local tissue level [120]. Endothelial apoptotic bodies can convey miR-126 to athero-sclerotic lesions, which demonstrate uniquely paracrine-signaling function for miRNA during atherosclerosis [33, 121]. miRNA-containing vesicles can regulate intercellular communication between ECs and SMCs by selective packing of miR-143/145 in endothelial-derived vesicles, which are then transported to SMCs to control their phenotype [118].

How miRNAs are taken up by target cells and remain biologically active is still unknown. We know little about the mechanisms of vesicle-mediated cargo transfer. In physiological conditions, extracellular vesicles may bind to the membrane proteins of the surface of target cells through receptor–ligand interaction, resulting in intracellular stimulation of genetic pathways. They can also fuse with cell–target membranes and release genetic content in a nonselective manner. Furthermore, vesicles can bind to surface receptors on target cells with endocytotic internalization by recipient cells, followed by fusion with the membranes, leading to a release of their content into the cytosol of target cells [122].

A key event in the initiation and promotion of VIC and SMC calcification is the release of extracellular vesicles [81, 123]. Treatment of SMCs with elevated calcium levels promotes the production of calcifying vesicles (MVs), and the loss of fetuin-A, an inhibitor of mineral nucleation [124]. These vesicles act as early nucleation sites for calcification. The phosphatidylserine-membrane complex from SMC-derived and macrophage-derived MVs redistributes and nucleates hydroxyapatite [125-127]. In addition, hydroxyapatite nanocrystals shed from vesicles may further promote mineralization via direct effects on SMC phenotype [128].

Insight into the underlying mechanism of selective packing of miRNAs into extracellular vesicles and selective uptake into the target cell will help increase understanding of the role of miRNA-containing vesicles in physiological intercellular communication, which may prevent calcification in the cardiovascular system.

6. miRNAs in the "calcification paradox"

Osteoporosis frequently associates with cardiovascular calcification, and the severity of aortic calcification associates positively with bone loss [2, 129, 130]. The "calcification paradox" could be explained by the shared molecular pathways in bone remodeling and cardiovascular calcification [3]. How these two processes associate with each other and whether osteoporosis leads to cardiovascular calcification - or whether both disorders just share common risk factors - is unclear. In this section, we link cardiovascular calcification and bone loss and show commonalities in the systems' miRNA pathways/patterns.

Studies of miRNA in patients with bone disease are lacking. A recent clinical study first reported miRNA as a potential biomarker for postmenopausal osteoporosis. Wang *et al.* demonstrated an association of miR-133a levels in circulating monocytes - osteoclast precursors - with postmenopausal osteoporosis [131]. Women with low bone mineral density showed higher circulating miR-133a levels [131], but the number of patients per group was small (n=10). Circulating miR-133a levels were also higher in patients with CAD [14]. Unfortunately, the study investigating bone mineral density in patients with osteoporosis did not mention characteristics of the cardiovascular patient population. miR-133a belongs to the Runx2-targeting miRNA cluster [77].

Additionally, miR-2861 contributes to osteoporosis in mice and humans by targeting histone deacethylase 5, and thereby increasing Runx2 [132]. No studies of miR-2861 in the cardiovascular system have been reported. Patients with rheumatoid arthritis also suffer from vascular calcification in different vessel beds, in addition to osteoporosis; the pathogenesis includes pro-inflammatory cytokines and site-specific inflammation (reviewed in detail elsewhere [133]). miR-146a, a negative regulator of inflammation and osteoclastogenesis, also associates with rheumatoid arthritis [134]. Similar to patients with CAD, in patients with rheumatoid arthritis, miR-146a is up-regulated in PBMCs [25].

7. Conclusion and perspectives

In vitro and *in vivo* studies have established miRNAs as biomarkers focusing on different aspects and providing circulating miRNA signatures for different diseases. But these circulating miRNAs may not have biological functions within the cell while circulating — instead, they act as intercellular communicators, and this communication may be disturbed by calcified vesicles. More studies are needed to fully exploit this potentially novel mechanism of cardiovascular calcification.

Moreover, miRNA biology is very complex. Multiple miRNAs can target the same gene (e.g., Runx2–miRNA cluster), and one miRNA may have several targets. Only a small amount of these fine-tuned targets may alter biological responses and phenotypes. Understanding the role of miRNA in vascular calcification may be helpful in considering the paradoxical clinical observations of the concurrence of cardiovascular calcification and osteoporosis. Despite its global clinical burden, no medical therapies are available to treat cardiovascular calcification. Targeting of miRNA represents a novel therapeutic opportunity for treating calcification disorders. As vascular calcification and bone remodeling share common mechanisms, we have to understand in greater detail the functions of miRNAs and their association with the molecular pathogenesis of osteoporosis and vascular/valvular calcification.

Author details

Claudia Goettsch[1] and Elena Aikawa[1,2]

*Address all correspondence to: eaikawa@partners.org

1 Center for Interdisciplinary Cardiovascular Sciences, Cardiovascular Medicine, Brigham and Women's Hospital, Harvard Medical School, Boston, MA, USA

2 Center for Excellence in Vascular Biology, Cardiovascular Medicine, Brigham and Women's Hospital, Harvard Medical School, Boston, MA, USA

References

[1] Hjortnaes J, Bouten CV, Van Herwerden LA, Grundeman PF, Kluin J. Translating autologous heart valve tissue engineering from bench to bed. Tissue engineering Part B, Reviews 2009;15(3):307-17.

[2] Rajamannan NM, Evans FJ, Aikawa E, Grande-Allen KJ, Demer LL, Heistad DD, et al. Calcific aortic valve disease: not simply a degenerative process: A review and agenda for research from the National Heart and Lung and Blood Institute Aortic Stenosis Working Group. Executive summary: Calcific aortic valve disease-2011 update. Circulation 2011;124(16):1783-91.

[3] Sage AP, Tintut Y, Demer LL. Regulatory mechanisms in vascular calcification. Nature reviews Cardiology 2010;7(9):528-36.

[4] Johnson RC, Leopold JA, Loscalzo J. Vascular calcification: pathobiological mechanisms and clinical implications. Circulation research 2006;99(10):1044-59.

[5] Ambros V. The functions of animal microRNAs. Nature 2004;431(7006):350-5.

[6] Bartel DP. MicroRNAs: target recognition and regulatory functions. Cell 2009;136(2): 215-33.

[7] Santovito D, Mezzetti A, Cipollone F. MicroRNAs and atherosclerosis: New actors for an old movie. Nutrition, metabolism, and cardiovascular diseases : NMCD 2012.

[8] Lee Y, Kim M, Han J, Yeom KH, Lee S, Baek SH, et al. MicroRNA genes are transcribed by RNA polymerase II. The EMBO journal 2004;23(20):4051-60.

[9] Lee Y, Ahn C, Han J, Choi H, Kim J, Yim J, et al. The nuclear RNase III Drosha initiates microRNA processing. Nature 2003;425(6956):415-9.

[10] Yi R, Qin Y, Macara IG, Cullen BR. Exportin-5 mediates the nuclear export of pre-microRNAs and short hairpin RNAs. Genes & development 2003;17(24):3011-6.

[11] Chendrimada TP, Gregory RI, Kumaraswamy E, Norman J, Cooch N, Nishikura K, et al. TRBP recruits the Dicer complex to Ago2 for microRNA processing and gene silencing. Nature 2005;436(7051):740-4.

[12] Hutvagner G, Zamore PD. A microRNA in a multiple-turnover RNAi enzyme complex. Science 2002;297(5589):2056-60.

[13] Aikawa E, Nahrendorf M, Figueiredo JL, Swirski FK, Shtatland T, Kohler RH, et al. Osteogenesis associates with inflammation in early-stage atherosclerosis evaluated by molecular imaging in vivo. Circulation 2007;116(24):2841-50.

[14] Fichtlscherer S, De Rosa S, Fox H, Schwietz T, Fischer A, Liebetrau C, et al. Circulating microRNAs in patients with coronary artery disease. Circulation research 2010;107(5):677-84.

[15] Li T, Cao H, Zhuang J, Wan J, Guan M, Yu B, et al. Identification of miR-130a, miR-27b and miR-210 as serum biomarkers for atherosclerosis obliterans. Clinica chimica acta; international journal of clinical chemistry 2011;412(1-2):66-70.

[16] Raitoharju E, Lyytikainen LP, Levula M, Oksala N, Mennander A, Tarkka M, et al. miR-21, miR-210, miR-34a, and miR-146a/b are up-regulated in human atherosclerotic plaques in the Tampere Vascular Study. Atherosclerosis 2011;219(1):211-7.

[17] Bidzhekov K, Gan L, Denecke B, Rostalsky A, Hristov M, Koeppel TA, et al. microRNA expression signatures and parallels between monocyte subsets and atherosclerotic plaque in humans. Thrombosis and haemostasis 2012;107(4):619-25.

[18] Vengrenyuk Y, Carlier S, Xanthos S, Cardoso L, Ganatos P, Virmani R, et al. A hypothesis for vulnerable plaque rupture due to stress-induced debonding around cellular microcalcifications in thin fibrous caps. Proceedings of the National Academy of Sciences of the United States of America 2006;103(40):14678-83.

[19] Hoshino T, Chow LA, Hsu JJ, Perlowski AA, Abedin M, Tobis J, et al. Mechanical stress analysis of a rigid inclusion in distensible material: a model of atherosclerotic calcification and plaque vulnerability. American journal of physiology Heart and circulatory physiology 2009;297(2):H802-10.

[20] Cipollone F, Felicioni L, Sarzani R, Ucchino S, Spigonardo F, Mandolini C, et al. A unique microRNA signature associated with plaque instability in humans. Stroke; a journal of cerebral circulation 2011;42(9):2556-63.

[21] Gao W, He HW, Wang ZM, Zhao H, Lian XQ, Wang YS, et al. Plasma levels of lipometabolism-related miR-122 and miR-370 are increased in patients with hyperlipidemia and associated with coronary artery disease. Lipids in health and disease 2012;11(1):55.

[22] Kirschner MB, Kao SC, Edelman JJ, Armstrong NJ, Vallely MP, van Zandwijk N, et al. Haemolysis during sample preparation alters microRNA content of plasma. PloS one 2011;6(9):e24145.

[23] Wu C, Gong Y, Sun A, Zhang Y, Zhang C, Zhang W, et al. The human MTHFR rs4846049 polymorphism increases coronary heart disease risk through modifying miRNA binding. Nutrition, metabolism, and cardiovascular diseases : NMCD 2012.

[24] Zhi H, Wang L, Ma G, Ye X, Yu X, Zhu Y, et al. Polymorphisms of miRNAs genes are associated with the risk and prognosis of coronary artery disease. Clinical research in cardiology : official journal of the German Cardiac Society 2012;101(4):289-96.

[25] Takahashi Y, Satoh M, Minami Y, Tabuchi T, Itoh T, Nakamura M. Expression of miR-146a/b is associated with the Toll-like receptor 4 signal in coronary artery disease: effect of renin-angiotensin system blockade and statins on miRNA-146a/b and Toll-like receptor 4 levels. Clin Sci (Lond) 2010;119(9):395-405.

[26] Tabuchi T, Satoh M, Itoh T, Nakamura M. MicroRNA-34a regulates the longevity-associated protein SIRT1 in coronary artery disease: effect of statins on SIRT1 and microRNA-34a expression. Clin Sci (Lond) 2012;123(3):161-71.

[27] Minami Y, Satoh M, Maesawa C, Takahashi Y, Tabuchi T, Itoh T, et al. Effect of atorvastatin on microRNA 221 / 222 expression in endothelial progenitor cells obtained from patients with coronary artery disease. European journal of clinical investigation 2009;39(5):359-67.

[28] Hoekstra M, van der Lans CA, Halvorsen B, Gullestad L, Kuiper J, Aukrust P, et al. The peripheral blood mononuclear cell microRNA signature of coronary artery disease. Biochemical and biophysical research communications 2010;394(3):792-7.

[29] Taurino C, Miller WH, McBride MW, McClure JD, Khanin R, Moreno MU, et al. Gene expression profiling in whole blood of patients with coronary artery disease. Clin Sci (Lond) 2010;119(8):335-43.

[30] Hulsmans M, Sinnaeve P, Van der Schueren B, Mathieu C, Janssens S, Holvoet P. Decreased miR-181a Expression in Monocytes of Obese Patients Is Associated with the Occurrence of Metabolic Syndrome and Coronary Artery Disease. The Journal of clinical endocrinology and metabolism 2012;97(7):E1213-8.

[31] Satoh M, Tabuchi T, Minami Y, Takahashi Y, Itoh T, Nakamura M. Expression of let-7i is associated with Toll-like receptor 4 signal in coronary artery disease: effect of statins on let-7i and Toll-like receptor 4 signal. Immunobiology 2012;217(5):533-9.

[32] Sondermeijer BM, Bakker A, Halliani A, de Ronde MW, Marquart AA, Tijsen AJ, et al. Platelets in patients with premature coronary artery disease exhibit upregulation of miRNA340* and miRNA624*. PloS one 2011;6(10):e25946.

[33] Zampetaki A, Kiechl S, Drozdov I, Willeit P, Mayr U, Prokopi M, et al. Plasma microRNA profiling reveals loss of endothelial miR-126 and other microRNAs in type 2 diabetes. Circulation research 2010;107(6):810-7.

[34] Balasubramanyam M, Aravind S, Gokulakrishnan K, Prabu P, Sathishkumar C, Ranjani H, et al. Impaired miR-146a expression links subclinical inflammation and insulin resistance in Type 2 diabetes. Molecular and cellular biochemistry 2011;351(1-2): 197-205.

[35] Meng S, Cao JT, Zhang B, Zhou Q, Shen CX, Wang CQ. Downregulation of microRNA-126 in endothelial progenitor cells from diabetes patients, impairs their functional properties, via target gene Spred-1. Journal of molecular and cellular cardiology 2012;53(1):64-72.

[36] Kong L, Zhu J, Han W, Jiang X, Xu M, Zhao Y, et al. Significance of serum microRNAs in pre-diabetes and newly diagnosed type 2 diabetes: a clinical study. Acta diabetologica 2011;48(1):61-9.

[37] Neal CS, Michael MZ, Pimlott LK, Yong TY, Li JY, Gleadle JM. Circulating microRNA expression is reduced in chronic kidney disease. Nephrology, dialysis, trans-

plantation : official publication of the European Dialysis and Transplant Association - European Renal Association 2011;26(11):3794-802.

[38] Vickers KC, Palmisano BT, Shoucri BM, Shamburek RD, Remaley AT. MicroRNAs are transported in plasma and delivered to recipient cells by high-density lipoproteins. Nature cell biology 2011;13(4):423-33.

[39] Feng B, Chen S, McArthur K, Wu Y, Sen S, Ding Q, et al. miR-146a-Mediated extracellular matrix protein production in chronic diabetes complications. Diabetes 2011;60(11):2975-84.

[40] Aikawa E, Aikawa M, Libby P, Figueiredo JL, Rusanescu G, Iwamoto Y, et al. Arterial and aortic valve calcification abolished by elastolytic cathepsin S deficiency in chronic renal disease. Circulation 2009;119(13):1785-94.

[41] Krupa A, Jenkins R, Luo DD, Lewis A, Phillips A, Fraser D. Loss of MicroRNA-192 promotes fibrogenesis in diabetic nephropathy. Journal of the American Society of Nephrology : JASN 2010;21(3):438-47.

[42] Wang B, Komers R, Carew R, Winbanks CE, Xu B, Herman-Edelstein M, et al. Suppression of microRNA-29 expression by TGF-beta1 promotes collagen expression and renal fibrosis. Journal of the American Society of Nephrology : JASN 2012;23(2): 252-65.

[43] Wang Q, Wang Y, Minto AW, Wang J, Shi Q, Li X, et al. MicroRNA-377 is up-regulated and can lead to increased fibronectin production in diabetic nephropathy. FASEB journal : official publication of the Federation of American Societies for Experimental Biology 2008;22(12):4126-35.

[44] Nigam V, Sievers HH, Jensen BC, Sier HA, Simpson PC, Srivastava D, et al. Altered microRNAs in bicuspid aortic valve: a comparison between stenotic and insufficient valves. The Journal of heart valve disease 2010;19(4):459-65.

[45] Yanagawa B, Lovren F, Pan Y, Garg V, Quan A, Tang G, et al. miRNA-141 is a novel regulator of BMP-2-mediated calcification in aortic stenosis. The Journal of thoracic and cardiovascular surgery 2012.

[46] Nakasa T, Shibuya H, Nagata Y, Niimoto T, Ochi M. The inhibitory effect of microRNA-146a expression on bone destruction in collagen-induced arthritis. Arthritis and rheumatism 2011;63(6):1582-90.

[47] Ichii O, Otsuka S, Sasaki N, Namiki Y, Hashimoto Y, Kon Y. Altered expression of microRNA miR-146a correlates with the development of chronic renal inflammation. Kidney international 2012;81(3):280-92.

[48] Donners MM, Wolfs IM, Stoger LJ, van der Vorst EP, Pottgens CC, Heymans S, et al. Hematopoietic miR155 deficiency enhances atherosclerosis and decreases plaque stability in hyperlipidemic mice. PloS one 2012;7(4):e35877.

[49] Zhu N, Zhang D, Chen S, Liu X, Lin L, Huang X, et al. Endothelial enriched micro-
      RNAs regulate angiotensin II-induced endothelial inflammation and migration.
      Atherosclerosis 2011;215(2):286-93.

[50] Jia G, Stormont RM, Gangahar DM, Agrawal DK. Role of Matrix Gla Protein in An-
      giotensin II-Induced Exacerbation of Vascular Stiffness. American journal of physiol-
      ogy Heart and circulatory physiology 2012.

[51] O'Brien KD, Shavelle DM, Caulfield MT, McDonald TO, Olin-Lewis K, Otto CM, et
      al. Association of angiotensin-converting enzyme with low-density lipoprotein in
      aortic valvular lesions and in human plasma. Circulation 2002;106(17):2224-30.

[52] Armstrong ZB, Boughner DR, Drangova M, Rogers KA. Angiotensin II type 1 recep-
      tor blocker inhibits arterial calcification in a pre-clinical model. Cardiovascular re-
      search 2011;90(1):165-70.

[53] Shavelle DM, Takasu J, Budoff MJ, Mao S, Zhao XQ, O'Brien KD. HMG CoA reduc-
      tase inhibitor (statin) and aortic valve calcium. Lancet 2002;359(9312):1125-6.

[54] Taipaleenmaki H, Bjerre Hokland L, Chen L, Kauppinen S, Kassem M. Mechanisms
      in endocrinology: micro-RNAs: targets for enhancing osteoblast differentiation and
      bone formation. European journal of endocrinology / European Federation of Endo-
      crine Societies 2012;166(3):359-71.

[55] New SE, Aikawa E. Molecular imaging insights into early inflammatory stages of ar-
      terial and aortic valve calcification. Circulation research 2011;108(11):1381-91.

[56] Hjortnaes J, Butcher J, Figueiredo JL, Riccio M, Kohler RH, Kozloff KM, et al. Arterial
      and aortic valve calcification inversely correlates with osteoporotic bone remodel-
      ling: a role for inflammation. European heart journal 2010;31(16):1975-84.

[57] Geng Y, Hsu JJ, Lu J, Ting TC, Miyazaki M, Demer LL, et al. Role of cellular choles-
      terol metabolism in vascular cell calcification. The Journal of biological chemistry
      2011;286(38):33701-6.

[58] Rajamannan NM, Subramaniam M, Rickard D, Stock SR, Donovan J, Springett M, et
      al. Human aortic valve calcification is associated with an osteoblast phenotype. Cir-
      culation 2003;107(17):2181-4.

[59] Fadini GP, Rattazzi M, Matsumoto T, Asahara T, Khosla S. Emerging Role of Circu-
      lating Calcifying Cells in the Bone-Vascular Axis. Circulation 2012;125(22):2772-81.

[60] Doehring LC, Heeger C, Aherrahrou Z, Kaczmarek PM, Erdmann J, Schunkert H, et
      al. Myeloid CD34+CD13+ precursor cells transdifferentiate into chondrocyte-like cells
      in atherosclerotic intimal calcification. The American journal of pathology
      2010;177(1):473-80.

[61] Naik V, Leaf EM, Hu JH, Yang HY, Nguyen NB, Giachelli CM, et al. Sources of cells that contribute to atherosclerotic intimal calcification: an in vivo genetic fate mapping study. Cardiovascular research 2012;94(3):545-54.

[62] Elia L, Quintavalle M, Zhang J, Contu R, Cossu L, Latronico MV, et al. The knockout of miR-143 and -145 alters smooth muscle cell maintenance and vascular homeostasis in mice: correlates with human disease. Cell death and differentiation 2009;16(12): 1590-8.

[63] Cordes KR, Sheehy NT, White MP, Berry EC, Morton SU, Muth AN, et al. miR-145 and miR-143 regulate smooth muscle cell fate and plasticity. Nature 2009;460(7256): 705-10.

[64] Boettger T, Beetz N, Kostin S, Schneider J, Kruger M, Hein L, et al. Acquisition of the contractile phenotype by murine arterial smooth muscle cells depends on the Mir143/145 gene cluster. The Journal of clinical investigation 2009;119(9):2634-47.

[65] Ji R, Cheng Y, Yue J, Yang J, Liu X, Chen H, et al. MicroRNA expression signature and antisense-mediated depletion reveal an essential role of MicroRNA in vascular neointimal lesion formation. Circulation research 2007;100(11):1579-88.

[66] Cheng Y, Liu X, Yang J, Lin Y, Xu DZ, Lu Q, et al. MicroRNA-145, a novel smooth muscle cell phenotypic marker and modulator, controls vascular neointimal lesion formation. Circulation research 2009;105(2):158-66.

[67] Steitz SA, Speer MY, Curinga G, Yang HY, Haynes P, Aebersold R, et al. Smooth muscle cell phenotypic transition associated with calcification: upregulation of Cbfa1 and downregulation of smooth muscle lineage markers. Circulation research 2001;89(12):1147-54.

[68] Yoshida T, Yamashita M, Hayashi M. Kruppel-like factor 4 contributes to high phosphate-induced phenotypic switching of vascular smooth muscle cells into osteogenic cells. The Journal of biological chemistry 2012.

[69] Xin M, Small EM, Sutherland LB, Qi X, McAnally J, Plato CF, et al. MicroRNAs miR-143 and miR-145 modulate cytoskeletal dynamics and responsiveness of smooth muscle cells to injury. Genes & development 2009;23(18):2166-78.

[70] Torella D, Iaconetti C, Catalucci D, Ellison GM, Leone A, Waring CD, et al. MicroRNA-133 controls vascular smooth muscle cell phenotypic switch in vitro and vascular remodeling in vivo. Circulation research 2011;109(8):880-93.

[71] Li Z, Hassan MQ, Volinia S, van Wijnen AJ, Stein JL, Croce CM, et al. A microRNA signature for a BMP2-induced osteoblast lineage commitment program. Proceedings of the National Academy of Sciences of the United States of America 2008;105(37): 13906-11.

[72] Komori T. Regulation of bone development and extracellular matrix protein genes by RUNX2. Cell and tissue research 2010;339(1):189-95.

[73] Byon CH, Javed A, Dai Q, Kappes JC, Clemens TL, Darley-Usmar VM, et al. Oxidative stress induces vascular calcification through modulation of the osteogenic transcription factor Runx2 by AKT signaling. The Journal of biological chemistry 2008;283(22):15319-27.

[74] Sun Y, Byon C, Yuan K, Chen J, Mao X, Heath JM, et al. Smooth Muscle Cell-Specific Runx2 Deficiency InhibitsVascular Calcification. Circulation research 2012.

[75] Speer MY, Li X, Hiremath PG, Giachelli CM. Runx2/Cbfa1, but not loss of myocardin, is required for smooth muscle cell lineage reprogramming toward osteochondrogenesis. Journal of cellular biochemistry 2010;110(4):935-47.

[76] Miller JD, Weiss RM, Serrano KM, Castaneda LE, Brooks RM, Zimmerman K, et al. Evidence for active regulation of pro-osteogenic signaling in advanced aortic valve disease. Arteriosclerosis, thrombosis, and vascular biology 2010;30(12):2482-6.

[77] Zhang Y, Xie RL, Croce CM, Stein JL, Lian JB, van Wijnen AJ, et al. A program of microRNAs controls osteogenic lineage progression by targeting transcription factor Runx2. Proceedings of the National Academy of Sciences of the United States of America 2011;108(24):9863-8.

[78] Lim K, Lu TS, Molostvov G, Lee C, Lam FT, Zehnder D, et al. Vascular Klotho deficiency potentiates the development of human artery calcification and mediates resistance to fibroblast growth factor 23. Circulation 2012;125(18):2243-55.

[79] Gui T, Zhou G, Sun Y, Shimokado A, Itoh S, Oikawa K, et al. MicroRNAs that target Ca(2+) transporters are involved in vascular smooth muscle cell calcification. Laboratory investigation; a journal of technical methods and pathology 2012.

[80] Cui RR, Li SJ, Liu LJ, Yi L, Liang QH, Zhu X, et al. MicroRNA-204 Regulates Vascular Smooth Muscle Cell Calcification in vitro and in vivo. Cardiovascular research 2012.

[81] Shanahan CM, Crouthamel MH, Kapustin A, Giachelli CM. Arterial calcification in chronic kidney disease: key roles for calcium and phosphate. Circulation research 2011;109(6):697-711.

[82] Mizuno Y, Yagi K, Tokuzawa Y, Kanesaki-Yatsuka Y, Suda T, Katagiri T, et al. miR-125b inhibits osteoblastic differentiation by down-regulation of cell proliferation. Biochemical and biophysical research communications 2008;368(2):267-72.

[83] Goettsch C, Rauner M, Pacyna N, Hempel U, Bornstein SR, Hofbauer LC. miR-125b regulates calcification of vascular smooth muscle cells. The American journal of pathology 2011;179(4):1594-600.

[84] Albinsson S, Suarez Y, Skoura A, Offermanns S, Miano JM, Sessa WC. MicroRNAs are necessary for vascular smooth muscle growth, differentiation, and function. Arteriosclerosis, thrombosis, and vascular biology 2010;30(6):1118-26.

[85] Bostrom KI, Rajamannan NM, Towler DA. The regulation of valvular and vascular sclerosis by osteogenic morphogens. Circulation research 2011;109(5):564-77.

[86] Bostrom K, Watson KE, Horn S, Wortham C, Herman IM, Demer LL. Bone morphogenetic protein expression in human atherosclerotic lesions. The Journal of clinical investigation 1993;91(4):1800-9.

[87] Dhore CR, Cleutjens JP, Lutgens E, Cleutjens KB, Geusens PP, Kitslaar PJ, et al. Differential expression of bone matrix regulatory proteins in human atherosclerotic plaques. Arteriosclerosis, thrombosis, and vascular biology 2001;21(12):1998-2003.

[88] Seya K, Yu Z, Kanemaru K, Daitoku K, Akemoto Y, Shibuya H, et al. Contribution of bone morphogenetic protein-2 to aortic valve calcification in aged rat. Journal of pharmacological sciences 2011;115(1):8-14.

[89] Itoh T, Nozawa Y, Akao Y. MicroRNA-141 and -200a are involved in bone morphogenetic protein-2-induced mouse pre-osteoblast differentiation by targeting distal-less homeobox 5. The Journal of biological chemistry 2009;284(29):19272-9.

[90] Monroe DG, McGee-Lawrence ME, Oursler MJ, Westendorf JJ. Update on Wnt signaling in bone cell biology and bone disease. Gene 2012;492(1):1-18.

[91] Miller JD, Chu Y, Brooks RM, Richenbacher WE, Pena-Silva R, Heistad DD. Dysregulation of antioxidant mechanisms contributes to increased oxidative stress in calcific aortic valvular stenosis in humans. Journal of the American College of Cardiology 2008;52(10):843-50.

[92] Al-Aly Z, Shao JS, Lai CF, Huang E, Cai J, Behrmann A, et al. Aortic Msx2-Wnt calcification cascade is regulated by TNF-alpha-dependent signals in diabetic Ldlr-/- mice. Arteriosclerosis, thrombosis, and vascular biology 2007;27(12):2589-96.

[93] Cheng SL, Shao JS, Halstead LR, Distelhorst K, Sierra O, Towler DA. Activation of vascular smooth muscle parathyroid hormone receptor inhibits Wnt/beta-catenin signaling and aortic fibrosis in diabetic arteriosclerosis. Circulation research 2010;107(2): 271-82.

[94] Faverman L, Mikhaylova L, Malmquist J, Nurminskaya M. Extracellular transglutaminase 2 activates beta-catenin signaling in calcifying vascular smooth muscle cells. FEBS letters 2008;582(10):1552-7.

[95] Glinka A, Wu W, Delius H, Monaghan AP, Blumenstock C, Niehrs C. Dickkopf-1 is a member of a new family of secreted proteins and functions in head induction. Nature 1998;391(6665):357-62.

[96] Mukhopadhyay M, Shtrom S, Rodriguez-Esteban C, Chen L, Tsukui T, Gomer L, et al. Dickkopf1 is required for embryonic head induction and limb morphogenesis in the mouse. Developmental cell 2001;1(3):423-34.

[97] Thambiah S, Roplekar R, Manghat P, Fogelman I, Fraser WD, Goldsmith D, et al. Circulating sclerostin and Dickkopf-1 (DKK1) in predialysis chronic kidney disease

(CKD): relationship with bone density and arterial stiffness. Calcified tissue international 2012;90(6):473-80.

[98]   Beazley KE, Deasey S, Lima F, Nurminskaya MV. Transglutaminase 2-mediated activation of beta-catenin signaling has a critical role in warfarin-induced vascular calcification. Arteriosclerosis, thrombosis, and vascular biology 2012;32(1):123-30.

[99]   Bai XY, Ma Y, Ding R, Fu B, Shi S, Chen XM. miR-335 and miR-34a Promote renal senescence by suppressing mitochondrial antioxidative enzymes. Journal of the American Society of Nephrology : JASN 2011;22(7):1252-61.

[100] Boon RA, Seeger T, Heydt S, Fischer A, Hergenreider E, Horrevoets AJ, et al. MicroRNA-29 in aortic dilation: implications for aneurysm formation. Circulation research 2011;109(10):1115-9.

[101] Zhang J, Tu Q, Bonewald LF, He X, Stein G, Lian J, et al. Effects of miR-335-5p in modulating osteogenic differentiation by specifically downregulating Wnt antagonist DKK1. Journal of bone and mineral research : the official journal of the American Society for Bone and Mineral Research 2011;26(8):1953-63.

[102] Kapinas K, Kessler C, Ricks T, Gronowicz G, Delany AM. miR-29 modulates Wnt signaling in human osteoblasts through a positive feedback loop. The Journal of biological chemistry 2010;285(33):25221-31.

[103] Kapinas K, Kessler CB, Delany AM. miR-29 suppression of osteonectin in osteoblasts: regulation during differentiation and by canonical Wnt signaling. Journal of cellular biochemistry 2009;108(1):216-24.

[104] Jones JA, Stroud RE, O'Quinn EC, Black LE, Barth JL, Elefteriades JA, et al. Selective microRNA suppression in human thoracic aneurysms: relationship of miR-29a to aortic size and proteolytic induction. Circulation Cardiovascular genetics 2011;4(6): 605-13.

[105] Chen NX, O'Neill KD, Chen X, Kiattisunthorn K, Gattone VH, Moe SM. Activation of arterial matrix metalloproteinases leads to vascular calcification in chronic kidney disease. American journal of nephrology 2011;34(3):211-9.

[106] Freeman RV, Otto CM. Spectrum of calcific aortic valve disease: pathogenesis, disease progression, and treatment strategies. Circulation 2005;111(24):3316-26.

[107] Mohammadpour AH, Shamsara J, Nazemi S, Ghadirzadeh S, Shahsavand S, Ramezani M. Evaluation of RANKL/OPG Serum Concentration Ratio as a New Biomarker for Coronary Artery Calcification: A Pilot Study. Thrombosis 2012;2012:306263.

[108] Kiechl S, Schett G, Schwaiger J, Seppi K, Eder P, Egger G, et al. Soluble receptor activator of nuclear factor-kappa B ligand and risk for cardiovascular disease. Circulation 2007;116(4):385-91.

[109] Dombkowski AA, Sultana Z, Craig DB, Jamil H. In silico analysis of combinatorial microRNA activity reveals target genes and pathways associated with breast cancer metastasis. Cancer informatics 2011;10:13-29.

[110] Mizoguchi F, Izu Y, Hayata T, Hemmi H, Nakashima K, Nakamura T, et al. Osteoclast-specific Dicer gene deficiency suppresses osteoclastic bone resorption. Journal of cellular biochemistry 2010;109(5):866-75.

[111] Wang K, Zhang S, Weber J, Baxter D, Galas DJ. Export of microRNAs and microRNA-protective protein by mammalian cells. Nucleic acids research 2010;38(20): 7248-59.

[112] Arroyo JD, Chevillet JR, Kroh EM, Ruf IK, Pritchard CC, Gibson DF, et al. Argonaute2 complexes carry a population of circulating microRNAs independent of vesicles in human plasma. Proceedings of the National Academy of Sciences of the United States of America 2011;108(12):5003-8.

[113] Turchinovich A, Weiz L, Langheinz A, Burwinkel B. Characterization of extracellular circulating microRNA. Nucleic acids research 2011;39(16):7223-33.

[114] Diehl P, Fricke A, Sander L, Stamm J, Bassler N, Htun N, et al. Microparticles: major transport vehicles for distinct microRNAs in circulation. Cardiovascular research 2012;93(4):633-44.

[115] Pigati L, Yaddanapudi SC, Iyengar R, Kim DJ, Hearn SA, Danforth D, et al. Selective release of microRNA species from normal and malignant mammary epithelial cells. PloS one 2010;5(10):e13515.

[116] Chen TS, Lai RC, Lee MM, Choo AB, Lee CN, Lim SK. Mesenchymal stem cell secretes microparticles enriched in pre-microRNAs. Nucleic acids research 2010;38(1): 215-24.

[117] Kosaka N, Iguchi H, Yoshioka Y, Takeshita F, Matsuki Y, Ochiya T. Secretory mechanisms and intercellular transfer of microRNAs in living cells. The Journal of biological chemistry 2010;285(23):17442-52.

[118] Hergenreider E, Heydt S, Treguer K, Boettger T, Horrevoets AJ, Zeiher AM, et al. Atheroprotective communication between endothelial cells and smooth muscle cells through miRNAs. Nature cell biology 2012;14(3):249-56.

[119] Creemers EE, Tijsen AJ, Pinto YM. Circulating microRNAs: novel biomarkers and extracellular communicators in cardiovascular disease? Circulation research 2012;110(3):483-95.

[120] Valadi H, Ekstrom K, Bossios A, Sjostrand M, Lee JJ, Lotvall JO. Exosome-mediated transfer of mRNAs and microRNAs is a novel mechanism of genetic exchange between cells. Nature cell biology 2007;9(6):654-9.

[121] Zernecke A, Bidzhekov K, Noels H, Shagdarsuren E, Gan L, Denecke B, et al. Delivery of microRNA-126 by apoptotic bodies induces CXCL12-dependent vascular protection. Science signaling 2009;2(100):ra81.

[122] Meckes DG, Jr., Raab-Traub N. Microvesicles and viral infection. Journal of virology 2011;85(24):12844-54.

[123] Wuthier RE, Lipscomb GF. Matrix vesicles: structure, composition, formation and function in calcification. Frontiers in bioscience : a journal and virtual library 2011;16:2812-902.

[124] Reynolds JL, Joannides AJ, Skepper JN, McNair R, Schurgers LJ, Proudfoot D, et al. Human vascular smooth muscle cells undergo vesicle-mediated calcification in response to changes in extracellular calcium and phosphate concentrations: a potential mechanism for accelerated vascular calcification in ESRD. Journal of the American Society of Nephrology : JASN 2004;15(11):2857-67.

[125] Chen NX, O'Neill KD, Chen X, Moe SM. Annexin-mediated matrix vesicle calcification in vascular smooth muscle cells. Journal of bone and mineral research : the official journal of the American Society for Bone and Mineral Research 2008;23(11): 1798-805.

[126] Kapustin AN, Davies JD, Reynolds JL, McNair R, Jones GT, Sidibe A, et al. Calcium regulates key components of vascular smooth muscle cell-derived matrix vesicles to enhance mineralization. Circulation research 2011;109(1):e1-12.

[127] New SE, Marchini JF, Aikawa M, Shanahan CM, Croce K, Aikawa E. Novel Role of Macrophage-derived Matrix Vesicles in Arterial Microcalcification Circulation 2011;124(21 Supplement):A10866.

[128] Sage AP, Lu J, Tintut Y, Demer LL. Hyperphosphatemia-induced nanocrystals upregulate the expression of bone morphogenetic protein-2 and osteopontin genes in mouse smooth muscle cells in vitro. Kidney international 2011;79(4):414-22.

[129] Naves M, Rodriguez-Garcia M, Diaz-Lopez JB, Gomez-Alonso C, Cannata-Andia JB. Progression of vascular calcifications is associated with greater bone loss and increased bone fractures. Osteoporosis international : a journal established as result of cooperation between the European Foundation for Osteoporosis and the National Osteoporosis Foundation of the USA 2008;19(8):1161-6.

[130] Jensky NE, Hyder JA, Allison MA, Wong N, Aboyans V, Blumenthal RS, et al. The association of bone density and calcified atherosclerosis is stronger in women without dyslipidemia: the multi-ethnic study of atherosclerosis. Journal of bone and mineral research : the official journal of the American Society for Bone and Mineral Research 2011;26(11):2702-9.

[131] Wang Y, Li L, Moore BT, Peng XH, Fang X, Lappe JM, et al. MiR-133a in human circulating monocytes: a potential biomarker associated with postmenopausal osteoporosis. PloS one 2012;7(4):e34641.

[132] Li H, Xie H, Liu W, Hu R, Huang B, Tan YF, et al. A novel microRNA targeting HDAC5 regulates osteoblast differentiation in mice and contributes to primary osteoporosis in humans. The Journal of clinical investigation 2009;119(12):3666-77.

[133] Paccou J, Brazier M, Mentaverri R, Kamel S, Fardellone P, Massy ZA. Vascular calcification in rheumatoid arthritis: Prevalence, pathophysiological aspects and potential targets. Atherosclerosis 2012.

[134] Pauley KM, Satoh M, Chan AL, Bubb MR, Reeves WH, Chan EK. Upregulated miR-146a expression in peripheral blood mononuclear cells from rheumatoid arthritis patients. Arthritis research & therapy 2008;10(4):R101.

Genetics, Proteomics and Metabolomics of Calcific Aortic Valve Disease

Chapter 6

Genetics of Bicuspid Aortic Valve and Calcific Aortic Valve Disease

Robert B. Hinton

Additional information is available at the end of the chapter

1. The clinical taxonomy: Malformation vs. disease

Aortic valve malformation is a spectrum including Bicuspid Aortic Valve. Aortic valve malformation has been appreciated since the Renaissance when artists advanced our understanding of anatomy and specifically, Leonardo da Vinci illustrated and described variants of aortic valve morphology [1]. Aortic valve malformation is the most common cardiovascular malformation (CVM), and bicuspid aortic valve (BAV, MIM#109730) is the most common type of aortic valve malformation. BAV is present at birth and is characterized by two rather than three cusps. The incidence of BAV is 1-2% in the general population and affects an estimated 3 million people [2,3]. BAV itself is subclinical and the valve is typically functional, making BAV an endophenotype. Two patterns of BAV morphology are commonly observed: ~70% of isolated cases have fusion of the right and left (RL) coronary cusps with the remainder consisting almost entirely of those with fusion of the right and non (RN) coronary cusps [4,5]. Rarely, cases have shown fusion of the left and non (LN) coronary cusps. In addition to BAV subtypes, there is a spectrum of aortic valve malformation (Figure 1), ranging from various types of unicuspid to quadricuspid aortic valves with the three BAV morphology patterns and a thickened tricommissural aortic valve representing intermediate phenotypes [7]. Presently, it remains unclear to what degree these variations of malformation represent true differences.

Calcific Aortic Valve Disease is a growing public health problem. Aortic valve disease is defined by abnormal valve function. Valve disease may manifest as *stenosis*, an obstruction to normal forward blood flow, or *insufficiency*, a defective closure resulting in backward blood flow. Valve disease tends to progress. Ultimately, ventricular function can be compromised. Aortic valve stenosis is the most common manifestation of CAVD and classically presents as angina, syncope and heart failure. The diagnosis can be made clinically and confirmed by echocardiography, which quantifies the severity, and, over time, the progression of disease [8].

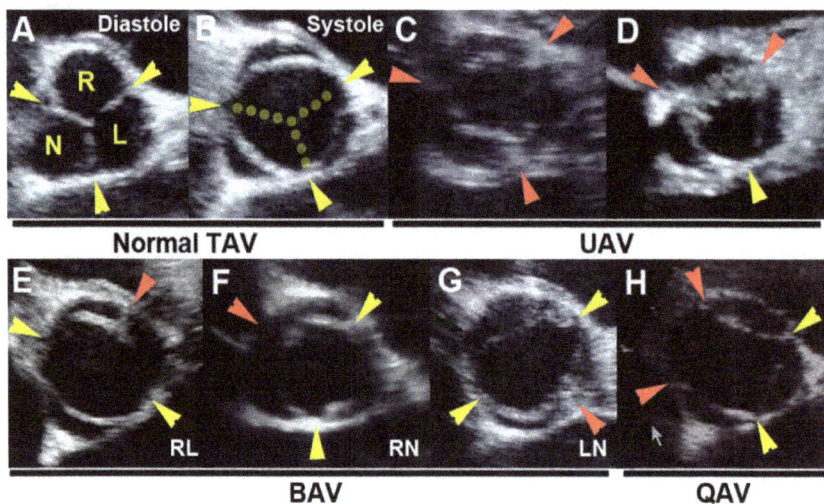

Figure 1. Phenotype definition: spectrum of aortic valve malformation. Aortic valve malformation Parasternal short axis echocardiographic views at the base of the heart showing the aortic valve en face (A-H). Normal tricommissural aortic valve (TAV) morphology is demonstrated in diastole (A) and systole (B). Distinct morphologies are based on fusion patterns of the commissures (dotted lines, B) as they relate to the right (R), left (L) and non (N) coronary sinuses of Valsalva (A). Aortic valve malformation ranges from unicuspid (UAV) to bicuspid (BAV) to a thickened tricuspid (not shown) to quadricuspid (QAV) morphology. Three normal commissures are demonstrated in panel A, and normal opening of the commissures results in complete cusp separation to the wall of the aorta at the sinotubular junction (yellow arrowheads). UAV manifests as either partial fusion of all three commissures (red arrowheads, C) or complete fusion of both the RN and RL commissures (D). Bicuspid aortic valve (BAV) may manifest as fusion of the RL (E), RN (F), and rarely LN (G) commissures. Rarely, a quadricuspid aortic valve (QAV, H) is identified. Adapted from [6].

Histopathology from diseased valves explanted at the time of surgery from patients with CAVD demonstrates large nodules of overt calcification, in addition to cell-matrix abnormalities (Figure 2). Research efforts have focused on the valve cusp, and as a result the valve annulus has been largely overlooked [4,7,9]. Human studies investigating valve disease have suggested that the base of the valve cusp and valve annulus regions is the origin of disease processes, including both sclerosis and calcification [10,11]. Greater than 2.5% of the population has AVD, causing more than 25,000 deaths annually in the US [12,13]. The actual direct cost for valve disease in the US alone has been estimated at 1 billion dollars per year [14]. Taken together, the public health impact and burden to society of CAVD is significant and underappreciated. The majority of valve disease at any age has an underlying valve malformation suggesting a genetic basis [15]. Aging is an independent risk factor for CAVD, resulting in a higher prevalence of disease as the population achieves greater longevity [16,17]. Aortic valve sclerosis, a marker of cardiovascular risk, and to a lesser extent valve disease, is present in more than 25% of the aged [18]. Therapy for CAVD remains primarily surgical and is restricted to late stage disease. Aortic valve replacement is the second most frequent cardiovascular surgical procedure [3,9], and the need for re-intervention is common [19]. Bioprosthetic replacement approaches are effective, but not durable [20,21]. Because there is a lack of pharmacologic treatments for CAVD, the indications for surgical intervention dominate the clinical landscape. Early disease processes and progression remain poorly understood, and there are presently no pharmacologic based treatment options for CAVD.

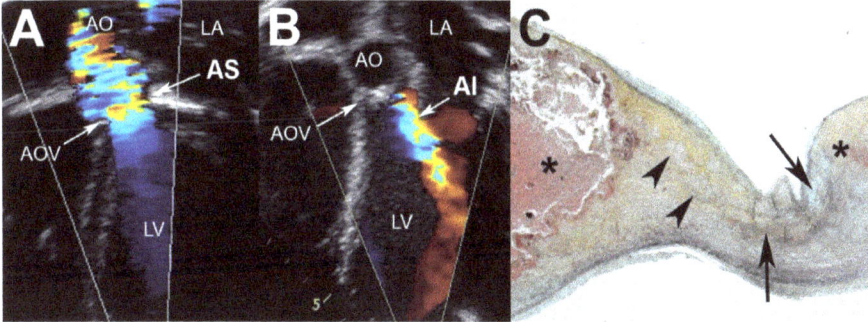

Figure 2. Phenotype definition: types of aortic valve disease. Color Doppler echocardiographic apical four chamber images demonstrate the two basic types of aortic valve disease. Aortic valve disease is characterized by a dysfunctional valve and is classified as stenosis (obstruction, A) and/or insufficiency (incompetence, B). Aortic stenosis (AS) and aortic insufficiency (AI) result in hemodynamic perturbations that lead to clinical disease states. Advanced calcific aortic valve disease is typically characterized by stenosis, and histopathology identifies gross calcific nodules in the fibrosa layer of the cusp (asterisks, C), clusters of cartilage like interstitial cells (arrowheads, C), and marked heterogeneity of extracellular matrix abnormalities (arrows, C). AO aorta; AOV aortic valve; LA left atrium; LV left ventricle.

Bicuspid Aortic Valve is an independent risk factor for Calcific Aortic Valve Disease. BAV is an established risk factor for CAVD [3,7,13]. The majority of CAVD cases at any age have an underlying BAV, and longitudinal studies in young adults with BAV have shown that >20% ultimately require surgical intervention [15,22,23]. In addition, those CAVD patients with an underlying BAV tend to develop calcification a decade earlier than those with normal aortic valve morphology [24]. Recently, a National Heart Lung and Blood Institute Executive Statement on CAVD identified a critical need to identify "clinical risk factors for the distinct phases of initiation and progression of AVD" [25], where standard cardiac risk factors including sclerosis have not yet been applicable. There has been avid interest and conflicting reports regarding the potential use of BAV morphology as a specific predictor of CAVD. Fernandes et al identified an association between RN BAV and AVD in a pediatric population, while Tzemos et al found no association in an adult population [5,22]. Exploring AVD in a pediatric population allows for examination of the disease process free from the confounding effects of cardiovascular comorbidities. Risk factors for AVD in children are poorly understood [23], but recently Calloway et al. reported that children with RN BAV and adults with RL BAV were more likely to develop AVD, suggesting BAV morphology may have predictive value for the time course of AVD [26]. It is unclear if AVD in children, which is not characterized by calcification, represents a different genetic type of disease or one end of a spectrum of the same disease.

Careful clinical phenotyping is critical for research, especially genetic discovery. Phenotype definition and stratification are necessary to advance our understanding of CAVD, especially in the context of genetic discovery. In addition to distinguishing malformation from disease, CAVD phenotyping needs to be detailed and comprehensive using all aspects of the clinical taxonomy, even those currently considered clinically inconsequential. The first step of any human genetic research study is to clearly and precisely define the phenotype. Studies that use too broad or too narrow a phenotype definition may fail to find association with an existing genetic variant or identify a pathologic one. Thus, identification of the phenotype most aligned with the underlying genetic etiology is essential for successful identification of associated genetic variants, a concept recently described as "deep phenotyping" [27]. Cardiovascular risk factors have been established for a variety of cardiovascular diseases, including substantial overlap for CAVD and coronary artery disease (CAD) or atherosclerosis [16,28,29]. While these disease processes often co-occur, as evidenced by the high frequency of concurrent coronary artery bypass grafting and aortic valve replacement surgery, only a small proportion of CAVD patients have CAD [30]. Likewise, there is an increased incidence of CAVD in patients with other cardiovascular disease, including systemic hypertension and chronic kidney disease [31,32]. Substantial investigation has established the adverse effects of common comorbid cardiovascular diseases on the progression of AVD; however, increasing attention on the underlying genetic and developmental processes will identify early mechanisms that incite disease processes. Emerging evidence suggests that both specific genetic factors and clinical cardiac risks may be necessary for disease initiation and progression.

Phenotype definition must expand to include non-clinical paradigms. Like many diseases, especially cardiovascular diseases, the clinical taxonomy of CAVD is based on anatomy and physiology. Classification schemes are organized with clinical standard of care, particularly surgical intervention, in mind [33,34]. The gold standard for diagnosis of cardiovascular diseases is imaging, such as echocardiography or magnetic resonance, modalities that define anatomy and physiology. While these approaches have been clinically useful, there is substantial phenotypic heterogeneity of unclear significance, including for example, the distinction between malformation and disease. Expanding phenotype to include an improved understanding of embryologic patterns underlying malformation will provide insight into pathogenesis [35-37]. Increasingly, combinations of phenotypes long held to be independent from a clinical perspective are now understood to be related from an etiologic perspective, challenging classic notions of disease classification. Molecular insights may inform new pharmacologic treatments the same way imaging informs surgical decision-making. Ultimately, identifying the genetic causes of disease will require reconciling clinical and molecular taxonomies of disease.

2. The genetic basis of BAV and CAVD

BAV has a strong genetic basis, but the precise causes remain unknown. Heritability estimates the proportion of a disease attributable to genetics. BAV heritability estimates are high, ranging from 75 to 89%, indicating that major genetic factors contribute to the development of BAV [38]. Pedigree and segregation analyses have consistently identified autosomal dominant inheritance with reduced penetrance and complex inheritance underlying BAV [38-41], acknowledging that BAV is subclinical and therefore may be underestimated. Interestingly, while BAV is highly heritable, AVD is not, suggesting the phenotypic variability of CAVD is determined largely by non-genetic factors [26]. Consistent with these human observations, an established hamster model of BAV also shows the same characteristics of complex inheritance [42,43]. An additional quantitative measure of familial risk is recurrence risk. The recurrence risk of a disease measures the proportion of relatives who have the disease. BAV recurrence risk in siblings has been estimated to be approximately 9% [44], identifying further evidence of a genetic basis. Linkage analysis determines whether susceptibility variant segregates with disease in families. Previous studies have supported a strong underlying genetic basis for isolated nonsyndromic BAV, including family-based studies that have identified numerous loci [44-46]. Combined, these loci harbor hundreds of genes that may contribute to BAV. Multiple loci identify BAV as a genetically heterogeneous trait. Missense mutations in *NOTCH1* have been identified in a small proportion of nonsyndromic CAVD patients with BAV [47,48]. NOTCH1 is an intriguing biological candidate gene. In animal systems, Notch loss of function recapitulates the AVD phenotype, and actively regulates the maladaptive development of associated calcification, further supporting a mechanistic role [49-51]. In addition, a recent report described copy number variants (CNVs) in 10% of left-sided CVM cases, including BAV and aortic stenosis, potentially identifying new causes and/ or modifiers of CAVD [52]. Association studies have not been used for BAV due to the large number of cases required to perform analyses (typically at least 1000), but combined linkage-association may be an excellent approach for discovery to leverage the strengths of each method. It is unclear how whole exome sequencing will impact discovery, but combining the various new tools for discovery promises to yield increasing insight into the genetic basis of BAV and CAVD.

BAV is a congenital malformation, a defect in cardiac development. Malformations present at birth often have strong genetic causes, if not monogenic etiology. Primary cardiac development occurs in humans from 2-8 weeks gestation, and semilunar valve (including the aortic valve) formation occurs in the seventh and eighth weeks. The heart is the first organ to form and continued survival of the organism is dependent on the circulation. The primitive heart tube is composed of a myocardial cell layer surrounding an endothelial cell layer. The formation of endocardial cushions is the first event of valve development. Endocardial cushion formation is accomplished by an early epithelial to mesenchymal transition (EMT) that generates a progenitor cell population embedded in a loosely organized extracellular matrix (ECM), followed by a late ECM remodeling stage that results in mature cusp organization (ventricularis, spongiosa, fibrosa) and valve interstitial cells [35-37]. Early defects in this process result in embryonic lethality, but late defects result in viable malformation and disease [53], hypothetically making the mechanisms of late developmental defects more applicable to human disease. It remains unknown why there are uneven frequencies of the different BAV types, but several developmental hypotheses have been proposed including a neural crest contribution that is not necessary but when present results in fusion of the right and left coronary cusps [42]. Further, the relatively rare unicuspid morphology underlies the majority of cases of critical aortic stenosis in the newborn and is associated with hypoplastic left heart syndrome (HLHS), suggesting genetic ("severe" malformation) and environmental (flow perturbations) factors combine to result in disease manifestation [15,54,55]. Elucidation of the genetic basis of both BAV and CAVD will result in a reconciled classification system that integrates the molecular basis of cardiac development with the pathologic basis of disease in a clinically meaningful manner.

Genetic factors contributing to CAVD are numerous and relatively small. Common complex traits are generally the result of numerous factors, each with a small additive effect and none necessary or sufficient to cause disease [56]. Coronary artery disease (CAD) and systemic hypertension (HTN) are well-described examples of this type of trait. While there is unequivocal evidence that BAV with CAVD is a complex trait, it is not nearly as common as CAD or HTN, and is more strongly linked to developmental processes, therefore it is likely that BAV/CAVD is an "intermediate" phenotype between the "rare single-gene" and "common complex" diseases. Importantly, this suggests that it is more likely to discover clinically useful patterns of variants associated with CAVD. Clinically, CAVD, CAD and HTN are considered discrete disease states, but there is a preponderance of epidemiologic and molecular evidence suggesting some pathogenesis is shared. Therefore, variants that have been identified studying individuals with CAD and HTN may inform risk assessment in patients with CAVD. Just as some clinical cardiovascular risk factors are common to all cardiovascular disease states, some genetic variants may pertain to predisposition of any cardiovascular disease depending on the aggregate risk (Figure 3). For example, the 10q24 locus has been identified in probands from BAV, CAD, HTN, thoracic aortic aneurysm (TAA) and intracranial aneurysm families [44, 57-60], suggesting the gene(s) in this region plays a role in each of these related cardiovascular phenotypes and therefore may be a general cardiovascular risk variant. It remains unclear whether a specified number of general cardiovascular risk variants are sufficient to cause any one disease, or more intuitively both *specific* and *general* disease variants are necessary.

CAVD is a latent phenotype, an injury or defect in valve maintenance. Typically, aortic valve disease does not manifest until the fourth or fifth decade of life and often does not progress to require surgical intervention until a decade later. How can developmental defects be functional for so long, only to fail in adulthood? The prevailing view is that individuals with a genetic predisposition for CAVD require an additional "second" insult to trigger disease initiation and progression that otherwise would not have occurred. While many of the genes that have been implicated in CAVD effect valve development [61,62], they may have additional distinct roles in valve maintenance [63], that is, how the tissue responds over time to the hemodynamic demands of constant motion and changing physiology. Similarly, there are genes that do not have a role in valve development but may be necessary for valve homeostasis [35,63]. Indeed, CAVD has been labeled a "degenerative" condition for decades, and age-related "wear and tear" contributes to valve failure. For example, elastic fiber degradation occurs with advanced age and predisposes the individual to inflammation, which may contribute to CAVD acceleration in later life [64,65]. Equally important, however, are comorbid conditions such as CAD that may serve to be an injury, or second hit, in vulnerable aortic valve tissue. For example, in an individual with genetic variants predisposing specifically for CAVD, the presence of CAD

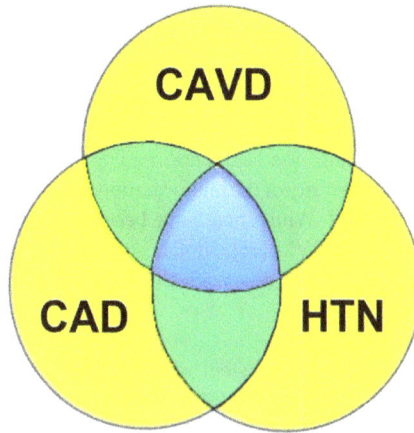

Figure 3. Shared predisposing genetic risk variants in common cardiovascular diseases. Cardiovascular diseases characterized by complex inheritance may have genetic variants specific to the clinical disease state, e.g., CAVD, CAD, HTN (yellow), as well as nonspecific genetic variants that may contribute to two (green) or three (blue) different cardiovascular diseases.

may initiate additional disease processes that incite CAVD (e.g. endothelial dysfunction). Taken together, a nonspecific cardiovascular insult in the context of a specific genetic predisposition for BAV may be necessary and sufficient for the manifestation of CAVD. As the genetic and developmental basis of valve malformation and disease is elucidated, opportunities for novel medical therapies will emerge and potentially preclude or delay the need for surgery. Defining regulation of valve tissue maintenance and homeostasis will provide exciting opportunities for cell-based or molecular therapies for valve disease.

Complex inheritance is characterized by a liability threshold. Polygenic conditions are characterized by a fixed number of susceptibility genes and a liability threshold, whereby a variety of combinations of predisposing variants may reach a specified level (e.g., 3 risk variants) to cause in combination the phenotype. In general, the importance of genetic modifiers and epigenetics is rapidly emerging, but little is known about these factors in the context of BAV/CAVD. Different BAV morphologies may reflect different combinations of shared genetic variants that carry different clinical risks, e.g. CAVD, thoracic aortic aneurysm and dissection, or associated CVM. It has been shown for example that RN BAV morphology is associated with a higher risk of developing valve disease and experiencing a cardiac event [5,22]. Together, patterns of predisposing genetic variants, which may be reflected in part by anatomical subtleties such as BAV morphology, may translate to variations in clinical disease states, suggesting major modifiers play a significant role in phenotype definition. Identifying these patterns may impact care, for example by facilitating the ability to consistently predict natural history [66,67].

3. The molecular taxonomy: Genes, pathways, and proteins

Genetic syndromes provide important biologic insights. Turner syndrome is associated with BAV and aorta abnormalities, and is the only monosomy compatible with life despite the fact that the vast majority of cases result in early spontaneous abortion. Turner syndrome can occur for a variety of reasons, including nondisjunction and mosaicism, and the exact genetic abnormality correlates with the severity of the malformations with 45,X more likely mosaicism less likely to have associated CVM. While there have been some studies examining possible maternal effects in nonsyndromic CVM [68], similar studies in Turner syndrome have not identified genomic imprinting in general or specifically with regard to BAV [69]. Interestingly, BAV morphology was RL in over 95% of cases, nearly uniform and significantly more disproportionate than the general ratio [70], suggesting a genotype-phenotype relationship of potential clinical significance. This is consistent with the observation that RL BAV is more commonly associated with aortic coarctation [5]. Little is known about long-term outcomes, e.g. the prevalence of CAVD requiring surgical aortic valve replacement or associated thoracic aneurysm that dissects, and there is not a mouse model to date that recapitulates the cardiac phenotype, but involvement of one of the sex chromosomes provides novel ways to explore specific genetic factors contributing to BAV.

The classic connective tissue disorders, Marfan and Ehlers-Danlos syndromes, caused by mutations in the FIBRILLIN-1 and COLLAGEN Type 3 genes respectively, are well-known to effect the aortic valve. While there is clearly reduced penetrance for BAV in these groups, there is a significantly increased incidence for BAV in both conditions of 10-30% [71,72]. Additional genetic syndromes that affect the connective tissue include Williams syndrome and osteogenesis imperfecta, caused by mutations in the ELASTIN and COLLAGEN Type 1 genes respectively, which also have an increased incidence of valve malformation and disease [73,74]. In addition, there are a number of genetic syndromes that are associated with BAV, often in the context of complex CVM. These include aneuploidies such as deletion 4p, deletion 10p, deletion 11q (Jacobsen syndrome), trisomy 18 (Edwards syndrome), deletion 20p12 (Alagille syndrome), as well as other genetic syndromes, including Adams-Oliver syndrome and Kabuki syndrome [75,76]. Trisomy 18 is a particularly interesting entity that is associated with polyvalvular disease, an unusual type of valve disease that is characterized by malformation, including BAV, and dysplasia of the valves, a poorly understood process that does not have a clear association with CAVD but challenges the malformation-disease distinction [77]. In addition, BAV is often one of multiple CVMs in the same individual and the patterns of co-occurrence can inform cause [78]. Taken together, there is a multitude of ways that valve tissue can be affected, and a molecular understanding of these conditions will inform CAVD.

Developmental signaling pathways identify basic regulatory factors in valvulogenesis. From a cardiac development perspective, there are three transcription factors that are considered the master regulators of basic heart development, NKX2.5, GATA4 and TBX5. Loss of function mutations in each of these genes has been associated with various forms of CVM [79-83]. While none of these genes has been associated with BAV, the Nkx2.5 mutant mouse is characterized by a variety of CVMs including BAV [84], suggesting like NOTCH1, NKX2.5

may account for a very small proportion of cases of BAV and therefore may contribute to the pathogenesis underlying CAVD. As the focus has shifted from early to late (post endothelial-mesenchymal transition) regulatory factors, the role of additional factors, such as Notch and Wnt have been studied in the context of ECM stratification in the mature cups [53,63,85]. The progression of CAVD includes activation of osteogenic gene regulatory pathways and calcification, generally localized to the fibrosa layer [25,86-88]. Atherosclerotic mechanisms have been implicated in valve calcification, and there are overlapping risk factors for CAVD and CAD as described above, suggesting endothelial injury and inflammation play a key role in disease progression [17,87,89]. However, it remains unclear if these are inciting causal factors or exacerbating factors. TGFB signaling dysregulation has been associated with CAVD and cardiovascular disease progression, especially as it pertains to fibrosis and inflammation [90-92]. During human aortic valve calcification, expression of several genes associated with osteogenesis, including *Runx2, osteocalcin, osteopontin, alkaline phophatase,* and *bone sialoprotein,* is induced [93-97]. There is increasing evidence that CAVD recapitulates gene regulatory interactions characteristic of osteogenesis.

The molecular basis of aberrant calcification is poorly understood. While physiologic mineralization in the context of bone development and maintenance has been used successfully as a paradigm to study aberrant calcification in CAVD [86,98], less is known about the genetic basis of disease phenotypes characterized by aberrant calcification. Vascular calcification and the calcification that can occur in advanced CAD has been studied extensively and forms some of the basis for the prevailing view that CAD and CAVD are related disease states. Using a rare genetic disease, alkaptonuria, Hannoush et al identified a metabolic link between vascular calcification and advanced CAVD in a cohort of nearly one hundred patients [99]. Importantly, CAVD in this population was present and advanced, often requiring surgery, independent of standard cardiac risk factors, suggesting a primary link in pathogenesis not related to common comorbidities. In vitro, studies have focused on vascular smooth muscle's role in calcification, especially in the context of clinical comorbidities of CAVD such as CAD and HTN, as well as the context of pathways regulating the associated inflammation and the renin-angiotensin system [92,100]. While vascular smooth muscle cells are not present in valve tissue, there are subsets of VICs that have smooth muscle cell-like properties [101,102] and the expression of smooth muscle actin is considered a marker of activated VICs, the cells implicated in CAVD progression [103].

Understanding valve tissue homeostasis or maintenance will require proteomics. Focusing on valve injury or defects in valve homeostasis or maintenance requires increasing attention to processes downstream from the transcriptional regulation that dominates cardiac development paradigms of CAVD. Proteomics is one emerging field that provides a compelling strategy to address the challenges of dynamic post-translational biology in valve tissue and will undoubtedly have significant impact on our understanding of healthy valve maintenance and CAVD pathogenesis [104]. Proteomics involves a sophisticated technical approach that requires in vitro validation and substantial bioinformatics support. Angel et al. have demonstrated a number of seminal observations by defining the semilunar valve proteome in the adult mouse using MALDI mass spectrometry [105,106]. Specifically, this rigorous and unbiased approach has yielded the identification and characterization of global protein expression and protein-protein networking provides a specific cell-matrix definition of valve maintenance that can be used further to explore the impact of aging, physiologic hemodynamic stresses due to constant motion, and systemic pathologic insults on specific signaling and metabolic dynamics. Importantly, this study provides proof of concept in mouse that will allow the approach to leverage the power of targeted mutagenesis [107]. Despite the difficulty of obtaining healthy controls, early observations have been made in human valve disease specimens, that when compared with control tissue, demonstrate misexpression of critical matrix proteins, including specific lipoproteins, inflammatory proteins, and proteases [108]. One study has focused this approach on VICs exposed to pro-calcific stimuli and has shown that specific chaperone proteins alter transport and cytoskeletal organization, providing insight into both valve homeostasis and CAVD [109]. Taken together, proteomics promises to generate novel insight into disease progression as well as potentially develop a new clinical tool that uses novel global proteomic analyses in plasma as a noninvasive comprehensive biomarker panel.

Dysregulation of structural proteins and remodeling enzymes is a common pathway. Normal valve function requires coordinated movement of complex structures. Gross and Kugel proposed nomenclature for valve tissue organization in 1931 that is now well established [110]. The mature valve structure is made up of highly organized ECM that is compartmentalized into three layers, the fibrosa, spongiosa, and ventricularis [9,53,111]. The annulus, composed primarily of fibrous collagens, provides a buttress for dispersion of forces, and tethering of the cusp in a crown-shape for tissue stabilization [112,113]. Studies examining ECM in valve tissue have focused by convention on structural properties, specifically durability (collagens) and flexibility (proteoglycans and elastic fibers). However, several studies have shown that ECM components reciprocally regulate growth factors and signaling pathways, in addition to causing architectural abnormalities, suggesting a primary rather than secondary role in pathogenesis [Reviewed in 53]. Studies in mouse models lacking ECM components critical for the mature aortic valve structure, including proteoglycans, collagens and elastic fiber components, demonstrate that the expression and organization of diverse ECM components are essential to the formation and structural integrity of the valves during development and after birth [114-123]. Further, mouse studies have shown that age and dietary manipulation can lead to ECM changes and CAVD [124-126].

During valve remodeling, the VICs regulate expression and organization of the valve ECM [127,128]. Additional ECM remodeling enzymes such as matrix metalloproteases (MMPs) and cathepsins also are expressed during valve maturation [128,129]. VICs from developing valves are highly synthetic, and extensive remodeling is required to achieve the mature organization [127,130]. In normal adult valves, the VICs are largely quiescent with little or no cell proliferation and maintain baseline levels of ECM gene expression necessary for valve homeostasis [103]. ECM enzyme dysregulation is established in the valve disease literature [131-135]. The elastin insufficient mouse demonstrates cartilage-like nodules in the valve annulus reminiscent of calcific nodules [119,136]. MMP misexpression malformation and more disease, suggesting malformation processes are due in part to remodeling defects and malformation and disease processes are shared [136]. Similar nodules are seen in the aortic valve annulus of the Adamts9 null mouse [137], confirming the importance of ECM remodeling enzymes. Elastolysis and associated elastic fiber fragments have been implicated as a trigger for myofibroblast mediated calcification [138,139]. Loss of balance between elastases and elastase inhibitors has been identified as one fundamental cause of elastolysis [140]. Interestingly, previous studies have shown that different elastic fiber fragments have different biologic functions, for example, some fragments induce calcification while others are chemo-attractants for endothelial cells [141,142].

The extracellular matrix is an interface between genetics and the environment. The heart valves function essentially to maintain unobstructed unidirectional blood flow. Valve structure-function relationships provide important insight in understanding mechanisms of valve homeostasis as well as developmental and disease processes. Valve ECM composition and biomechanics reflect underlying hemodynamics. There are three basic loading states that affect valve tissue during the cardiac cycle: flexure, shear and tension. Flexure occurs when the valve is actively opening or closing, shear occurs when blood is passing through the open valve, and tension occurs when the valve is closed [143]. Shear, compressive, and longitudinal stresses contribute to valve deformation, or displacement of the valve tissue during the constant motion of the cardiac cycle [144]. Valve tissue has exceptionally high strain because the tissue cycles to a completely unloaded state with each heart beat [145]. The heart beats more than 100,000 times per day handling approximately 5 liters of blood per minute. Over the average lifetime, there are greater than 3 billion heartbeats, or cardiac cycles. The long held appreciation of age-related degeneration and latent valve disease may in fact represent subtle defects in valve tissue maintenance.

CAVD is characterized by VIC activation, which in turn results in increased ECM and increased remodeling enzyme gene expression [103,127,128], and hemodynamic factors may activate VICs and therefore contribute to pathology. VIC activation is apparent by induction of myofibroblast markers, such as vimentin, smooth muscle actin, and embryonic non-muscle myosin heavy chain [129]. Some VICs have been shown to be dynamic and play an active role in ECM maintenance, as well as potentially regeneration and repair, and these VICs are progenitor cells with smooth muscle like properties [101,102,103,123,146,147]. Recently, two studies have demonstrated the complex interaction between developmental programs that predispose tissue to disease and shear stresses that trigger inflammation [148,149], providing examples of how these factors when combined may cause AVD. Research efforts are beginning to reconcile developmental and biomechanical considerations in an effort to more closely examine CAVD in vivo. A better understanding of hemodynamic-induced cell-matrix perturbations may inform the search for durable valve bioprostheses [150].

4. National Heart Lung and Blood Institute's research agenda for CAVD

New research agenda emphasizes genetics and development. Recently, the National Heart Lung and Blood Institute Aortic Stenosis Working Group defined a comprehensive research agenda for CAVD [25]. There are nine research priorities outlined in the statement that are summarized in Table 1. These priorities emphasize the identification of genetic factors that inform etiology, risk, and pharmacologic response, pointing to the clinical impact of these efforts being new diagnostic tests, biomarkers that may improve surveillance, and panels that may inform response to specific drugs. In addition, there is an emphasis on identifying genotype-phenotype relationships focusing on BAV. Improved understanding of valve biology, especially as it pertains to genetic predispositions for CAVD, is critical and will facilitate the identification of specific mechanisms involved in disease initiation and progression. The identification of molecular developmental processes and animal models of CAVD in vivo are needed to establish early pathogenesis and the effectiveness of new pharmacologic treatments for disease. In addition, genetic information will be increasingly important in the assessment of clinical studies that aim to refine clinical risk factors and identify new diagnostic and risk stratification tests.

---

1. Identify genetic, anatomic, and clinical risk factors for the distinct phases of initiation and progression of CAVD to identify individuals at higher risk, to determine interactions between risk factors, and to determine whether the severity of AS is a risk factor for surgical AV replacement.

---

2. Develop high-resolution and high-sensitivity imaging modalities that can identify early and subclinical CAVD, including molecular imaging and other innovative imaging approaches.

---

3. Understand the pathogenesis and pathophysiology of BAV, especially to establish correlations between phenotype and genotype, and to clarify the key features of this disease process that potentiate calcification.

---

4. Understand the basic valve biology (e.g., early events, mechanisms, and regulatory effects) of CAVD, including signaling pathways and the roles of valve interstitial and endothelial cells and the autocrine and paracrine signaling between them, the extracellular matrix and matrix stiffness, the role of age-related changes in both valve cells and extracellular matrix, the interacting mechanisms of cardiovascular calcification and physiological bone mineralization, and micro-scale mechanotransduction
and macro-scale hemodynamics.

---

5. Develop and validate suitable multi-scale in vitro, ex vivo, and animal models. Improved models are needed that realistically duplicate the conditions in which human CAVD develops.

---

6. Identify the relationship between calcification of the AV and bone and the reciprocal regulation of these processes.

---

7. Encourage, promote, or establish tissue banks that make valve tissue from surgery, pathology, and autopsy unsuitable or unneeded for transplantation, with and without CAVD, available for research.

---

8. Conduct clinical studies specific to CAVD to determine the feasibility of earlier pharmacological intervention in aortic AV sclerosis versus stenosis.

---

9. Determine the risk factors and optimal timing of surgical valve replacement in view of the current state of the data defining the biological mechanisms of CAVD.

Table 1. Current NHLBI Research Agenda for CAVD. Reproduced from [25].

There is an increasing need for networks and biorepositories. The current paradigm in translational human genetics research involves discovery (the identification of sequence variation associated with disease), mechanistic investigation (definition of pathogenesis), and finally development of new clinical approaches (application). Findings from human genetic studies are being taken into the laboratory where increasingly sophisticated animal models are providing the basis to define pathogenesis in a variety of diseases. The elucidation of pathogenesis subsequently results in the development of new diagnostic and therapeutic strategies, which can then be taken back to the patient. Taken together, this is referred to as the "bedside to bench to bedside" approach to disease and has led to numerous initiatives aiming to realize "translational" research goals, e.g., the NHLBI's Bench to Bassinet Program supporting excellence in pediatric cardiovascular translational research (http://www.bench-tobassinet.com), including CVMs such as BAV. Given the incidence of BAV and the sample size required to use new genetic discovery tools, it is necessary to combine cohorts. Genetic information is also impacting the understanding of pharmacology as it relates to drug indications and drug responses further facilitating improved care. Taken together, genetic information provides an impetus to shift the focus of medicine from treatment of end stage disease to strategies emphasizing primary prevention and early intervention.

Given some of the specific research priorities, for example the need to immortalize valve interstitial cell (VIC) lines, it will be important both to design biorepositories that are specifically built for cardiovascular disease needs and to organize virtual biobanks that can leverage combined resources from multiple centers. In effect, this will maximize translational impact and return on investment. The organization of biorepositories has advanced considerably in recent years, and significant strides have been made by international groups to coordinate resources. For example, the mission of the International Society for Biological and Environmental Repositories (ISBER) is to address technical, legal, ethical and managerial issues relevant to the governance of wide ranging biorepositories (http://www.isber.org) [151]. Several institutions have initiated biorepositories that include blood and tissue from CAVD patients. Virtual repositories, or multiple repositories that coordinate efforts to leverage sample size considerations, are becoming operational and the current funding climate is accelerating development of special rules to optimize tissue utility [152]. Funding bodies at the government and foundation levels need to recognize valve disease as a significant public health problem and establish valve specific funding opportunities. Further, valve biology and CAVD specific symposia are needed at large conferences, such as the American Heart Association.

5. Comprehensive counseling and genetic testing increasingly impact clinical care

A detailed family history remains a powerful tool and genetic testing will advance its impact. A detailed family history refers to questioning multiple individuals within a family and requires specific demographic information (e.g., age at disease onset) and documentation of disease and other pertinent health issues by medical record review [153]. The results of a detailed family history may warrant referral to a cardiovascular genetics service. A detailed family history is a powerful tool and can help establish a diagnosis and initiate comprehensive care in a timely fashion [154-158]. There are significant barriers to the optimal use of family history information, primarily a lack of awareness on the family's part and considerable time restrictions on the health care professional's part. Studies have shown that a majority of people do not know their family history and do not appreciate its relevance in medical management, and consequently the potential impact of family history information is diminished [159]. In an effort to increase family history awareness, tools have been developed and are available to the general public to generate and maintain a detailed family history. For example, the Health and Human Services Family History Initiative has designed a publicly available, web-based program providing a means to generate and maintain a detailed family history [160]. Genetics has transformed the use of family history information and has led to the reemergence of the detailed genetic family history. Detailed family history information is necessary for the optimal use of genetic screening and testing and this translates to the essential need of genetic counselors embedded in cardiology clinics.

Genetic testing is anticipated for BAV and CAVD. As the etiology of BAV is defined and the complex genetics of CAVD is elucidated, a variety of variants associated with BAV and CAVD will be identified, including variants associated with etiology as well as variants associated with specific types of subsequent risk. All variants pertaining to CAVD will have to be organized based on utility. Once a significant proportion of cases can be diagnosed using genetic testing, clinical testing may be warranted. Presently, there are no CLIA (Clinical Laboratory Improvement Amendments) approved tests for the diagnosis or stratification of BAV or CAVD. NOTCH1 screening is of too little yield to justify testing (<2%), but may be included in larger panels of tests at a future time. Presently, there is no diagnostic utility for genetic testing for BAV or CAVD, but given the rate of discovery and the various technological advances being made, it would appear that this will occur in the near term. It is imperative that cardiologists understand the indications and limitations of clinical genetic testing [161,162]. However, genetic testing is being used for various clinical management reasons, and several of these uses have cardiovascular applications. For example, sequence variants in CYP2C9 and VKORC1 are associated with an increased bleeding risk and drug resistance, respectively, in patients taking warfarin [163,164]. Because CAVD patients often require valve replacement, and mechanical prostheses require anticoagulation, this particular example may be directly useful for CAVD patients. Ultimately, diagnostic panels of genetic variants that identify cause, and may provide insight regarding natural history, and additional management panels that identify disease-specific risks may inform clinical decision-making. Taken together, panels of genetic variants may be used in a manner similar to newborn screening, becoming an important part of the working information for every patient.

The opportunities and challenges of genotype definition in the clinic. Genotype definition will empower individuals and families to further control their health, extending the paradigm shift that occurred when the medical field embraced preventive medicine [165]. Increasing genetic information in the clinic creates new opportunities to improve cardiovascular health. However, this development also creates new challenges, including ethical and legal issues that challenge the existing regulatory landscape and directly impact application in the clinic [166]. For example, the meaning of a negative test often will not be clear, in addition to the ambiguity variants of unknown significance present. Despite the passage of the Genetic Information Nondiscrimination Act (GINA), a law that protects the public from insurance companies using genetic information for underwriting purposes, there are increasing concerns about privacy issues. Public education, including physician awareness, will be critical to facilitate the anticipated clinical uses of genetic information. Genetic testing will play an increasing role in the clinical management of BAV and CAVD patients. Ultimately, genotype definition may be able to identify those patients with BAV that are at risk (or not at risk) of developing CAVD or other associated problems, impacting clinical management decisions. As more is learned about the genetic basis of BAV and CAVD, the yield of clinical genetic testing will be sufficient to warrant routine diagnostic testing. As the genotypes associated with BAV and CAVD are defined, there will be a need to expand Consensus Guidelines for BAV to include full consideration of genetic information, especially overlapping silent and/or latent disease processes. Clinical applications of genetic variant panels will potentially include refined diagnosis, risk stratification (early intervention, timing of surgery), pharmacogenomics (which drug, what dose, risk of adverse effects), and screening strategies for relatives.

The clinical implications of genotype definition: examples. Because CAVD remains essentially a surgical problem, early clinical impact may be realized first in surgical considerations. For example, the pulmonary artery dimension is increased in BAV patients [167,168], consistent with previously reported histopathologic abnormalities in the pulmonary artery of BAV patients [169]. This may be clinically relevant in BAV patients who require aortic valve replacement and may be candidates for the Ross procedure (autologous pulmonary valve placed in the aortic position). Some patients with apparently isolated CAVD undergoing surgical repair may be at risk for subsequently developing TAA, a not uncommon scenario that may be predicted by genotyping. McKellar et al recently described aorta complications in 1,286 aortic valve replacement patients with a median 12 year follow up, and reported that 10% demonstrate progressive aortic enlargement and only a minority of these lead to dissection or require further surgery [170]. However, in those patients, prophylactic replacement of the aorta would be warranted and would fundamentally change the overall approach to this group of patients. In addition, stratifying by genotype CAVD patients into those with and those without aorta abnormalities potentially informs type of surgical approach as well [171,172]. The ability to identify those patients at risk before the first surgery may substantially impact clinical decision-making, including for example a selective approach to combined valve and aorta replacement.

Genotype phenotype information will have important implications for clinical surveillance. For example, current recommendations for functional BAV patients include screening echocardiograms every 5 years for all first-degree relatives [13]. Recently it was shown that surveillance may be modified by morphology such that pediatric patients with RN morphology are screened every 2 years because they are at higher risk of developing new AVD, while individuals with RL BAV could be monitored less aggressively in early childhood as the risk of having AVD at this time is relatively low [26]. Family members of BAV patients may be at risk for TAA or other cardiovascular disease (even if they don't have BAV), underscoring the importance of thoughtful monitoring. Since CAVD is a latent phenotype, continued surveillance is required. Since some individuals with BAV have progressive CAVD and others never develop disease, there is reason to think that genetic insights will clarify this phenomenon. Overall, refined screening strategies promise to provide opportunities for improved care.

Ultimately, genetic information will inform the identification of new pharmacologic based therapies for CAVD [173]. Genetics research in CAVD will lead to further basic research in animal models that can define the early pathogenesis and natural history of disease and therefore identify new therapeutic targets. This paradigm will have increasing significance as bioinformatics approaches overcome the challenges of extraordinary amounts of data. There has been considerable interest in applying CAD treatment paradigms to valve disease. However, while statin therapy showed early in vitro evidence of a potentially beneficial effect, a large clinical trial demonstrated that statin therapy does not positively impact either aortic valve disease progression or the need for surgery [174]. Recently, a strategy to use pediatric valve disease patients as a means to identify early genetic aspects of CAVD has been advanced because this population provides insight into the disease process that is not confounded by the common comorbidities of adulthood, such as CAD and HTN [127,175]. Increasingly, developmental paradigms will inform the search for etiology, new treatments and better bioprostheses. New therapies are likely to emerge from molecular biology fields, and innovative approaches to studying the genetic basis of CAVD will be needed to realize this goal.

Author details

Robert B. Hinton

Address all correspondence to: robert.hinton@cchmc.org

The Heart Institute, Division of Cardiology, Cincinnati Children's Hospital Medical Center, USA

References

[1] Clayton M. Leonardo's anatomy years. Nature 2012;484:314-316.

[2] Hoffman JI, Kaplan S. The incidence of congenital heart disease. J Am Coll Cardiol 2002;39:1890-1900.

[3] Roger VL, Go AS, Lloyd-Jones DM, Adams RJ, Berry JD, Brown TM, Carnethon MR, Dai S, De Simone G, Ford ES, Fox CS, Fullerton HJ, Gillespie C, Greenlund KJ, Hailpern SM, Heit JA, Ho M, Howard VJ, Kissela BM, Kittner SJ, Lackland DT, Lichtman JH, Lisabeth LD, Makuc DM, Marcus GM, Marelli A. Heart disease and stroke statis-

tics--2011 update: A report from the American Heart Association. Circulation 2011;123:e18-e209.

[4] Roberts WC. The congenitally bicuspid aortic valve. A study of 85 autopsy cases. Am J Cardiol 1970;26:72-83.

[5] Fernandes SM, Sanders SP, Khairy P, Jenkins KJ, Gauvreau K, Lang P, Simonds H, Colan SD. Morphology of bicuspid aortic valve in children and adolescents. J Am Coll Cardiol 2004;44:1648-1651.

[6] Hinton RB. Bicuspid aortic valve and thoracic aortic aneurysm: three patient populations, two disease phenotypes, and one shared genotype. Cardiol Res Pract 2012;2012:926975.

[7] Ward C. Clinical significance of the bicuspid aortic valve. Heart 2000;83:81-85.

[8] Otto CM. Valvular aortic stenosis: disease severity and timing of intervention. J Am Coll Cardiol 2006;47:2141-2151.

[9] Schoen FJ. Evolving concepts of cardiac valve dynamics: the continuum of development, functional structure, pathobiology, and tissue engineering. Circulation 2008;118:1864-1880.

[10] Otto CM, Kuusisto J, Reichenbach DD, Gown AM, O'Brien KD. Characterization of the early lesion of 'degenerative' valvular aortic stenosis. Histological and immuno-histochemical studies. Circulation 1994;90:844-853.

[11] Thubrikar MJ, Aouad J, Nolan SP. Patterns of calcific deposits in operatively excised stenotic or purely regurgitant aortic valves and their relation to mechanical stress. Am J Cardiol 1986;58:304-308.

[12] Nkomo VT, Gardin JM, Skelton TN, Gottdiener JS, Scott CG, Enriquez-Sarano M. Burden of valvular heart diseases: a population-based study. Lancet 2006;368:1005-1011.

[13] Bonow RO, Carabello BA, Chatterjee K, de Leon AC Jr, Faxon DP, Freed MD, Gaasch WH, Lytle BW, Nishimura RA, O'Gara PT, O'Rourke RA, Otto CM, Shah PM, Shanewise JS. Focused update incorporated into the ACC/AHA 2006 guidelines for the management of patients with valvular heart disease: a report of the American College of Cardiology/American Heart Association Task Force on Practice Guidelines. Circulation 2008;118:e523-661.

[14] Rajamannan NM, Gersh B, Bonow RO. Calcific aortic stenosis: from bench to the bedside--emerging clinical and cellular concepts. Heart 2003;89:801-805.

[15] Roberts WC, Ko JM. Frequency by decades of unicuspid, bicuspid, and tricuspid aortic valves in adults having isolated aortic valve replacement for aortic stenosis, with or without associated aortic regurgitation. Circulation 2005;111:920-925.

[16] Stewart BF, Siscovick D, Lind BK, Gardin JM, Gottdiener JS, Smith VE, Kitzman DW, Otto CM. Clinical factors associated with calcific aortic valve disease. Cardiovascular Health Study. J Am Coll Cardiol 1997;29:630-634.

[17] Owens DS, Katz R, Takasu J, Kronmal R, Budoff MJ, O'Brien KD. Incidence and progression of aortic valve calcium in the Multi-ethnic Study of Atherosclerosis (MESA). Am J Cardiol 2010;105:701-708.

[18] Otto CM, Lind BK, Kitzman DW, Gersh BJ, Siscovick DS. Association of aortic-valve sclerosis with cardiovascular mortality and morbidity in the elderly. N Engl J Med 1999;341:142-147.

[19] Keane JF, Driscoll DJ, Gersony WM, Hayes CJ, Kidd L, O'Fallon WM, Pieroni DR, Wolfe RR, Weidman WH. Second natural history study of congenital heart defects: Results of treatment of patients with aortic valvar stenosis. Circulation 1993;87:I16-27.

[20] Schoen FJ. Mechanisms of function and disease of natural and replacement heart valves. Annu Rev Pathol 2012;7:161-183.

[21] Gallegos RP. Selection of Prosthetic Heart Valves. Curr Treat Options Cardiovasc Med 2006;8:443-452.

[22] Tzemos N, Therrien J, Yip J, Thanassoulis G, Tremblay S, Jamorski MT, Webb GD, Siu SC. Outcomes in adults with bicuspid aortic valves. JAMA 2008;300:1317-1325.

[23] Mahle WT, Sutherland JL, Frias PA. Outcome of Isolated Bicuspid Aortic Valve in Childhood. J Pediatr 2010;157:445-449.

[24] Collins MJ, Butany J, Borger MA, Strauss BH, David TE. Implications of a congenitally abnormal valve: a study of 1025 consecutively excised aortic valves. J. Clin. Pathol 2008;61:530-536.

[25] Rajamannan NM, Evans FJ, Aikawa E, Grande-Allen KJ, Demer LL, Heistad DD, Simmons CA, Masters KS, Mathieu P, O'Brien KD, Schoen FJ, Towler DA, Yoganathan AP, Otto CM. Calcific aortic valve disease: not simply a degenerative process: A review and agenda for research from the National Heart and Lung and Blood Institute Aortic Stenosis Working Group. Executive summary: Calcific aortic valve disease. Circulation 2011;124:1783-1791.

[26] Calloway TJ, Martin LJ, Zhang X, Tandon A, Benson DW, Hinton RB. Risk factors for aortic valve disease in bicuspid aortic valve: a family-based study. Am J Med Genet A 2011;155:1015-1020.

[27] Lanktree MB, Hassell RG, Lahiry P, Hegele RA. Phenomics: expanding the role of clinical evaluation in genomic studies. J Investig Med 2010;58:700-706.

[28] Rajamannan NM. Calcific aortic stenosis: lessons learned from experimental and clinical studies. Arterioscler Thromb Vasc Biol 2009;29:162-168.

[29] Mohler ER, Sheridan MJ, Nichols R, Harvey WP, Waller BF. Development and progression of aortic valve stenosis: atherosclerosis risk factors--a causal relationship? A clinical morphologic study. Clin Cardiol 1991;14:995-999.

[30] Rapp AH, Hillis LD, Lange RA, Cigarroa JE. Prevalence of coronary artery disease in patients with aortic stenosis with and without angina pectoris. Am J Cardiol 2001;87:1216-1217.

[31] Aronow WS, Schwartz KS, Koenigsberg M. Correlation of serum lipids, calcium, and phosophorus, diabetes mellitus and history of systemic hypertension with presence or absence of calcified or thickened aortic cusps or root in elderly patients. Am J Cardiol 1987;59:998-999.

[32] Piers LH, Touw HRW, Gansevoort R, Franssen CFM, Oudkerk M, Zijlstra F, Tio RA. Relation of aortic valve and coronary artery calcium in patients with chronic kidney disease to the stage and etiology of the renal disease. Am J Cardiol 2009;103:1473-1477.

[33] Botto LD, Lin AE, Riehle-Colarusso T, Malik S, Correa A. Seeking causes: Classifying and evaluating congenital heart defects in etiologic studies. Birth Defects Res A Clin Mol Teratol 2007;79:714-727.

[34] Luo AK, Jefferson BK, Garcia MJ, Ginsburg GS, Topol EJ. Challenges in the phenotypic characterisation of patients in genetic studies of coronary artery disease. J Med Genet 2007;44:161-165.

[35] Markwald RR, Norris RA, Moreno-Rodriguez R, Levine RA. Developmental basis of adult cardiovascular diseases: valvular heart diseases. Ann N Y Acad Sci 2010;1188:177-183.

[36] Bruneau BG. The developmental genetics of congenital heart disease. Nature 2008;451:943-948.

[37] Schoen FJ. Evolving concepts of cardiac valve dynamics: the continuum of development, functional structure, pathobiology, and tissue engineering. Circulation 2008;118:1864-1880.

[38] Cripe L, Andelfinger G, Martin LJ, Shooner K, Benson DW. Bicuspid aortic valve is heritable. J Am Coll Cardiol 2004;44:138-143.

[39] Loscalzo ML, Goh DL, Loeys B, Kent KC, Spevak PJ, Dietz HC. Familial thoracic aortic dilation and bicommissural aortic valve: a prospective analysis of natural history and inheritance. Am J Med Genet A 2007;143A:1960-1967.

[40] Huntington K, Hunter AG, Chan KL. A prospective study to assess the frequency of familial clustering of congenital bicuspid aortic valve. J Am Coll Cardiol 1997;30:1809-1812.

[41] McBride KL, Marengo L, Canfield M, Langlois P, Fixler D, Belmont JW. Epidemiology of noncomplex left ventricular outflow tract obstruction malformations (aortic

valve stenosis, coarctation of the aorta, hypoplastic left heart syndrome) in Texas, 1999-2001. Birth Defects Res A Clin Mol Teratol 2005;73:555-561.

[42] Fernandez B, Duran AC, Fernandez-Gallego T, Fernández MC, Such M, Arqué JM, Sans-Coma V. Bicuspid aortic valves with different spatial orientations of the leaflets are distinct etiological entities. J Am Coll Cardiol 2009;54:2312-2318.

[43] Sans-Coma V, Carmen Fernández M, Fernández B, Durán AC, Anderson RH, Arqué JM. Genetically alike Syrian hamsters display both bifoliate and trifoliate aortic valves. J Anat 2012;220:92-101.

[44] Hinton RB, Martin LJ, Rame-Gowda S, Tabangin ME, Cripe LH, Benson DW. Hypoplastic left heart syndrome links to chromosomes 10q and 6q and is genetically related to bicuspid aortic valve. J Am Coll Cardiol 2009;53:1065-1071.

[45] Martin LJ, Ramachandran V, Cripe LH, Hinton RB, Andelfinger G, Tabangin M, Shooner K, Keddache M, Benson DW. Evidence in favor of linkage to human chromosomal regions 18q, 5q and 13q for bicuspid aortic valve and associated cardiovascular malformations. Hum Genet 2007;121:275-284.

[46] McBride KL, Zender GA, Fitzgerald-Butt SM, Koehler D, Menesses-Diaz A, Fernbach S, Lee K, Towbin JA, Leal S, Belmont JW. Linkage analysis of left ventricular outflow tract malformations (aortic valve stenosis, coarctation of the aorta, and hypoplastic left heart syndrome). Eur J Hum Genet 2009;17:811-819.

[47] Garg V, Muth AN, Ransom JF, Schluterman MK, Barnes R, King IN, Grossfeld PD, Srivastava D. Mutations in NOTCH1 cause aortic valve disease. Nature 2005;437:270-274.

[48] Mohamed SA, Aherrahrou Z, Liptau H, Erasmi AW, Hagemann C, Wrobel S, Borzym K, Schunkert H, Sievers HH, Erdmann J. Novel missense mutations (p.T596M and p.P1797H) in NOTCH1 in patients with bicuspid aortic valve. Biochem Biophys Res Commun 2006;345:1460-1465.

[49] Nus M, MacGrogan D, Martínez-Poveda B, Benito Y, Casanova JC, Fernández-Avilés F, Bermejo J, de la Pompa JL. Diet-induced aortic valve disease in mice haploinsufficient for the Notch pathway effector RBPJK/CSL. Arterioscler Thromb Vasc Biol 2011;31:1580-1588.

[50] Acharya A, Hans CP, Koenig SN, Nichols HA, Galindo CL, Garner HR, Merrill WH, Hinton RB, Garg V. Inhibitory role of Notch1 in calcific aortic valve disease. PLoS One 2011;6:e27743.

[51] Nigam V, Srivastava D. Notch1 represses osteogenic pathways in aortic valve cells. J Mol Cell Cardiol 2009;47:828-834.

[52] Hitz MP, Lemieux-Perreault LP, Marshall C, Feroz-Zada Y, Davies R, Yang SW, Lionel AC, D'Amours G, Lemyre E, Cullum R, Bigras JL, Thibeault M, Chetaille P, Montpetit A, Khairy P, Overduin B, Klaassen S, Hoodless P, Nemer M, Stewart AF,

Boerkoel C, Scherer SW, Richter A, Dubé MP, Andelfinger G. Rare copy number variants contribute to congenital left-sided heart disease. PLoS Genet 2012;8(9):e1002903.

[53] Hinton RB, Yutzey KE. Heart Valve Structure and Function in Development and Disease. Annual Review of Physiology 2011;73:29-46.

[54] Hinton RB, Jr., Martin LJ, Tabangin ME, Mazwi ML, Cripe LH, Benson DW. Hypoplastic left heart syndrome is heritable. J Am Coll Cardiol 2007;50:1590-1595.

[55] Novaro GM, Mishra M, Griffin BP. Incidence and echocardiographic features of congenital unicuspid aortic valve in an adult population. J Heart Valve Dis 2003;12:674-678.

[56] Kathiresan S, Srivastava D. Genetics of human cardiovascular disease. Cell 2012;148:1242-1257.

[57] Guo DC, Papke CL, Tran-Fadulu V, Regalado ES, Avidan N, Johnson RJ, Kim DH, Pannu H, Willing MC, Sparks E, Pyeritz RE, Singh MN, Dalman RL, Grotta JC, Marian AJ, Boerwinkle EA, Frazier LQ, LeMaire SA, Coselli JS, Estrera AL, Safi HJ, Veeraraghavan S, Muzny DM, Wheeler DA, Willerson JT, Yu RK, Shete SS, Scherer SE, Raman CS, Buja LM, Milewicz DM. Mutations in smooth muscle alpha-actin (ACTA2) cause coronary artery disease, stroke, and Moyamoya disease, along with thoracic aortic disease. Am J Hum Genet 2009;84:617-627.

[58] Takeuchi F, Isono M, Katsuya T, Yamamoto K, Yokota M, Sugiyama T, Nabika T, Fujioka A, Ohnaka K, Asano H, Yamori Y, Yamaguchi S, Kobayashi S, Takayanagi R, Ogihara T, Kato N. Blood pressure and hypertension are associated with 7 loci in the Japanese population. Circulation 2010;121:2302-2309.

[59] Schunkert H, König IR, Kathiresan S, Reilly MP, Assimes TL, Holm H, Preuss M, Stewart AF, Barbalic M, Gieger C, Absher D, Aherrahrou Z, Allayee H, Altshuler D, Anand SS, Andersen K, Anderson JL, Ardissino D, Ball SG, Balmforth AJ, Barnes TA, Becker DM, Becker LC, Berger K, Bis JC, Boekholdt SM, Boerwinkle E, Braund PS, Brown MJ, Burnett MS, Buysschaert I; Cardiogenics, Carlquist JF, Chen L, Cichon S, Codd V, Davies RW, Dedoussis G, Dehghan A, Demissie S, Devaney JM, Diemert P, Do R, Doering A, Eifert S, Mokhtari NE, Ellis SG, Elosua R, Engert JC, Epstein SE, de Faire U, Fischer M, Folsom AR, Freyer J, Gigante B, Girelli D, Gretarsdottir S, Gudnason V, Gulcher JR, Halperin E, Hammond N, Hazen SL, Hofman A, Horne BD, Illig T, Iribarren C, Jones GT, Jukema JW, Kaiser MA, Kaplan LM, Kastelein JJ, Khaw KT, Knowles JW, Kolovou G, Kong A, Laaksonen R, Lambrechts D, Leander K, Lettre G, Li M, Lieb W, Loley C, Lotery AJ, Mannucci PM, Maouche S, Martinelli N, McKeown PP, Meisinger C, Meitinger T, Melander O, Merlini PA, Mooser V, Morgan T, Mühleisen TW, Muhlestein JB, Münzel T, Musunuru K, Nahrstaedt J, Nelson CP, Nöthen MM, Olivieri O, Patel RS, Patterson CC, Peters A, Peyvandi F, Qu L, Quyyumi AA, Rader DJ, Rallidis LS, Rice C, Rosendaal FR, Rubin D, Salomaa V, Sampietro ML, Sandhu MS, Schadt E, Schäfer A, Schillert A, Schreiber S, Schrezenmeir J, Schwartz SM, Siscovick DS, Sivananthan M, Sivapalaratnam S, Smith A, Smith TB, Snoep JD,

Soranzo N, Spertus JA, Stark K, Stirrups K, Stoll M, Tang WH, Tennstedt S, Thorgeirsson G, Thorleifsson G, Tomaszewski M, Uitterlinden AG, van Rij AM, Voight BF, Wareham NJ, Wells GA, Wichmann HE, Wild PS, Willenborg C, Witteman JC, Wright BJ, Ye S, Zeller T, Ziegler A, Cambien F, Goodall AH, Cupples LA, Quertermous T, März W, Hengstenberg C, Blankenberg S, Ouwehand WH, Hall AS, Deloukas P, Thompson JR, Stefansson K, Roberts R, Thorsteinsdottir U, O'Donnell CJ, McPherson R, Erdmann J; CARDIoGRAM Consortium, Samani NJ. Large-scale association analysis identifies 13 new susceptibility loci for coronary artery disease. Nat Genet 2011;43:333-338.

[60] Yasuno K, Bilguvar K, Bijlenga P, Low SK, Krischek B, Auburger G, Simon M, Krex D, Arlier Z, Nayak N, Ruigrok YM, Niemelä M, Tajima A, von und zu Fraunberg M, Dóczi T, Wirjatijasa F, Hata A, Blasco J, Oszvald A, Kasuya H, Zilani G, Schoch B, Singh P, Stüer C, Risselada R, Beck J, Sola T, Ricciardi F, Aromaa A, Illig T, Schreiber S, van Duijn CM, van den Berg LH, Perret C, Proust C, Roder C, Ozturk AK, Gaál E, Berg D, Geisen C, Friedrich CM, Summers P, Frangi AF, State MW, Wichmann HE, Breteler MM, Wijmenga C, Mane S, Peltonen L, Elio V, Sturkenboom MC, Lawford P, Byrne J, Macho J, Sandalcioglu EI, Meyer B, Raabe A, Steinmetz H, Rüfenacht D, Jääskeläinen JE, Hernesniemi J, Rinkel GJ, Zembutsu H, Inoue I, Palotie A, Cambien F, Nakamura Y, Lifton RP, Günel M. Genome-wide association study of intracranial aneurysm identifies three new risk loci. Nat Genet 2010;42:420-425.

[61] Armstrong EJ, Bischoff J. Heart valve development: endothelial cell signaling and differentiation. Circ Res 2004;95:459-470.

[62] Olson EN. Gene regulatory networks in the evolution and development of the heart. Science 2006;313:1922-1927.

[63] Combs MD, Yutzey KE. Heart valve development: regulatory networks in development and disease. Circ Res 2009;105:408-421.

[64] Antonicelli F, Bellon G, Debelle L, Hornbeck W. Elastin-elastases and Inflamm-Aging. Current Topics in Dev Biol 2007;79:99-138.

[65] Stephens EH, de Jonge N, McNeill MP, Durst CA, Grande-Allen KJ. Age-related changes in material behavior of porcine mitral and aortic valves and correlation to matrix composition. Tissue Eng Part A 2010;16:867-878.

[66] Michelena HI, Desjardins VA, Avierinos JF, Russo A, Nkomo VT, Sundt TM, Pellikka PA, Tajik AJ, Enriquez-Sarano M. Natural history of asymptomatic patients with normally functioning or minimally dysfunctional bicuspid aortic valve in the community. Circulation 2008;117:2776-2784.

[67] Beroukhim RS, Kruzick TL, Taylor AL, Gao D, Yetman AT. Progression of aortic dilation in children with a functionally normal bicuspid aortic valve. Am J Cardiol 2006;98:828-830.

[68] Whittemore R, Hobbins JC, Engle MA. Pregnancy and its outcome in women with and without surgical treatment of congenital heart disease. Am J Cardiol 1982;50:641-651.

[69] Bondy CA, Matura LA, Wooten N, Troendle J, Zinn AR, Bakalov VK. The physical phenotype of girls and women with Turner syndrome is not X-imprinted. Hum Genet 2007;121:469-474.

[70] Sachdev V, Matura LA, Sidenko S, Ho VB, Arai AE, Rosing DR, Bondy CA. Aortic valve disease in Turner syndrome. J Am Coll Cardiol 2008;51:1904-1909.

[71] Roberts WC, Honig HS. The spectrum of cardiovascular disease in the Marfan syndrome: a clinico-morphologic study of 18 necropsy patients and comparison to 151 previously reported necropsy patients. Am Heart J 1982;104:115-135.

[72] Atzinger CL, Meyer RA, Khoury PR, Gao Z, Tinkle BT. Cross-sectional and longitudinal assessment of aortic root dilation and valvular anomalies in hypermobile and classic Ehlers-Danlos syndrome. J Pediatr 2011;158:826-830.

[73] Eronen M, Peippo M, Hiippala A, Raatikka M, Arvio M, Johansson R, Kahkonen M. Cardiovascular manifestations in 75 patients with Williams syndrome. J Med Genet 2002;39:554-558.

[74] Radunovic Z, Wekre LL, Diep LM, Steine K. Cardiovascular abnormalities in adults with osteogenesis imperfecta. Am Heart J 2011;161:523-529.

[75] Pierpont ME, Basson CT, Benson DW, Gelb BD, Giglia TM, Goldmuntz E, McGee G, Sable CA, Srivastava D, Webb CL. Genetic basis for congenital heart defects: current knowledge: a scientific statement from the American Heart Association Congenital Cardiac Defects Committee, Council on Cardiovascular Disease in the Young: endorsed by the American Academy of Pediatrics. Circulation 2007;115:3015-3038.

[76] Goldmuntz E, Lin AE. Genetics of Congenital heart defects. In: Moss and Adams' Heart Disease in Infants, Children and Adolescents, 7th edition (Editors: Allen HD, Driscoll DJ, Feltes TF, Shaddy RE). p 545-572.

[77] Bharati S, Lev M. Congenital polyvalvular disease. Circulation 1973;47:575-586.

[78] Duran AC, Frescura C, Sans-Coma V, Angelini A, Basso C, Thiene G. Bicuspid aortic valves in hearts with other congenital heart disease. J Heart Valve Dis 1995;4:581-590.

[79] Schott JJ, Benson DW, Basson CT, Pease W, Silberbach GM, Moak JP, Maron BJ, Seidman CE, Seidman JG. Congenital heart disease caused by mutations in the transcription factor NKX2-5. Science 1998;281:108-111.

[80] McElhinney DB, Geiger E, Blinder J, Benson DW, Goldmuntz E. NKX2.5 mutations in patients with congenital heart disease. J Am Coll Cardiol 2003;42:1650-1655.

[81] Garg V, Kathiriya IS, Barnes R, Schluterman MK, King IN, Butler CA, Rothrock CR, Eapen RS, Hirayama-Yamada K, Joo K, Matsuoka R, Cohen JC, Srivastava D. GATA4

mutations cause human congenital heart defects and reveal an interaction with TBX5. Nature 2003;424:443-447.

[82] Rajagopal SK, Ma Q, Obler D, Shen J, Manichaikul A, Tomita-Mitchell A, Boardman K, Briggs C, Garg V, Srivastava D, Goldmuntz E, Broman KW, Benson DW, Smoot LB, Pu WT. Spectrum of heart disease associated with murine and human GATA4 mutation. J Mol Cell Cardiol 2007;43:677-685.

[83] Basson CT, Cowley GS, Solomon SD, Weissman B, Poznanski AK, Traill TA, Seidman JG, Seidman CE. The clinical and genetic spectrum of the Holt-Oram syndrome (heart-hand syndrome). N Engl J Med 1994;330:885-891.

[84] Biben C, Weber R, Kesteven S, Stanley E, McDonald L, Elliott DA, Barnett L, Köentgen F, Robb L, Feneley M, Harvey RP. Cardiac septal and valvular dysmorphogenesis in mice heterozygous for mutations in the homeobox gene Nkx2-5. Circ Res 2000;87:888-895.

[85] Jain R, Engleka KA, Rentschler SL, Manderfield LJ, Li L, Yuan L, Epstein JA. Cardiac neural crest orchestrates remodeling and functional maturation of mouse semilunar valves. J Clin Invest 2011;121:422-430.

[86] Miller JD, Weiss RM, Heistad DD. Calcific aortic valve stenosis: Methods, models, and mechanisms. Circ. Res 2011;108:1392-1412.

[87] Bostrom K, Rajamannan NM, Towler DA. The regulation of valvular and vascular sclerosis by osteogenic morphogens. Circ. Res 2011;109:564-577.

[88] Simmons CA, Grant GR, Manduchi E, Davies PF. Spatial heterogeneity of endothelial phenotypes correlates with side-specific vulnerability to calcification in normal porcine aortic valves. Circ Res 2005;96:792-799.

[89] Hans CP, Koenig SN, Huang N, Cheng J, Beceiro S, Guggilam A, Kuivaniemi H, Partida-Sánchez S, Garg V. Inhibition of notch1 signaling reduces abdominal aortic aneurysm in mice by attenuating macrophage-mediated inflammation. Arterioscler Thromb Vasc Biol 2012;32:3012-3023.

[90] Jian B, Narula N, Li QY, Mohler ER 3rd, Levy RJ. Progression of aortic valve stenosis: TGF-beta1 is present in calcified aortic valve cusps and promotes aortic valve interstitial cell calcification via apoptosis. Ann Thorac Surg 2003;75:457-465.

[91] Chen JH, Chen WL, Sider KL, Yip CY, Simmons CA. β-catenin mediates mechanically regulated, transforming growth factor-β1-induced myofibroblast differentiation of aortic valve interstitial cells. Arterioscler Thromb Vasc Biol 2011;31:590-597.

[92] Xu S, Liu AC, Gotlieb AI. Common pathogenic features of atherosclerosis and calcific aortic stenosis: role of transforming growth factor-beta. Cardiovasc Pathol 2010;19:236-247.

[93] Caira FC, Stock SR, Gleason TG, McGee EC, Huang J, Bonow RO, Spelsberg TC, McCarthy PM, Rahimtoola SH, Rajamannan NM. Human degenerative valve disease is

associated with up-regulation of low-density lipoprotein-related protein 5 receptor-mediated bone formation. J Am Coll Cardiol 2006;47:1707-1712.

[94] Rajamannan NM, Subramaniam M, Rickard DJ, Stock SR, Donovan J, Springett M, Orszulak T, Fullerton DA, Tajik AJ, Bonow RO, Spelsberg TC. Human aortic valve calcification is associated with an osteoblast phenotype. Circulation 2003;107:2181-2184.

[95] Rajamannan NM, Nealis TB, Subramaniam M, Pandya S, Stock SR, Ignatiev CI, Sebo TJ, Rosengart TK, Edwards WD, McCarthy PM, Bonow RO, Spelsberg TC. Calcified rheumatic valve neoangiogenesis is associated with vascular endothelial growth factor expression and osteoblast-like bone formation. Circulation 2005;111:3296-3301.

[96] Mohler ER, Gannon F, Reynolds C, Zimmerman R, Keane MG, Kaplan FS. Bone formation and inflammation in cardiac valves. Circulation 2001;103:1522-1528.

[97] Steiner I, Kasparová P, Kohout A, Dominik J. Bone formation in cardiac valves: a histopathological study of 128 cases. Virchows Arch 2007;450:653-657.

[98] Lincoln J, Lange AW, Yutzey KE. Hearts and bones: shared regulatory mechanisms in heart valve, cartilage, tendon, and bone development. Dev Biol 2006;294:292-302.

[99] Hannoush H, Introne WJ, Chen MY, Lee SJ, O'Brien K, Suwannarat P, Kayser MA, Gahl WA, Sachdev V. Aortic stenosis and vascular calcifications in alkaptonuria. Mol Genet Metab 2012;105:198-202.

[100] Aikawa E, Aikawa M, Libby P, Figueiredo JL, Rusanescu G, Iwamoto Y, Fukuda D, Kohler RH, Shi GP, Jaffer FA, Weissleder R. Arterial and aortic valve calcification abolished by elastolytic cathepsin S deficiency in chronic renal disease. Circulation 2009;119:1785-1794.

[101] Filip DA, Radu A, Simionescu M. Interstitial cells of the heart valves possess characteristics similar to smooth muscle cells. Circ Res 1986;59:310-320.

[102] Walker GA, Masters KS, Shah DN, Anseth KS, Leinwand LA. Valvular myofibroblast activation by transforming growth factor-beta: implications for pathological extracellular matrix remodeling in heart valve disease. Circ Res 2004;95:253-260.

[103] Liu AC, Joag VR, Gotlieb AI. The emerging role of valve interstitial cell phenotypes in regulating heart valve pathobiology. Am J Pathol 2007;171:1407-18.

[104] Zerkowski HR, Grussenmeyer T, Matt P, Grapow M, Engelhardt S, Lefkovits I. Proteomics strategies in cardiovascular research. J Proteome Res 2004;3:200-208.

[105] Chaurand P, Cornett DS, Angel PM, Caprioli RM. From whole-body sections down to cellular level, multiscale imaging of phospholipids by MALDI mass spectrometry. Mol Cell Proteomics 2011;10:O110.004259.

[106]   Angel PM, Nusinow D, Brown CB, Violette K, Barnett JV, Zhang B, Baldwin HS, Caprioli RM. Networked-based characterization of extracellular matrix proteins from adult mouse pulmonary and aortic valves. J Proteome Res 2011;10: 812-823.

[107]   Yutzey KE, Robbins J. Principles of genetic murine models for cardiac disease. Circulation 2007;115:792-799.

[108]   Martín-Rojas T, Gil-Dones F, Lopez-Almodovar LF, Padial LR, Vivanco F, Barderas MG. Proteomic profile of human aortic stenosis: insights into the degenerative process. J Proteome Res 2012;11:1537-1550.

[109]   Bertacco E, Millioni R, Arrigoni G, Faggin E, Iop L, Puato M, Pinna LA, Tessari P, Pauletto P, Rattazzi M. Proteomic analysis of clonal interstitial aortic valve cells acquiring a pro-calcific profile. J Proteome Res 2010;9:5913-5921.

[110]   Gross L, Kugel MA. Topographic anatomy and histology of the valves in the human heart. Am J Path 1931;7:445-456.

[111]   Misfeld M, Sievers HH. Heart valve macro- and microstructure. Philos Trans R Soc Lond B Biol Sci 2007;362:1421-1436.

[112]   Anderson RH. Clinical anatomy of the aortic root. Heart 2000;84:670-673.

[113]   Yacoub MH, Kilner PJ, Birks EJ, Misfeld M. The aortic outflow and root: a tale of dynamism and crosstalk. Ann Thorac Surg 1999;68:S37-43.

[114]   Mjaatvedt CH, Yamamura H, Capehart AA, Turner D, Markwald RR. The Cspg2 gene, disrupted in the hdf mutant, is required for right cardiac chamber and endocardial cushion formation. Dev Biol 1998;202:56-66.

[115]   George EL, Georges-Labouesse EN, Patel-King RS, Rayburn H, Hynes RO. Defects in mesoderm, neural tube and vascular development in mouse embryos lacking fibronectin. Development 1993;119:1079-1091.

[116]   Löhler J, Timpl R, Jaenisch R. Embryonic lethal mutation in mouse collagen I gene causes rupture of blood vessels and is associated with erythropoietic and mesenchymal cell death. Cell 1984;38:597-607.

[117]   Liu X, Wu H, Byrne M, Krane S, Jaenisch R. Type III collagen is crucial for collagen I fibrillogenesis and for normal cardiovascular development. Proc Natl Acad Sci U S A 1997;94:1852-1856.

[118]   Ng CM, Cheng A, Myers LA, Martinez-Murillo F, Jie C, Bedja D, Gabrielson KL, Hausladen JMW, Mecham RP, Judge DP, Dietz HC. TGF-b-dependent pathogenesis of mitral valve prolapse in a mouse model of Marfan syndrome. J Clin Invest 2004;114:1586-1592.

[119]   Hinton RB, Adelman-Brown J, Witt S, Krishnamurthy VK, Osinska H, Sakthivel B, James JF, Li DY, Narmoneva DA, Mecham RP, Benson DW. Elastin haploinsufficien-

cy results in progressive aortic valve malformation and latent valve disease in a mouse model. Circ Res 2010;107:549-557.

[120] Cheek JD, Wirrig EE, Alfieri CM, James JF, Yutzey KE. Differential activation of valvulogenic, chondrogenic, and osteogenic pathways in mouse models of myxomatous and calcific aortic valve disease. J Mol Cell Cardiol 2012;52:689-700.

[121] Snider P, Hinton RB, Moreno-Rodriguez R, Wang J, Rogers R, Lindsley A, Li F, Ingram DA, Menick D, Field L, Firulli AB, Molkentin JD, Markwald RR, Conway SJ. Periostin is required for maturation and extracellular matrix stabilization of noncardiomyocyte lineages of the heart. Circ Res 2008;102:752-760.

[122] Lincoln J, Florer JB, Deutsch GH, Wenstrup RJ, Yutzey KE. ColVa1 and ColXIa1 are required for ventricular chamber morphogenesis and heart valve development. Dev Dyn 2006;235:3295-3305.

[123] Schroeder JA, Jackson LF, Lee DC, Camenisch TD. Form and function of developing heart valves: coordination by extracellular matrix and growth factor signaling. J Mol Med 2003;81:392-403.

[124] Drolet MC, Roussel E, Deshaies Y, Couet J, Arsenault M. A high fat/high carbohydrate diet induces aortic valve disease in C57BL/6J mice. J Am Coll Cardiol 2006;47:850-855.

[125] Weiss RM, Ohashi M, Miller JD, Young SG, Heistad DD. Calcific aortic valve stenosis in old hypercholesterolemic mice. Circulation 2006;114:2065-2069.

[126] Towler DA, Bidder M, Latifi T, Coleman T, Semenkovich CF. Diet-induced diabetes activates an osteogenic gene regulatory program in the aortas of low density lipoprotein receptor-deficient mice. J Biol Chem 1998;273:30427-30434.

[127] Hinton RB, Lincoln J, Deutsch GH, Osinska H, Manning PB, Benson DW, Yutzey KE. Extracellular matrix remodeling and organization in developing and diseased aortic valves. Circ Res 2006;98:1431-1438.

[128] Aikawa E, Whittaker P, Farber M, Mendelson K, Padera RF, Aikawa M, Schoen FJ. Human semilunar cardiac valve remodeling by activated cells from fetus to adult. Circulation 2006;113:1344-1352.

[129] Rabkin E, Aikawa M, Stone JR, Fukumoto Y, Libby P, Schoen FJ. Activated interstitial myofibroblasts express catabolic enzymes and mediate matrix remodeling in myxomatous heart valves. Circulation 2001;104:2525-2532.

[130] Lincoln J, Alfieri CM, Yutzey KE. Development of heart valve leaflets and supporting apparatus in chicken and mouse embryos. Dev Dyn 2004;230:239-250.

[131] Fedak PW, de Sa MP, Verma S, Nili N, Kazemian P, Butany J, Strauss BH, Weisel RD, David TE. Vascular matrix remodeling in patients with bicuspid aortic valve malfor-

mations: implications for aortic dilatation. J Thorac Cardiovasc Surg. 2003;126:797-806.

[132] Fondard O, Detaint D, Lung B, Choqueux C, Adle-Biassette H, Jarraya M, Hvass U, Couetil JP, Henin D, Michel JB, Vahanian A, Jacob MP. Extracellular matrix remodelling in human aortic valve disease: the role of matrix metalloproteinases and their tissue inhibitors. Eur Heart J 2005;26:1333-1341.

[133] Dreger SA, Taylor PM, Allen SP, Yacoub MH. Profile and localization of matrix metalloproteinases (MMPs) and their tissue inhibitors (TIMPs) in human heart valves. J Heart Valve Dis 2002;11:875-880.

[134] Edep ME, Shirani J, Wolf P, Brown DL. Matrix metalloproteinase expression in nonrheumatic aortic stenosis. Cardiovasc Pathol 2000;9:281-286.

[135] Jian B, Jones PL, Li Q, Mohler ER 3rd, Schoen FJ, Levy RJ. Matrix metalloproteinase-2 is associated with tenascin-C in calcific aortic stenosis. Am J Pathol 2001;159:321-327.

[136] Krishnamurthy VK, Opoka AM, Kern CB, Guilak F, Narmoneva DA, Hinton RB. Maladaptive matrix remodeling and regional biomechanical dysfunction in a mouse model of aortic valve disease. Matrix Biol 2012;31:197-205.

[137] Kern CB, Wessels A, McGarity J, Dixon LJ, Alston E, Argraves WS, Geeting D, Nelson CM, Menick DR, Apte SS. Reduced versican cleavage due to Adamts9 haploinsufficiency is associated with cardiac and aortic anomalies. Matrix Biol 2010;29:304-316.

[138] Perrotta I, Russo E, Camastra C, Filice G, Di Mizio G, Colosimo F, Ricci P, Tripepi S, Amorosi A, Triumbari F, Donato G. New evidence for a critical role of elastin in calcification of native heart valves: immunohistochemical and ultrastructural study with literature review. Histopathology 2011;59:504-513.

[139] Aikawa E, Aikawa M, Libby P, Figueiredo JL, Rusanescu G, Iwamoto Y, Fukuda D, Kohler RH, Shi GP, Jaffer FA, Weissleder R. Arterial and aortic valve calcification abolished by elastolytic cathepsin S deficiency in chronic renal disease. Circulation 2009;119:1785-1794.

[140] Jacob MP. Extracellular matrix remodeling and matrix metalloproteinases in the vascular wall during aging and in pathological conditions. Biomed Pharmacother 2003;57:195-202.

[141] Long MM, King VJ, Prasad KU, Freeman BA, Urry DW. Elastin repeat peptides as chemoattractants for bovine aortic endothelial cells. J Cell Physiol 1989;140:512-518.

[142] Hollinger JO, Schmitz JP, Yaskovich R, Long MM, Prasad KU, Urry DW. A synthetic polypentapeptide of elastin for initiating calcification. Calcif Tissue Int 1988;42:231-236.

[143] Sacks MS, David Merryman W, Schmidt DE. On the biomechanics of heart valve function. J Biomech 2009;42:1804-1824.

[144] Grande KJ, Cochran RP, Reinhall PG, Kunzelman KS. Stress variations in the human aortic root and valve: the role of anatomic asymmetry. Ann Biomed Eng 1998;26:534-545.

[145] Sacks MS, Yoganathan AP. Heart valve function: a biomechanical perspective. Philos Trans R Soc Lond B Biol Sci 2007;362:1369-1391.

[146] Visconti RP, Ebihara Y, LaRue AC, Fleming PA, McQuinn TC, Masuya M, Minamiguchi H, Markwald RR, Ogawa M, Drake CJ. An in vivo analysis of hematopoietic stem cell potential: hematopoietic origin of cardiac valve interstitial cells. Circ Res 2006;98:690-6.

[147] Li C, Xu S, Gotlieb AI. The response to valve injury. A paradigm to understand the pathogenesis of heart valve disease. Cardiovasc Pathol 2011;20:183-90.

[148] Hakuno D, Kimura N, Yoshioka M, Mukai M, Kimura T, Okada Y, Yozu R, Shukunami C, Hiraki Y, Kudo A, Ogawa S, Fukuda K. Periostin advances atherosclerotic and rheumatic cardiac valve degeneration by inducing angiogenesis and MMP production in humans and rodents. J Clin Invest 2010;120:2292-306.

[149] Woo KV, Qu X, Babaev VR, Linton MF, Guzman RJ, Fazio S, Baldwin HS. Tie1 attenuation reduces murine atherosclerosis in a dose-dependent and shear stress-specific manner. J Clin Invest. 2011;121:1624-35.

[150] Schoen FJ. Mechanisms of function and disease of natural and replacement heart valves. Annu Rev Pathol. 2012;7:161-83.

[151] Campbell LD, Betsou F, Garcia DL, Giri JG, Pitt KE, Pugh RS, Sexton KC, Skubitz APN, Somiari SB, Astrin J, Baker S, Barr TJ, Benson E, Cada M, Campbell L, Hugo A, Froes J, Campos M, Carpentieri D, Clement O, Coppola D, De Souza Y, Fearn P, Feil K, Garcia D, Giri J, Grizzle WE, Groover K, Harding K, Kaercher E, Kessler J, Loud S, Maynor H, McCluskey K, Meagher K, Michels C, Miranda L, Muller-Cohn J, Muller R, O'Sullivan J, Pitt K, Pugh R, Ravid R, Sexton K, Silva RLA, Simione F, Skubitz A, Somiari S, van der Horst F, Welch G, Zaayenga A. 2012 Best Practices for Repositories: Collection, Storage, Retrieval, and Distribution of Biological Materials for Research. Biopreserv Biobank 2012;10:79-161.

[152] McCarty CA, Chisholm RL, Chute CG, Kullo IJ, Jarvik GP, Larson EB, Li R, Masys DR, Ritchie MD, Roden DM, Struewing JP, Wolf WA; eMERGE Team. The eMERGE Network: a consortium of biorepositories linked to electronic medical records data for conducting genomic studies. BMC Med Genomics 2011;4:13.

[153] Bennett R. The Practical Guide to the Genetic Family History. Wiley-Liss, Inc, 1999.

[154] Yoon PW, Scheuner MT, Peterson-Oehlke KL, Gwinn M, Faucett A, Khoury MJ. Can family history be used as a tool for public health and preventive medicine? Genet Med 2002;4:304-10.

[155] Williams RR, Hunt SC, Heiss G, Province MA, Bensen JT, Higgins M, Chamberlain RM, Ware J, Hopkins PN. Usefulness of cardiovascular family history data for population-based preventive medicine and medical research (the Health Family Tree Study and the NHLBI Family Heart Study). Am J Cardiol 2001;87:129-35.

[156] Greendale K, Pyeritz RE. Empowering primary care health professionals in medical genetics: how soon? How fast? How far? Am J Med Genet 2001;106:223-232.

[157] Hinton RB. The family history: reemergence of an established tool. Crit Care Nurs Clin North Am 2008;20:149-58.

[158] O'Neill SM, Rubinstein WS, Wang C, Yoon PW, Acheson LS, Rothrock N, Starzyk EJ, Beaumont JL, Galliher JM, Ruffin MT 4th; Family Healthware Impact Trial group. Familial risk for common diseases in primary care: the Family Healthware Impact Trial. Am J Prev Med 2009;36:506-14.

[159] Collins FS, Bochm K. Avoiding casualties in the genetic revolution: the urgent need to educate physicians about genetics. Acad Med 1999;74:48-49.

[160] Guttmacher AE, Collins FS, Carmona RH. The family history--more important than ever. N Engl J Med 2004;351:2333-2336.

[161] Robin NH, Tabereaux PB, Benza R, Korf BR. Genetic testing in cardiovascular disease. J Am Coll Cardiol 2007;50:727-737.

[162] Rogowski WH, Grosse SD, Khoury MJ. Challenges of translating genetic tests into clinical and public health practice. Nat Rev Genet 2009;10:489-495.

[163] Aithal GP, Day CP, Kesteven PJ, Daly AK. Association of polymorphisms in the cytochrome P450 CYP2C9 with warfarin dose requirement and risk of bleeding complications. Lancet 1999;353:717-719.

[164] Rost S, Fregin A, Ivaskevicius V, Conzelmann E, Hörtnagel K, Pelz HJ, Lappegard K, Seifried E, Scharrer I, Tuddenham EG, Müller CR, Strom TM, Oldenburg J. Mutations in VKORC1 cause warfarin resistance and multiple coagulation factor deficiency type 2. Nature 2004;427:537-541.

[165] Rose G. Strategy of prevention: lessons from cardiovascular disease. Br Med J 1981;282:1847-1851.

[166] Ashley EA, Hershberger RE, Caleshu C, Ellinor PT, Garcia JG, Herrington DM, Ho CY, Johnson JA, Kittner SJ, Macrae CA, Mudd-Martin G, Rader DJ, Roden DM, Scholes D, Sellke FW, Towbin JA, Van Eyk J, Worrall BB; American Heart Association Advocacy Coordinating Committee. Genetics and cardiovascular disease: a policy statement from the American Heart Association. Circulation 2012;126:142-157.

[167] Loscalzo ML, Goh DL, Loeys B, Kent KC, Spevak PJ, Dietz HC. Familial thoracic aortic dilation and bicommissural aortic valve: a prospective analysis of natural history and inheritance. Am J Med Genet A 2007;143A:1960-1967.

[168] Martin LJ, Hinton RB, Zhang X, Cripe LH, Benson DW. Aorta Measurements are Heritable and Influenced by Bicuspid Aortic Valve. Front Genet 2011;2:61.

[169] de Sa M, Moshkovitz Y, Butany J, David TE. Histologic abnormalities of the ascending aorta and pulmonary trunk in patients with bicuspid aortic valve disease: clinical relevance to the Ross procedure. J Thorac Cardiovasc Surg 1999;118:588-594.

[170] McKellar SH, Michelena HI, Li Z, Scharr HV, Sundt TM. Long-Term Risk of Aortic Events Following Aortic Valve Replacement in Patients with Bicuspid Aortic Valves. Am J Cardiol 2010;106:1626-1633.

[171] David TE, Armstrong S, Ivanov J, Feindel CM, Omran A, Webb G. Results of aortic valve-sparing operations. J Thorac Cardiovasc Surg 2001;122:39-46.

[172] Bethea BT, Fitton TP, Alejo DE, Barreiro CJ, Cattaneo SM, Dietz HC, Spevak PJ, Lima JA, Gott VL, Cameron DE. Results of aortic valve-sparing operations: experience with remodeling and reimplantation procedures in 65 patients. Ann Thorac Surg 2004;78:767-772.

[173] Conti R, Veenstra DL, Armstrong K, Lesko LJ, Grosse SD. Personalized medicine and genomics: challenges and opportunities in assessing effectiveness, cost-effectiveness, and future research priorities. Med Decis Making 2010;30:328-340.

[174] Rossebo AB, Pedersen TR, Boman K, Brudi P, Chambers JB, Egstrup K, Gerdts E, Gohlke-Barwolf C, Holme I, Kesaniemi YA, Malbecq W, Nienaber CA, Ray S, Skjaerpe T, Wachtell K, Willenheimer R. Intensive lipid lowering with simvastatin and ezetimibe in aortic stenosis. N Engl J Med 2008;359:1343-1356.

[175] Wirrig EE, Hinton RB, Yutzey KE. Differential expression of cartilage and bone-related proteins in pediatric and adult diseased aortic valves. J Mol Cell Cardiol 2011;50, 561-569.

Chapter 7

Proteomics and Metabolomics in Aortic Stenosis: Studying Healthy Valves for a Better Understanding of the Disease

L. Mourino-Alvarez, C.M. Laborde and
M.G. Barderas

Additional information is available at the end of the chapter

1. Introduction

1.1. Aortic stenosis

Aortic stenosis is characterized by the abnormal narrowing of the aortic valve (AV) opening, producing a blockage of the blood flow from the left ventricle into the aorta. Two different types of aortic stenosis can be distinguished. In congenital aortic stenosis an inherited abnormal formation of the AV exists. Otherwise, in acquired aortic stenosis external causes such as rheumatic fever or valve degeneration occur. Calcific aortic stenosis (AS) is the most common valvular disease in elder population and remain the main cause of aortic valve replacement in developed countries [1].

AS progresses from a primary stage of aortic sclerosis, with thickening and stiffness of the AV, to severe calcific stenosis. Its most common symptoms are dyspnea, angina and syncope, which predict the rapid deterioration of left ventricular function, the development of heart failure and, if the pathology progresses, the patient's death. Therefore, the appearance of any of these symptoms is considered as an indication for the treatment of this pathology. In these cases, surgery is recommended to replace the AV since there is not treatment to delay the progression of the disease.

Classically, this disease has been considered as a consequence of the aging process of the valve. However, recent studies have provided evidences that inflammation plays a key role in the physiopathology of AS as well as classical cardiovascular risk factors such as hypertension, hypercholesterolemia, diabetes, smoking, age or sex [2]. Degeneration of the valve begins with an endothelial dysfunction in the aortic side as a result of the abovementioned risk factors. Low density lipoproteins (LDLs) are accumulated in the subendothelial space of the valve, where they are oxidized, resulting in the activation of the endothelial cells. These cells express adhesion and chemotactic molecules, which attract inflammatory cells such as monocytes and T lymphocytes. Monocytes extravasate to the fibrous layer and differentiate into macrophages, which capture oxidized lipoproteins and become foam cells. Proinflammatory cytokines released by both cell types induce phenotypic differentiation of a subset of myofibroblasts to osteoblasts, which leads to the subsequent formation of calcium nodules [3]. These numerous similarities suggest a common relationship between atherosclerosis and AS.

1.2. Proteomic and metabolomic study of healthy valves

A complete knowledge of the structures involved in a disease it is important to understand its development. Previously, healthy tissue such as vasculature and myocardial have been succesfully studied to better understand the molecular mechanisms involved in vascular develepment and angiogenesis as well as biochemical changes that occur during physiological ageing [4, 5].

Histologically, AV consists of three layers: fibrosa, spongiosa and ventricularis. The fibrosa is located in the aortic side of the leaflets and it is mainly composed of fibroblasts and collagen fibers. The spongiosa is located below and it is formed by fibroblasts, mesenchymal cells and a polysaccharides-rich matrix. The ventricularis, found in the ventricular side of the leaflet, is made up of elastic fibers radially distributed. The AV is externally covered by several layers of endothelial cells. Collagen is responsible for the mechanical integrity of the valve, the spongiosa serves as a shock absorber and elastic fibers contract cusps during systole [3, 6].

However, it is also essential to perform studies at the molecular level of the tissue, looking for the discovery of tissue- and disease-specific markers. For this purpose, proteomic and metabolomic analyses can be ideally used since they allow the unbias analysis of hundreds or thousands of molecules at a time, detecting and identifying which molecules are present. In contrast to genomics and transcriptomics, proteomics and metabolomics study dynamic protein products, low molecular weight compounds and their interactions, which have a direct effect on the phenotype of the tissue (Figure 1).

Descriptive proteomics is a methodology that enables unbiased large-scale study of the set of all proteins in a biologic system at any given time. Thus, the expression, localization, interaction, structural domains and activity of these proteins, including splice isoforms and post-translational modifications (PTMs), can be studied [7]. Metabolomics is the study of a complete metabolome or a single group of particular metabolites, which are small molecules that participate in general metabolic reactions and that are required for the maintenance, growth and normal function of a cell [8]. The study of healthy valves through proteomic and metabolomic approaches and the subsequent integration of data, can provide molecular level information of the metabolic pathways that are more active in that tissue and will help to understand the mechanisms of physiological/pathological processes in aortic stenosis valves. This makes it easier the search for potential markers for early diagnosis of the disease, thus being able to predict which people may develop aortic stenosis in the future.

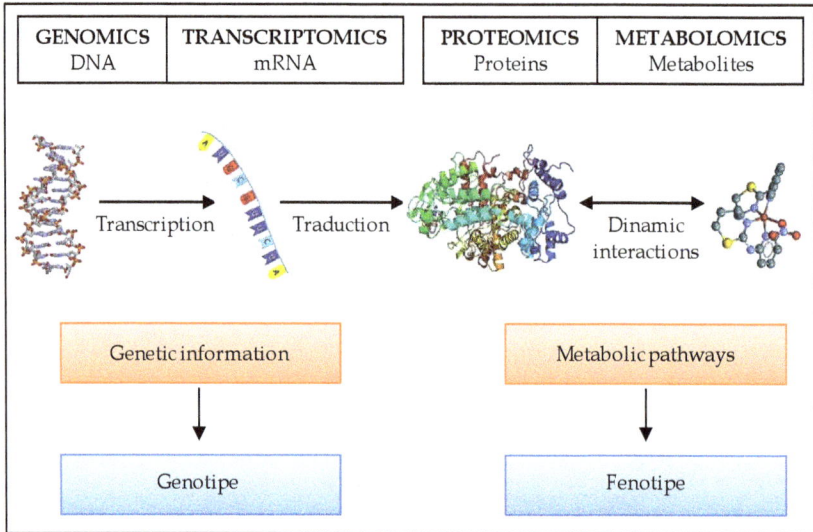

Figure 1. Dynamic study of the physiophatology of a disease through "-omics" technologies.

2. Proteomics

Proteomics is the large-scale study of the proteins content in a given sample (ie. biofluid or tissue) [9]. Since proteins are the final product of genes expression, proteomics constitutes a powerful tool for the study of biological systems thanks to proteome reflects the current state of the organism and it varies according to its functional situation [10]. These studies can be performed through a wide variety of techniques and methodologies, depending on the sample and the experimental design. In the case of descriptive proteomics, in which the most usually is the study of very complex samples, it is essential to perform certain steps to facilitate the study: 1) sample preparation, 2) protein separation and 3) analysis by mass spectrometry.

2.1. Sample preparation

Preparation of the samples prior to the analysis using proteomic techniques is an essential step for obtaining robust and reproducible data. Between the large number of standardized protocols, the selected one must be carefully chosen to suit the sample to be analyzed, as well as for the proteins of interest. In the case of the AV an effective and suitable protocol has been previously described [11] (Figure 2). Briefly, within 2 hours after surgery, valves were washed in PBS and then ground into a powder in liquid N2 with a mortar. 0.2 g of this powder was resuspended in 400 μl of protein extraction buffer (Tris 10 mM [pH 7.5], 500 mM NaCl, 0.1% Triton x-100, 1% β-mercaptoethanol, 1 mM PMSF) and then centrifuged to precipitate membranes and tissue debris [12]. Supernatant containing most of the soluble proteins was collected and pellet was solubilized in 7M urea, 2M thiourea, 4% CHAPS prior to another centrifugation [13, 14]. This second supernatant, which was rich in hydrophobic proteins, was also collected and stored at -20°. Depending on which is the fraction of interest, supernatants can be analyzed together or separately. Because of the nature of the extraction buffers, sample must be processed to eliminate interference substances with the downstream analyses. Samples must be filtered by centrifugation and dialyzed against Tris 2mM. Before proteomic analyses it is also recommended the use of the commercial kit 2D-Clean-Up (GE Healthcare), which precipitates proteins while leaving interfering substances, such as detergents, salts, lipids, phenolics, and nucleic acids, in solution. The pellet can then be solubilized in a proper buffer for further analyses.

Instead of solubilized the proteins of whole tissue, histology sections or specific cell types can be used for isolate different structures of the tissue as regions, cells or even subcellular fractions by means of laser microdissection (LMD) [15]. It consists in cutting microscopically selected tissue by laser using different systems [16]: 1) selected regions are transferred onto a film or to a special cap; 2) selected regions can be catapulted into a collection tube and 3) cut samples fall down into the lid of a collection tube by gravitation. The collected tissue has to be lysed and prepared for downstream analyses. The main disadvantage of this methodology in combination with proteomics is the scarce amount of protein that can be obtain, since the laser cannot be applied for a long time in order to avoid protein degradation. However, mass spectrometers have exponentially improved their sensitivity, so there are several interesting studies combining LMD and Proteomics in other cardiovascular tissues samples [17-20]. The application of LMD to the analysis of the AV tissue could provide specific data from the different layers/structures in the tissue, as well as from the behavior of the different cells in the tissue.

2.2. Protein separation

For complex mixtures, it is important to separate proteins according to their different charac-teristic to increase the efficiency of the study. For this purpose, the most usually used techni-ques are 2-dimensional electrophoresis (2-DE), off-gel fractionation, and 2-dimensional liquid chromatography (LC) [21-23] (Figure 3).

2.2.1. 2-Dimensional electrophoresis

This method stands out for its high applicability to a wide range of biological samples. In this case, a good protein separation can be reached through two simple steps: isoelectric focusing (IEF) and sodium dodecyl sulfate polyacrylamide gel electrophoresis (SDS-PAGE) [24, 25]. During the first phase, the protein mixture is separated on a pH gradient according to their isoelectric point (pI) using commercial strips covered by an acrylamide gel. To perform this separation, proteins are completely solubilized in a special buffer containing urea, a nonionic detergent (CHAPS) to prevent clustering, a reducing agent (DTT) to break the disulfide bonds and a mixture of ampholytes to minimize aggregations by charge interaction. In the second step, proteins are separated in a second dimension depending on their molecular mass and a two-dimensional protein spot map is obtained that can be visualized through different staining

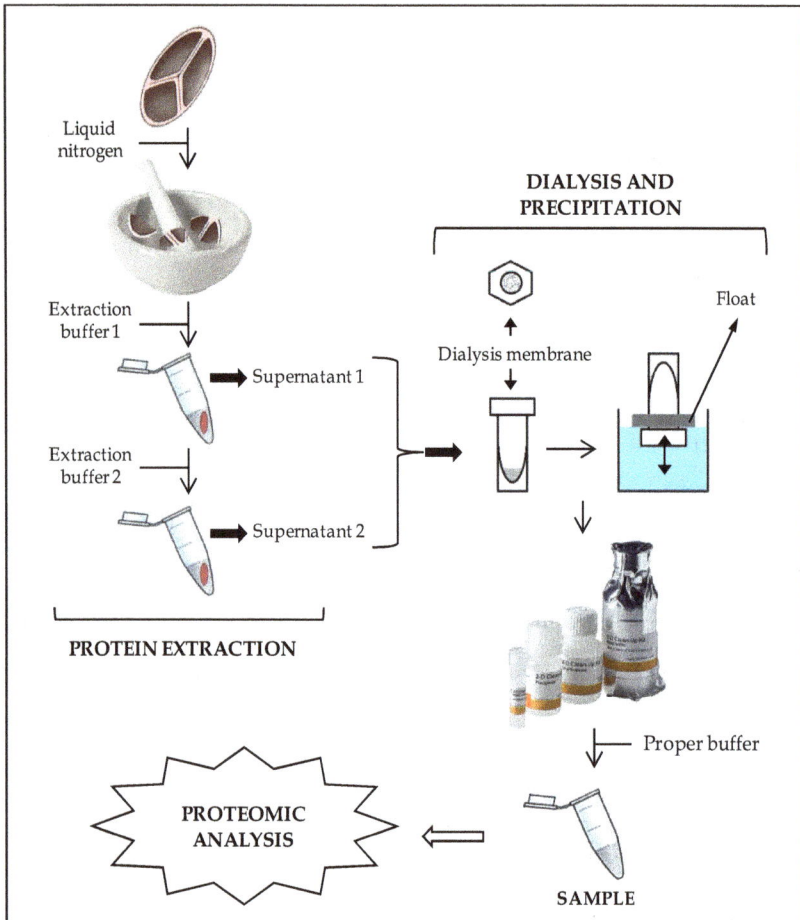

Figure 2. Protocol of aortic valve preparation for proteomic analyses

techniques as Coomassie blue, silver staining and Sypro Ruby [26]. Stained gels are scanned and digitalized using different computer programs to obtain an image of the gel and spots of interest will be identified by mass spectrometry techniques. There are three protein groups which are problematic: highly alkaline, extremely high and low molecular sizes and membrane-bound proteins. However, improving protein solubilization, pre-fractionation of protein groups of interest prior to 2DE, or adjustments to the 2-DE regime enhance separation of these more difficult-to-resolve proteins. The main advantage of 2-DE is that it delivers a map of intact proteins, which reflects changes in protein expression level, isoforms or post-translational modifications [27].

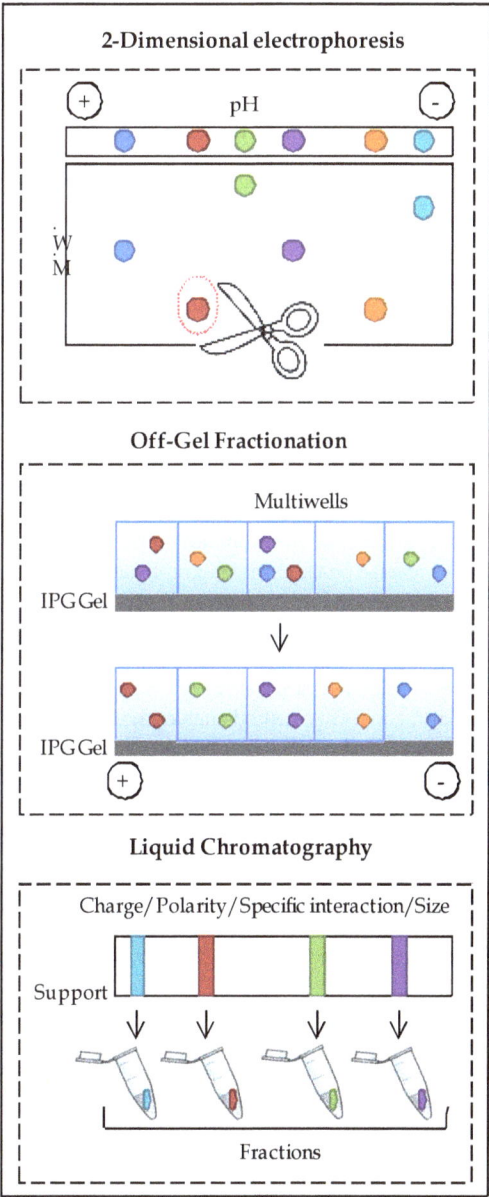

Figure 3. Most common used protein separation techniques

2.2.2. Off-gel fractionation

There is another protein fractionation technique which is based on off-gel IEF, where the proteins are separated according to their pI in a multiwell device. This separation is based on immobilized pH gradient (IPG) strips and permits to separate peptides and proteins according to their pI, but is realized in solution without the need of carrier ampholytes or buffers [28, 29]. The main advantage of this technique is that the fractions can be directly recovered in solution for further analysis and directly digested if necessary [28, 30]

2.2.3. Liquid chromatography

Liquid chromatography (LC) is a fractionation technique that can be applied to separate a wide range of molecules such as proteins or peptides according to their physical and/or chemical properties. Different types of chromatographic support can be distinguished: ion exchange (separation based on protein or peptide charge), reverse phase (according to their polarity), affinity (based on a highly specific interaction such as that between antigen and antibody, enzyme and substrate, or receptor and ligand) and molecular exclusion (depending on size). LC can be used before or after 2-DE [31-33] and can be directly coupled to a mass spectrometer for further identification [34, 35]. To increase the resolution of proteomics analyses, it is recommended the use several consecutive chromatographic methods. In this sense a combination of ion exchange and reverse phase chromatography allows a two-dimensional separation with the advantage that the second column can be directly coupled to MS, which enhances the automatization of the proteomic methodology. With this idea, multidimensional protein identification technology (MudPIT) has been developed. It consists of a column with two chromatographic supports in tandem: a cation exchange support in the proximal area followed by a reverse phase in the distal one. This method enables the two-dimensional LC using high-performance LC (HPLC) coupled to a mass spectrometer with electrospray ionization (ESI) source in an automated manner [36, 37]. This approach is more sensitivity and reproducibility than gel-based methodologies and allows the analyses of smaller quantities each time because of the development of new equipments which are able to work with sample volumes of the order of microliters and nanoliters. LC together with mass spectrometry has been successfully employed in a previous work in which the proteome of the coronary artery was described [17].

2.3. Protein analyses by mass spectrometry

Once our sample is separated, these fractions or spots must be analyzed to identify the different proteins. Since the development of matrix-assisted laser desorption ionization (MALDI) and ESI, two ionization methods that allows the analysis of proteins and peptides using MS, this technique have become indispensable for protein identification [38-40]. Mass spectrometers consist of three essential elements: ionization source, mass analyzer and detector (Figure 4). The ionization source ionizes and vaporizes the sample. Different ionization sources are MALDI, ESI or surface-enhanced laser desorption/ionization (SELDI) [41-43]. ESI allows the identification of many volatile and thermolabile compounds of a wide range of molecular weight with high sensitivity. MALDI and SELDI are very similar methods but they are used for low and high complex mixtures, respectively [44]. The mass analyzer separates the ions according to their relation m/z. There are also different types of mass analyzer, such as quadrupole (Q), time of flight (TOF), ion trap (IT), Fourier transform ion cyclotron resonance (FT-ICR) and Orbitrap. The ion stream reaches to the detector and it is transformed into an electrical signal. These signals are then integrated by a computer system which generates a mass spectrum which represents the abundance of the different generated ions.

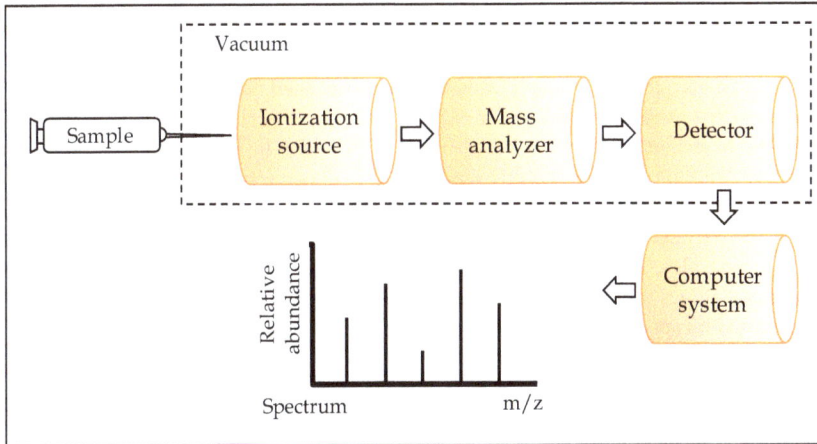

Figure 4. Different elements of a mass spectrometer

There are two different ways to identify the molecules included in a complex mix using MS: peptide mass fingerprinting (PMF) and tandem mass spectrometry (MS/MS or MS2). Briefly, identification based on PMF identifies proteins according to the peptides generated after digestion with specific endoproteases, usually trypsine. Experimentally obtained peptide masses are compared to theoretical peptide masses of proteins stored in databases through mass search engines such as MASCOT (Matrix Science Ltd.) [45], MS-Fit [46] or Profound [47, 48]. These samples usually come from gel bands, 2-DE spots or LC fractions with low complexity and are analyzed through MALDI-TOF or ESI-TOF [48, 49]. In the case of MS/MS, two mass analyzers are used in tandem. The first one allows the measurement of the m/z values of the peptides and the second one, after the fragmentation of some peptides, allows the measurement of the m/z values of these fragments. Thus, a partial or even total sequence of the peptide can be obtained. Most usually used mass spectrometer for this purpose are MALDI-TOF-TOF (for low complex mixtures) and ESI coupled to different analyzers (Q3, Q-TOF, IT, Q-Q-LIT, FT y Orbitrap).

2.4. Tissue sections analysis: MALDI imaging mass spectrometry

MALDI imaging mass spectrometry (IMS) is a powerful tool for investigating the distribution of proteins and small molecules present in thin tissue sections. This technique generates molecular profiles and two-dimensional ion density maps of peptide and protein signals directly from the surface of these sections [50]. For this analyses, it is indispensable a correct sample preparation in terms of chemical and structural integrity [51]. Preparation methods must avoid delocalization and degradation of the analytes so it is important to take into account several parameters such as treatment of tissue immediately after sample procurement, sectioning, sample transfer to the MALDI target plate, matrix application, and tissue storage after sectioning [52]. It is advisable the used of fresh tissue sections though sometimes it is necessary embedding the sample in gelatine or agarose to facilitate its manipulation [53-55]. One of the important aspects of tissue profiling is the comparison of histological features obtained from stained sections using light microscopy with molecular images obtained by mass spectrometry [56]. Previously, this was accomplished using two separate adjacent sections, one for histology and one for MALDI-IMS [57, 58]. However, visual registration between both sections it is difficult because of differences in tissue architecture. Ideally, histology and protein profiling should be performed on the same tissue section. For this reason, several commonly used histological dyes have been tested for compatibility with MS analysis. It was found that hematoxilin and eosin interfered with MS but, on the other hand, cresyl violet and methylene blue, between others, do not compromise mass spectra quality [56]. This methodology allows the study of the entire tissue, maintaining its structure, so MS analysis can be focused on specific morphological regions of interest.

3. Metabolomics

Metabolomics is the study of the set of final products and by-products of many metabolic pathways, called metabolites, which exist in humans and other living systems [8]. In order to perform a descriptive analysis of healthy valves, an untargeted approach, not focused on a specific group of metabolites, is the most recommended methodology. This method, also called metabolomic fingerprinting, permits to detect the largest number of metabolites optimizing different experimental conditions such as sample preparation and chromatographic and MS parameters. This approach usually compromises the sensitivity and specificity for identification of individual metabolites [59, 60]. Additionally, metabolomic fingerprinting involves less up-front method development when compared with targeted approaches but requires an exhaustive analysis due to the large number of identified metabolites. As well as in proteomics analyses, there are three main steps when performing a metabolomic study: [1] sample preparation; [2] metabolite detection and [3] data analysis.

3.1. Sample preparation

Optimization of sample-preparation protocol is extremely important in metabolomic studies because it affects both metabolite profile and quality data, leading to possible erroneous conclusions [61, 62]. An ideal sample-preparation method for metabolomic fingerprinting should have the following characteristics [1] non-selective to ensure adequate metabolite coverage; [2] simple and fast, with the minimum number of steps possible to minimize metabolite loss and/or degradation of the sample and enable high-throughput; [3] reproducible and [4] incorporate a metabolism-quenching step (low temperatures, addition of acid, or fast heating) to represent true metabolome composition at the time of sampling (Figure 5) [63]. For tissue metabolomics, the protocol includes a previous step of manual homogenization at low temperatures follow by a quenching step in liquid nitrogen [64]. Although the tissue disruption technique can altered the precision and metabolite coverage, the selection of the extraction solvent have a stronger effect on the number of extracted metabolites [65]. Several aqueous and organic solvents can be used, such us methanol [66, 67], methanol/water [68], isopropanol/acetonitrile/water [69], acetonitrile/methanol/water [70], acidic acetonitrile/water [71] or methanol/acetonitrile/acetone [72] between others. However, there is no an established protocol for aortic valve so it is important the development of an adequate method before metabolic fingerprinting.

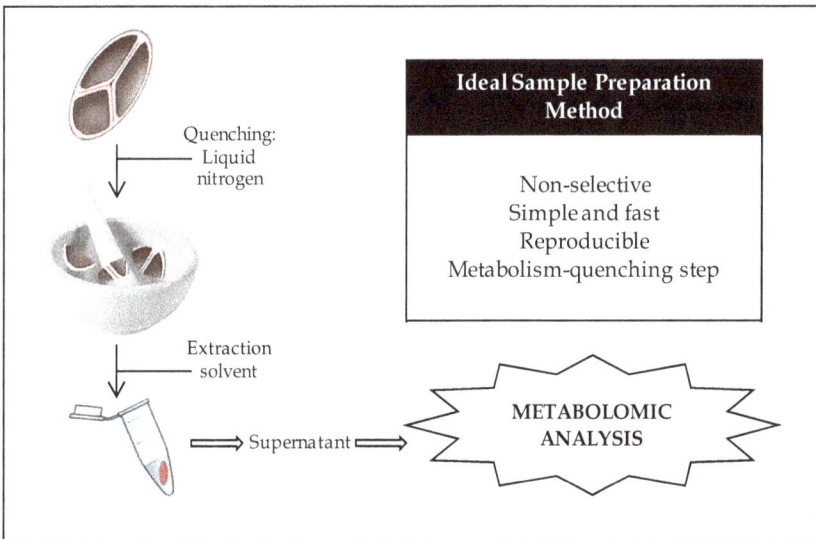

Figure 5. Protocol of tissue preparation for metabolomic analyses.

3.2. Metabolite detection

There is a great variability of metabolites in terms of polarity, solubility, and volatility with a wide dynamic range of concentration in biological samples. Therefore it is necessary to combine different chromatographic platforms for covering the largest range of metabolite possible. The two main platforms used in metabolomics analysis are nuclear magnetic resonance (NMR) and MS, usually coupled with a separation method for metabolites (LC or gas chromatography (GC)-MS) [73, 74]. The platform of choice will depend on the physico-chemical characteristics of the metabolites of interest. As it is explained below, CG-MS is a high-quality technique for analyzing hydrophobic compounds while LC-MS permits to determine a larger number of metabolites. Finally, NMR shows superior capability for determining the structure of unknown metabolites. Therefore, each platform has inherent advantages and disadvantages for the metabolomic analysis of different compounds and only through their combined use the best understanding of the physiopathology of AV will be achieved (Table 1).

Advantages	PLATFORM	Disadvantages
Minimal sample preparation Non-destructive Reproducible Structural information	NMR	Sensitivity Spectral resolution
No derivatization required Variety of metabolites	LC-MS	No comprehensive spectral libraries
Sensitivity Robust Reproducible Comprehensive spectral libraries	CG-MS	Derivatization required Limited mass range

Table 1. Comparison of the most common analytical methods used for metabolomics

3.2.1. Nuclear magnetic resonance

NMR is a spectroscopic analysis technique that exploits the specific magnetic spin or resonance frequency of the protons within atomic nuclei of specific molecules. When nuclei in a magnetic field are exposed to a radiofrequency pulse their protons temporarily move to a higher energy state, and then release a characteristic radiowave when they return to their normal energy state [75]. The resulting NMR spectrum is a collection of characteristic peaks and intensities of each compound that allow its identification [76]. NMR requires minimal sample preparation, it is a nondestructive and very reproducible technique and provides structural information of metabolites. These particular advantages confers NMR superior ability for the identification of unknown metabolites and constitutes a valuable approach for identification of unknown metabolites [77]. However, NMR is limited in terms of sensitivity and spectral resolution so it is not a good technology to identify metabolites that are found in low concentration [78].

NMR also allows the analyses of intact tissue using a technique called high-resolution magic angle spinning (HRMAS) NMR. The sample is spun at high speed about an axis at an angle of 54°44′(the so-called "magic angle") [79]. This rapid spinning at this precise angle has the effect of reducing dipolar coupling effects and narrowing of the broad lines found in this tissue. HRMAS-NMR has been applied successfully to analyze different intact cells and tissues [80-85], so it seems to be a powerful tool for the analyses of aortic valve tissue.

3.2.2. Mass spectrometry

As well as in proteomic studies, MS uses m/z value to identify metabolites. When coupled with chromatographic methods, MS can analyze a wide number of metabolites with enhanced sensitivity. The two main strategies for metabolite separation are LC (for nonvolatile compounds in solution) or GC (for volatile samples or when the expected compounds can be easily made volatile by derivatization). LC-MS using ESI as ionization source is the most currently used platform for metabolomic studies since it permits the analysis of a wider variety of metabolites than GC-MS [86, 87]. Also, derivatization step prior the analysis is no necessary reducing losses of compounds during the sample preparation. Single quadrupole, ion trap and TOF analyzers are the most commonly used mass analyzers. GC-MS is a first-rate choice for the analysis of volatile compounds such as fatty acids and organic acids [88]. In most cases, it is necessary a prior step for chemical derivatization of non-volatile and thermally stable metabolites. The two more used derivatization reagents include BSTFA (N, O-Bis (trimethyl-silyl) trifluoroacetamide) and MSTFA (N-Methyl-N-(trimethylsilyl) trifluoroacetamide) [89-91]. Advantages of GC include higher resolution and more robust and reproducible retention times than LC, besides the existence of mass spectral libraries, which facilitates the identification process.

In the course of the study of the physiopathology of AS the better comprehension of implicated and altered biochemical pathways will be acquired through the metabolomic study of biological samples, specially plasma and tissue. For this purpose NMR and MS represent the two most valuable techniques for metabolite identification thus the information that both techniques provide will suppose a cornerstone for the study of this disease.

3.3. Identification and data analysis

The data processing challenges in metabolomics are quite unique and often require specialized (and/or expensive) data analysis software and a complete knowledge of cheminformatics, bioinformatics and statistics for a correct interpretation of data. Ideally, data analysis softwares must be able to remove noise from the spectra, properly identify which metabolite generates every chromatographic peak and make a correct alignment of the peaks corresponding to the same compound in several successive samples [92, 93].

There are several commercial softwares available free such as MSFacts, MetAlign or Metab-oAnalyst which automatically import, reformat, align, correct the baseline, and export large chromatographic data sets to allow more rapid visualization of metabolomics data [94, 95]. However, most companies usually generate data that can be only read with own softwares which use mass spectral libraries for peak detection, identification and integration [96].

4. Towards a global understanding of physiology

The large number of genomes, including human, that have been mapped and the knowledge of the genetic code, have increased the interest in other –OMICS technologies, such as proteomics and metabolomics. Both proteomics and metabolomics differ from genomics in terms of complexity and dynamic variability. Proteome and metabolome are constantly changing according to the genome and the environment, therefore the ultimate phenotype of cell, organ, and organism is reflected in proteomic and metabolomic profiles. This variability, enhanced by the using of different methodologies and equipments, usually impedes obtaining reliable and reproducible results when comparing patients and healthy controls. The study of a large number of healthy valves using a standardized protocol may provide useful information about the heterogeneity of its profiles. Thus, different profiles could be assigned to different states such as sex, age or risk factors. This way, the creation of a protein atlas unmasking the expression and localization of proteins coupled to metabolomic results would function as a global knowledgebase with valuable information about normal cellular function [97, 98]. All these information can be storage in conventional web-based databases, in order to obtain a reference material to be used in further studies, when studying different valve diseases, helping to deepen the understanding of the beginning and development of the disease. It would also be possible to find some variation involving metabolic predisposition to develop the disease in the future. This will exponentially increase the possibilities to discover potential therapeutic targets and will open the door to develop a personalized medicine in this disease.

The major challenge of generating a complete database of AV tissue is obtaining enough biological material to be described, since it is not an easily accessible specimen. It is necessary a complex coordination of basic research activities, facilities and infrastructures, as well as the creation of an integrated and multidisciplinary environment with the participation of several different specialists in cardiovascular diseases, i.e. basic researchers, cardiologists, surgeons, pathologists, epidemiologists, patients, patient advocacy groups, funding agencies and industrial partners. Issues related to sample collection, handling and storage, standardization of protocols, common references, number of patients, availability of normal controls, access to bio-banks, tissue arrays, clinical information, follow-up clinical data, computational and statistical analysis, as well as ethical considerations are critical, and must be carefully considered and dealt with from the beginning [99]. With such a big collaborating work, there will be a more effective translation of basic discoveries into clinical applications.

No matter how much ambitious and complete the descriptive study is, it is essential integration of the results through a system biology approach. This consists of placing proteins and molecules from experimental analysis in the context of a network of biological interactions, such as gene–gene, gene–protein or protein–protein interactions, followed by different 'guilt-by-association' analyses [100]. Usually, these networks are deduced from previously published interactions or from computational prediction models. Different tools exist to perform these analyses, most of them based on Cytoscape Web, a freely available network visualization tool for integrating biomolecular interaction networks with high-throughput expression data and other molecular states into a unified conceptual framework [101-103]. Using an integrative approach, we can obtain a more holistic picture of the molecular mechanisms that occurs in normal aortic valves.

5. Conclusion

The study of healthy valves through proteomic and metabolomic approaches and the subsequent integration of data can provide molecular level information of the metabolic pathways that are more active in AV. The characterization of physiological proteins and metabolites in this tissue and the creation of a complete database with the results from the descriptive studies, may serve as a reference material for further studies. This would facilitate the searching for potential markers for early diagnosis of the disease, thus being able to predict which people may develop aortic stenosis in the future.

Acknowledgements

This work was supported by grants from the Instituto de Salud Carlos III (FIS PI070537, PI11/02239), Fondos Feder-Redes temáticas de Investigación Cooperativa en Salud (RD06/0014/1015), grants from Fundación para la Investigación Sanitaria de Castilla-La Mancha (FISCAM PI2008-08, PI2008-28, PI2008-52).

Author details

L. Mourino-Alvarez[1], C.M. Laborde[1,2] and M.G. Barderas[1,3]

1 Department of Vascular Physiopathology, Hospital Nacional de Paraplejicos, SESCAM, Toledo, Spain

2 Laboratory of Biochemistry, Hospital Nacional de Paraplejicos, SESCAM, Toledo, Spain

3 Proteomic Unit, Hospital Nacional de Paraplejicos, SESCAM, Toledo, Spain

References

[1] Goldbarg SH, Elmariah S, Miller MA, Fuster V. Insights Into Degenerative Aortic Valve Disease. J Am Coll Cardiol. 2007;50(13):1205-13.

[2] Helske S, Kupari M, Lindstedt KA, Kovanen PT. Aortic valve stenosis: an active athe‐ roinflammatory process. Curr Opin Lipidol. 2007;18(5):483-91 10.1097/MOL. 0b013e3282a66099.

[3] Freeman RV, Otto CM. Spectrum of calcific aortic valve disease: Pathogenesis , dis‐ ease progression, and treatment strategies. Circulation. 2005 June 21, 2005;111(24): 3316-26.

[4] Li Y, Yu J, Wang Y, Griffin NM, Long F, Shore S, et al. Enhancing Identifications of Lipid-embedded Proteins by Mass Spectrometry for Improved Mapping of Endothe‐ lial Plasma Membranes in Vivo. Mol Cell Proteomics. 2009 June 1, 2009;8(6):1219-35.

[5]   Grant JE, Bradshaw AD, Schwacke JH, Baicu CF, Zile MR, Schey KL. Quantification of Protein Expression Changes in the Aging Left Ventricle of Rattus norvegicus. J Proteome Res. 2009 2012/10/08;8(9):4252-63.

[6]   Schoen FJ. Evolving Concepts of Cardiac Valve Dynamics. Circulation. 2008 October 28, 2008;118(18):1864-80.

[7]   Anderson N, Anderson N. Proteome and proteomics: new technologies, new concepts, and new words. Electrophoresis. 1998;Aug;19(11):1853-61.

[8]   Pasikanti KK, Ho PC, Chan ECY. Gas chromatography/mass spectrometry in metabolic profiling of biological fluids. J Chromatogr B. 2008;871(2):202-11.

[9]   Pandey A, Mann M. Proteomics to study genes and genomes. Nature. 2000;405(6788): 837-46.

[10] Marshall T, Williams KM. Proteomics and its impact upon biomedical science. British journal of biomedical science. 2002;59(1):47-64.

[11] Gil-Dones F, Martin-Rojas T, Lopez-Almodovar LF, Cuesta Fdl, Darde VM, Alvarez-Llamas G, et al. Valvular Aortic Stenosis: A Proteomic Insight. Clin Med Insights Cardiol. 2010;4;4:1-7.

[12] Barderas MG, Wigdorovitz A, Merelo F, Beitia F, Alonso C, Borca MV, et al. Serodiagnosis of African swine fever using the recombinant protein p30 expressed in insect larvae. J Virol Methods. 2000;89(1-2):129-36.

[13] Gonzalez-Barderas M, Gallego-Delgado J, Mas S, Duran MC, Lázaro A, Hernandez-Merida S, et al. Isolation of circulating human monocytes with high purity for proteomic analysis. Proteomics. 2004;4(2):432-7.

[14] Duran MC, Mas S, Martin-Ventura JL, Meilhac O, Michel JB, Gallego-Delgado J, et al. Proteomic analysis of human vessels: Application to atherosclerotic plaques. Proteomics. 2003;3(6):973-8.

[15] Emmert-Buck M, Bonner R, Smith P, Chuaqui R, Zhuang Z, Goldstein S, et al. Laser capture microdissection Science. 1996;274(5289):998-1001.

[16] Rabien A. Laser microdissection. Methods Mol Biol. 2010;576:39-47.

[17] Bagnato C, Thumar J, Mayya V, Hwang S-I, Zebroski H, Claffey KP, et al. Proteomics Analysis of Human Coronary Atherosclerotic Plaque. Mol Cell Proteomics. 2007 June 2007;6(6):1088-102.

[18] De la Cuesta F, Alvarez-Llamas G, Maroto AS, Donado A, Juarez-Tosina R, Rodriguez-Padial L, et al. An optimum method designed for 2-D DIGE analysis of human arterial intima and media layers isolated by laser microdissection. Proteomics Clin Appl. 2009;Oct;3(10):1174-84.

[19] de la Cuesta F, Alvarez-Llamas G, Maroto AS, Donado A, Zubiri I, Posada M, et al. A proteomic focus on the alterations occurring at the human atherosclerotic coronary intima. Mol Cell Proteomics. [Article]. 2011 Apr;10(4):13.

[20] De Souza AI, McGregor E, Dunn MJ, Rose ML. Preparation of human heart for laser microdissection and proteomics. Proteomics. 2004;4(3):578-86.

[21] Waller LN, Shores K, Knapp DR. Shotgun Proteomic Analysis of Cerebrospinal Fluid Using Off-Gel Electrophoresis as the First-Dimension Separation. J Proteome Res. 2008 2012/10/08;7(10):4577-84.

[22] Nägele E, Vollmer M, Hörth P, Vad C. 2D-LC/MS techniques for the identification of proteins in highly complex mixtures. Expert Rev Proteomics. 2004 2012/10/08;1(1): 37-46.

[23] Hey J, Posch A, Cohen A, Liu N, Harbers A. Fractionation of complex protein mixtures by liquid-phase isoelectric focusing. Methods Mol Biol. 2008;424:225-39.

[24] Görg A, Obermaier C, Boguth G, Harder A, Scheibe B, Wildgruber R, et al. The current state of two-dimensional electrophoresis with immobilized pH gradients. Electrophoresis. 2000;21(6):1037-53.

[25] Gygi SP, Corthals GL, Zhang Y, Rochon Y, Aebersold R. Evaluation of two-dimensional gel electrophoresis-based proteome analysis technology. Proc Natl Acad Sci U S A. 2000 August 15, 2000;97(17):9390-5.

[26] Chevalier F, Rofidal V, Rossignol M. Visible and fluorescent staining of two-dimensional gels. Methods Mol Biol. 2007;355:145-56.

[27] Görg A, Weiss W, Dunn MJ. Current two-dimensional electrophoresis technology for proteomics. Proteomics. 2004;4(12):3665-85.

[28] Michel PE, Reymond F, Arnaud IL, Josserand J, Girault HH, Rossier JS. Protein fractionation in a multicompartment device using Off-Gel™ isoelectric focusing. Electrophoresis. 2003;24(1-2):3-11.

[29] Heller M, Michel PE, Morier P, Crettaz D, Wenz C, Tissot J-D, et al. Two-stage Off-Gel™ isoelectric focusing: Protein followed by peptide fractionation and application to proteome analysis of human plasma. Electrophoresis. 2005;26(6):1174-88.

[30] Hörth P, Miller CA, Preckel T, Wenz C. Efficient Fractionation and Improved Protein Identification by Peptide OFFGEL Electrophoresis. Mol Cell Proteomics. 2006 October 2006;5(10):1968-74.

[31] Medzihradszky K, Leffler H, Baldwin M, Burlingame A. Protein identification by in-gel digestion, high-performance liquid chromatography, and mass spectrometry: Peptide analysis by complementary ionization techniques. J Am Soc Mass Spectrom. 2001;12(2):215-21.

[32] Pieper R, Gatlin C, Makusky A, Russo P, Schatz C, Miller S, et al. The human serum proteome: display of nearly 3700 chromatographically separated protein spots on

two-dimensional electrophoresis gels and identification of 325 distinct proteins. Proteomics. 2003;Jul;3(7):1345-64.

[33] Badock V, Steinhusen U, Bommert K, Otto A. Prefractionation of protein samples for proteome analysis using reversed-phase high-performance liquid chromatography. Electrophoresis. 2001;Aug;22(14):2856-64.

[34] Issaq HJ. The role of separation science in proteomics research. Electrophoresis. 2001;22(17):3629-38.

[35] Lesley SA. High-Throughput Proteomics: Protein Expression and Purification in the Postgenomic World. Protein Expr Purif. 2001;22(2):159-64.

[36] Washburn M, Wolters D, 3rd YJ. Large-scale analysis of the yeast proteome by multi-dimensional protein identification technology. Nat Biotechnol. 2001;Mar;19(3):242-7.

[37] Delahunty C, 3rd YJ. MudPIT: multidimensional protein identification technology. Biotechniques. 2007;43(5):563, 5, 7 passim.

[38] Domon B, Aebersold R. Mass spectrometry and protein analysis. Science. 2006;312(5771):212-7.

[39] Karas M, Hillenkamp F. Laser desorption ionization of proteins with molecular masses exceeding 10,000 daltons. Anal Chem. 1988;60(20):2299-301.

[40] Fenn J, Mann M, Menq C, Wong S, Whitehouse C. Electrospray for mass spectrometry of large biomolecules. Science. 1989;246(4926):64-71.

[41] Kinter M, Sherman NE. Fundamental Mass Spectrometry. Protein Sequencing and Identification Using Tandem Mass Spectrometry: John Wiley & Sons, Inc.; 2005. p. 29-63.

[42] Merchant M, Weinberger SR. Recent advancements in surface-enhanced laser desorption/ionization-time of flight-mass spectrometry. ELECTROPHORESIS. 2000;21(6):1164-77.

[43] Issaq HJ, Veenstra TD, Conrads TP, Felschow D. The SELDI-TOF MS Approach to Proteomics: Protein Profiling and Biomarker Identification. Biochem Biophys Res Commun. 2002;292(3):587-92.

[44] Issaq HJ, Conrads TP, Prieto DA, Tirumalai R, D.Veenstra T. SELDI-TOF MS for Diagnostic Proteomics. Anal Chem. 2003 2012/10/16;75(7):148 A-55 A.

[45] Perkins DN, Pappin DJC, Creasy DM, Cottrell JS. Probability-based protein identification by searching sequence databases using mass spectrometry data. ELECTROPHORESIS. 1999;20(18):3551-67.

[46] Clauser K, Baker P, Burlingame A. Role of accurate mass measurement (+/- 10 ppm) in protein identification strategies employing MS or MS/MS and database searching. Anal Chem. 1999;71(14):2871-82.

[47] Zhang W, Chait B. ProFound: an expert system for protein identification using mass spectrometric peptide mapping information. Anal Chem. 2000;72(11):2482-9.

[48] Aebersold R, Goodlett D. Mass spectrometry in proteomics. Chem Rev. 2001;101(2): 269-95.

[49] Aebersold R, Mann M. Mass spectrometry-based proteomics. Nature. 2003;422(6928): 198-207.

[50] Chaurand P, Stoeckli M, Caprioli RM. Direct Profiling of Proteins in Biological Tissue Sections by MALDI Mass Spectrometry. Anal Chem. 1999 2012/09/05;71(23):5263-70.

[51] McDonnell LA, Heeren RMA. Imaging mass spectrometry. Mass Spectrom Rev. 2007;26(4):606-43.

[52] Caldwell RL, Caprioli RM. Tissue Profiling by Mass Spectrometry. Mol Cell Proteomics. 2005 April 1, 2005;4(4):394-401.

[53] Altelaar AFM, van Minnen J, Jiménez CR, Heeren RMA, Piersma SR. Direct Molecular Imaging of Lymnaea stagnalis Nervous Tissue at Subcellular Spatial Resolution by Mass Spectrometry. Anal Chem. 2004 2012/10/08;77(3):735-41.

[54] Kruse R, Sweedler J. Spatial profiling invertebrate ganglia using MALDI MS. J Am Soc Mass Spectrom. 2003;14(7):752-9.

[55] Schwartz SA, Reyzer ML, Caprioli RM. Direct tissue analysis using matrix-assisted laser desorption/ionization mass spectrometry: practical aspects of sample preparation. J Mass Spectrom. 2003;38(7):699-708.

[56] Chaurand P, Schwartz SA, Billheimer D, Xu BJ, Crecelius A, Caprioli RM. Integrating Histology and Imaging Mass Spectrometry. Analytical Chemistry. 2004 2012/09/05;76(4):1145-55.

[57] Fournier I, Day R, Salzet M. Direct analysis of neuropeptides by in situ MALDI-TOF mass spectrometry in the rat brain. Neuro Endocrinol Lett. 2003;24(1-2):9-14.

[58] Yanagisawa K, Shyr Y, Xu BJ, Massion PP, Larsen PH, White BC, et al. Proteomic patterns of tumour subsets in non-small-cell lung cancer. Lancet. 2003;362(9382):433-9.

[59] Garcia DE, Baidoo EE, Benke PI, Pingitore F, Tang YJ, Villa S, et al. Separation and mass spectrometry in microbial metabolomics. Curr Opin Microbiol. 2008;11(3):233-9.

[60] Nordstrom A, Want E, Northen T, Lehtio J, Siuzdak G. Multiple Ionization Mass Spectrometry Strategy Used To Reveal the Complexity of Metabolomics. Anal Chem. 2007 2012/10/08;80(2):421-9.

[61] Bruce SJ, Tavazzi I, Parisod Vr, Rezzi S, Kochhar S, Guy PA. Investigation of Human Blood Plasma Sample Preparation for Performing Metabolomics Using Ultrahigh Performance Liquid Chromatography/Mass Spectrometry. Anal Chem. 2009 2012/10/08;81(9):3285-96.

[62] Duportet X, Aggio R, Carneiro S, Villas-Bôas S. The biological interpretation of metabolomic data can be misled by the extraction method used. Metabolomics. 2012;8(3):410-21.

[63] Vuckovic D. Current trends and challenges in sample preparation for global metabolomics using liquid chromatography–mass spectrometry. Anal Bioanal Chem. 2012;403(6):1523-48.

[64] Rammouz RE, Létisse F, Durand S, Portais J-C, Moussa ZW, Fernandez X. Analysis of skeletal muscle metabolome: Evaluation of extraction methods for targeted metabolite quantification using liquid chromatography tandem mass spectrometry. Anal Biochem. 2010;398(2):169-77.

[65] Geier FM, Want EJ, Leroi AM, Bundy JG. Cross-Platform Comparison of Caenorhabditis elegans Tissue Extraction Strategies for Comprehensive Metabolome Coverage. Anal Chem. 2011 2012/10/08;83(10):3730-6.

[66] Xu Y, Cheung W, Winder CL, Dunn WB, Goodacre R. Metabolic profiling of meat: assessment of pork hygiene and contamination with Salmonella typhimurium. Analyst. 2011;136(3):508-14.

[67] Ji B, Ernest B, Gooding J, Das S, Saxton A, Simon J, et al. Transcriptomic and metabolomic profiling of chicken adipose tissue in response to insulin neutralization and fasting. BMC Genomics. 2012;13(1):441.

[68] Koek M, van der Kloet F, Kleemann R, Koistra T, Verheij E, Hankemeier T. Semi-automated non-target processing in GC × GC-MS metabolomics analysis: applicability for biomedical studies. Metabolomics. 2011;7(1):1-14.

[69] Budczies J, Denkert C, Muller B, Brockmoller S, Klauschen F, Gyorffy B, et al. Remodeling of central metabolism in invasive breast cancer compared to normal breast tissue - a GC-TOFMS based metabolomics study. BMC Genomics. 2012;13(1):334.

[70] Ellinger JJ, Miller DC, Lewis IA, Markley JL. Semiautomated Device for Batch Extraction of Metabolites from Tissue Samples. Analytical Chemistry. 2012 2012/09/07;84(4): 1809-12.

[71] Hallows WC, Yu W, Smith BC, Devires MK, Ellinger JJ, Someya S, et al. Sirt3 Promotes the Urea Cycle and Fatty Acid Oxidation during Dietary Restriction. Mol Cell. 2011;41(2):139-49.

[72] Tan G, Lou Z, Liao W, Zhu Z, Dong X, Zhang W, et al. Potential Biomarkers in Mouse Myocardium of Doxorubicin-Induced Cardiomyopathy: A Metabonomic Method and Its Application. PLoS ONE. 2011;6(11):e27683.

[73] Dunn WB, Bailey NJC, Johnson HE. Measuring the metabolome: current analytical technologies. Analyst. 2005;130(5):606-25.

[74] Issaq HJ, Abbott E, Veenstra TD. Utility of separation science in metabolomic studies. J Sep Sci. 2008;31(11):1936-47.

[75] Trock BJ. Application of metabolomics to prostate cancer. Urol Oncol. 2011;29(5): 572-81.

[76] Nicholson J, Wilson I. Opinion: understanding 'global' systems biology: metabonomics and the continuum of metabolism. Nat Rev Drug Discov. 2003;2(8):668-76.

[77] Raamsdonk LM, Teusink B, Broadhurst D, Zhang N, Hayes A. A functional genomics strategy that uses metabolome data to reveal the phenotype of silent mutations. Nat Biotechnol. 2001;19:45.

[78] Pan Z, Raftery D. Comparing and combining NMR spectroscopy and mass spectrometry in metabolomics. Anal Bioanal Chem. 2007;387(2):525-7.

[79] Martínez-Bisbal M, Esteve V, Martínez-Granados B, Celda B. Magnetic resonance microscopy contribution to interpret high-resolution magic angle spinning metabolomic data of human tumor tissue. J Biomed Biotechnol. 2011;2011.

[80] Cheng LL, Ma MJ, Becerra L, Ptak T, Tracey I, Lackner A, et al. Quantitative neuropathology by high resolution magic angle spinning proton magneticâ€‰resonanceâ€‰â€‰spectroscopy. Proc Natl Acad Sci U S A. 1997 June 10, 1997;94(12):6408-13.

[81] Hu JZ, Rommereim DN, Minard KR, Woodstock A, Harrer BJ, Wind RA, et al. Metabolomics in Lung Inflammation:A High-Resolution 1H NMR Study of Mice Exposedto Silica Dust. Toxicol Mech Methods. 2008;18(5):385-98.

[82] Bollard ME, Murray AJ, Clarke K, Nicholson JK, Griffin JL. A study of metabolic compartmentation in the rat heart and cardiac mitochondria using high-resolution magic angle spinning 1H NMR spectroscopy. FEBS letters. 2003;553(1):73-8.

[83] Tate AR, Foxall PJD, Holmes E, Moka D, Spraul M, Nicholson JK, et al. Distinction between normal and renal cell carcinoma kidney cortical biopsy samples using pattern recognition of 1H magic angle spinning (MAS) NMR spectra. NMR Biomed. 2000;13(2):64-71.

[84] Righi V, Mucci A, Schenetti L, Tosi MR, Grigioni WF, Corti B, et al. Ex vivo HR-MAS Magnetic Resonance Spectroscopy of Normal and Malignant Human Renal Tissues. Anticancer Res. 2007 September-October 2007;27(5A):3195-204.

[85] Chen J-H, Wu YV, DeCarolis P, O'Connor R, Somberg CJ, Singer S. Resolution of creatine and phosphocreatine 1H signals in isolated human skeletal muscle using HR-MAS 1H NMR. Magn Reson Med. 2008;59(6):1221-4.

[86] Grandori R, Santambrogio C, Brocca S, Invernizzi G, Lotti M. Electrospray-ionization mass spectrometry as a tool for fast screening of protein structural properties. Biotechnol J. 2009;4(1):73-87.

[87] Ho C, Lam C, Chan M, Cheung R, Law L, Lit L, et al. Electrospray ionisation mass spectrometry: principles and clinical applications. Clin Biochem Rev. 2003;24(1):3-12.

[88] Kuhara T. Noninvasive human metabolome analysis for differential diagnosis of inborn errors of metabolism. J Chromatogr B. 2007;855(1):42-50.

[89] Chen M, Zhao L, Jia W. Metabonomic Study on the Biochemical Profiles of A Hydrocortisone-Induced Animal Model. J Proteome Res. 2005 2012/10/08;4(6):2391-6.

[90] Dettmer K, Aronov PA, Hammock BD. Mass spectrometry-based metabolomics. Mass Spectrom Rev. 2007;26(1):51-78.

[91] Lee SH, Woo HM, Jung BH, Lee J, Kwon OS, Pyo HS, et al. Metabolomic Approach To Evaluate the Toxicological Effects of Nonylphenol with Rat Urine. Anal Chem. 2007 2012/10/08;79(16):6102-10.

[92] Issaq HJ, Van QN, Waybright TJ, Muschik GM, Veenstra TD. Analytical and statistical approaches to metabolomics research. J Sep Sci. 2009;32(13):2183-99.

[93] Lange E, Tautenhahn R, Neumann S, Gropl C. Critical assessment of alignment procedures for LC-MS proteomics and metabolomics measurements. BMC Bioinformatics. 2008;9(1):375.

[94] Hansen MAE, Villas-Bôas SG, Roessner U, Smedsgaard J, Nielsen J. Data Analysis. Metabolome Analysis: John Wiley & Sons, Inc.; 2006. p. 146-87.

[95] Duran AL, Yang J, Wang L, Sumner LW. Metabolomics spectral formatting, alignment and conversion tools (MSFACTs). Bioinformatics. 2003 November 22, 2003;19(17):2283-93.

[96] Sturm M, Bertsch A, Gropl C, Hildebrandt A, Hussong R, Lange E, et al. OpenMS - An open-source software framework for mass spectrometry. BMC Bioinformatics. 2008;9(1):163.

[97] Teraishi T, Miura K. Toward an in situ phospho-protein atlas: phospho- and site-specific antibody-based spatio-temporally systematized detection of phosphorylated proteins in vivo. BioEssays. 2009;31(8):831-42.

[98] Persson A, Hober S, Uhlen M. A human protein atlas based on antibody proteomics. Curr Opin Mol Ther. 2006;8(3):185-90.

[99] Celis JE, Moreira JMA, Gromova I, Cabezon T, Ralfkiaer U, Guldberg P, et al. Towards discovery-driven translational research in breast cancer. FEBS J. 2005;272(1): 2-15.

[100] Merico D, Gfeller D, Bader G. How to visually interpret biological data using networks. Nat Biotechnol. 2009;Oct;27(10):921-4.

[101] Shannon P, Markiel A, Ozier O, Baliga NS, Wang JT, Ramage D, et al. Cytoscape: a software environment for integrated models of biomolecular interaction networks. Genome Res. 2003 November 1, 2003;13(11):2498-504.

[102] Cline MS, Smoot M, Cerami E, Kuchinsky A, Landys N, Workman C, et al. Integration of biological networks and gene expression data using Cytoscape. Nat Protoc. 2007;2(10):2366-82.

[103] Smoot ME, Ono K, Ruscheinski J, Wang P-L, Ideker T. Cytoscape 2.8: new features for data integration and network visualization. Bioinformatics. 2011 February 1, 2011;27(3):431-2.

New Strategies in Heart Valve Tissue Engineering and Regenerative Medicine

Cutting-Edge Regenerative Medicine Technologies for the Treatment of Heart Valve Calcification

Laura Iop and Gino Gerosa

Additional information is available at the end of the chapter

1. Introduction

An early attempt of designing a valvular device was made already in 1513 by Leonardo da Vinci, who depicted the appearance of a prosthetic aortic valve to be reproduced in glass material [1].

The first real manufacture of valve substitutes goes back to the '50s of the previous century, when the application in heterotopic position of an aortic mechanical valve by Hufnagel and colleagues triggered the beginning of the surgical therapeutic era of valvulopathies [2]. It was however the contribution of Harken, Starr and Edwards to demonstrate the feasibility of orthotopic valve replacement with these early devices [3]. Since then, several mechanical and bioprosthetic replacements have been proposed as valve substitutes. Still, these solutions are not meeting important prerequisites.

Heart valve tissue engineering and, later, tissue-guided regeneration have been proposed to overcome the limitations associated to current valve substitutes. Principles, preclinical and clinical models of each approach are discussed in this chapter, together to the diverse improving strategies for the final achievement of viable and functional aortic valve substitutes.

2. Tissue engineering

The different drawbacks related to commercial replacement devices compromise their durability once in the patient and have shift the attention of cardiac surgeons and biomedical engineers towards a new therapeutic concept: heart valve tissue engineering. The first general definition of this approach has been proposed by Langer and Vacanti, as the *in vitro* creation of a viable tissue by combining separate elements, i.e. cells plus an extracellular matrix (ECM), properly conditioned to attain the correct mature function [4]. This universal paradigm has to be applied also to the reconstruction of the valve tissue. The rationale is to achieve the ability to construct *in vitro* a valve with adequate biomechanical properties, good hemodynamic performance, vital competence, growth/remodelling permissiveness and lack of inflammatory/immunological reactions. Such researches have required the synergistic application of different scientific disciplines, from cell biology to engineering and surgery. *In vitro* valve creation is commonly pursued via two different methods diverging for the starter matrix.

2.1. Biomaterial scaffolds

2.1.1. Polymeric materials

The choice of the ECM scaffold is not only a distinction parameter among diverse approaches, but also essential for the successful realization of tissue-engineered heart valves (TEHVs). ECM is able to establish the necessary 3D configuration and guides cell attachment and structural development of the new tissue.

Synthetic materials have often represented the privileged option in TEHV formulations. Biopolymers as aliphatic polyesters, polyhydroxyalcanoates or different polyurethane compounds have been preferentially employed, providing scaffolds with controllable chemo-physical characteristics as reproducibility, porousness and biodegradability rate. The chosen biomaterials have to respond to important requirements, as good cell-affinity and adequate structural architecture able to sustain the organ mechanics. To enable cell adhesion and spreading in the selected biopolymeric mesh, the modulation of porousness until 90% achievement is recommended [5].

In particular, most of these materials offer a further regenerative advantage also thanks to the good immunotolerance induced in the host body. In fact, after an initial guiding effect, the non-natural material is progressively degraded by colonizing cells, which in turn operate a new matrix synthesis. The process results in a newly produced tissue of completely autologous origin.

First generation polymeric heart valves were designed to overcome the poor durability and excessive wear shown by Teflon fabric-composed substitutes. These more rigid valves, with caged-ball or low-profile design, were based either on metals, like titanium or stellite 21, or on silicone with fixed fabric sewing rings. While metallic devices mostly presented difficulties in the insertion phase, elastomeric ball valves demonstrated less stability in the mid/long-term evaluation [6]. Polyurethanes were lately proposed for their relatively good haemodynamic behaviour especially in contact with blood cells and indeed for their easy manipulable chemical structure [7,8].

Again, biostability represented the major drawback associated to these elastomers together to the high calcification potential: polyester, polyether and polycarbonate urethanes were sequentially suggested for valve fabrication with minor biodegradation, but still insufficient stability [9]. The introduction of further chemical groups and other modifications in the polymer segments has been carried out and is still under study to improve the durability of polyurethane-based devices *in vivo* [8, 10]. In particular, when modified with polyhedral oligomeric silsesquioxanes (POSS), polycarbonate urethane-composed polymeric substitutes offer improved biological and hydrodynamic functioning in respect to bioprosthetic valves [11].

Shinoka et al. firstly reported in 1995 the application of aliphatic polyesters in TEHV formulation. The constructs were composed of polyglactin, polyglycolic acid (PGA) or polylactic acid (PLA) [12-14]. The scarce pliability of these biomaterials did not allow, however, a perfect shape modelling [15]. Conversely, polyhydroxyalcanoates, as polyhydroxyoctanoate (PHA) mixed or not with poly-4-hydroxybutyrate (PH4B), have demonstrated better thermoplastic proficiencies: a polyester group combined with bacterial-derived hydroxyacids is the chemical composition of these last polymers [16,17].

Polystyrene/polyisobutylene compounds were also developed for cardiovascular structure fabrication, showing superior resistance to the high environmental heart valve stresses [18].

Novel promising biopolymers are currently tested to better mimic chemo-physical properties of native heart valves: *inter alia*, polyvinyl alcohol-bacterial cellulose-based hydrogels can be opportunely modelled for a broad range of tuneable mechanical properties [19].

Contemporary procedures for polymeric aortic heart valve fabrication must rely on optimal tricuspid design, used as template for successive valve production. Multiple dip-coatings into poorly concentrated polymeric solutions have as major drawback inhomogeneous tissue thickness.

Another manufacturing technique combines the use of solvent and thermal treatment to properly shape polymeric films in a desired arrangement. Tri-dimensional models, additionally created through direct laser 'recording' in photo-sensitive polymers, act as blueprint for successive casting of hot biopolymers, which will assume the chosen conformation during chilling [20]. Similarly, injection systems assisted by hot/cold baths can be applied to the same aim [21].

2.1.2. Decellularized extracellular matrices

Despite the evident ability of these biopolymers to undergo cell remodelling, a proper mature, cell-operated tissue architectural reconstitution might require a chemo-mechanical stimulation for a long time. Often, to the best of their biostability and mechanical behaviour, biopolymeric heart valves do not develop a trilaminate structure and remarkably, the elastin network in leaflet layer *ventricularis* and wall *media* can be inconsistently achieved.

On this account, another research stream inside the heart valve tissue engineering approach prefers the usage of animal-derived decellularized scaffolds. A suitable decellularization procedure allows the removal of xenogeneic cells, maintaining all the fibre composition and distribution of the natural ECM. In addition, as further advantage in respect to commonly produced bioprostheses, the treatment with glutaraldehyde can be skipped following the absence of xenogeneic cells. The avoidance of this cytotoxic agent enables remodelling processes to occur by providing a cell-friendly milieu, where viable engrafting elements are able to accomplish synthetic and contractile functions with extracellular matrix continuous remodelling.

Cell-freed natural matrices can be realised by means of several methods: trypsin-based enzymatic and detergent decellularization procedures are only two examples of the proposed treatments. Most decellularizing protocols take advantage of a combined mechanical and chemical tissue handling to ease cell removal.

Grauss and colleagues interestingly compared various protocols currently applied to decellularize porcine aortic heart valves and verified that the combination of trypsin and Triton X-100, an anionic detergent, could be able to provoke a loss of matrix integrity [22]. Not only the enzymatic treatment with trypsin can induce elastin defragmentation, but also the use of sodium dodecyl sulphate can end out with a similar deleterious effect [23]. Conversely, the adoption of sodium cholate- and deoxycholate-based methods allows the achievement of fully nude matrices, able to be cell-recolonized *in vitro* and/or *in vivo* even for clinical implantation [23-28].

Besides native heart valves, another natural tissue has been regarded with attention for the production of animal-derived acellular scaffolds. Pericardium has been extensively applied in bioprosthetic manufacturing thanks to its biocompatible, mechanical and biological properties, entirely suitable for long-lasting heart valve substitutes. More often of bovine origin, this tissue partially differs from a native heart valve for its low cellularity and extremely compacted ECM, raising the question on which decellularization process can best convey the optimal outcome [29]. With regards to this tissue, the comparative analysis developed by Yang et al. revealed a superior decellularizing and preserving effect of enzymatic/detergent treatment or trypsin alone on Triton X100/sodium-deoxycholate-based extraction.

Sodium cholate demonstrates instead a less aggressive behaviour towards the pericardial tissue providing analogous results to its application on native semilunar heart valves [30].

Together to the elimination of xenogeneic cells, a variable depletion in the glycosaminoglycan (GAG) content is usually observed after decellularization procedure. GAGs play a significant viscoelastic role by mitigating valve stress during flexion: their highly hydrophilic nature allows, in fact, the hydration of the *spongiosa* layer in this cycle phase. Indeed, several biological processes appear to be modulated by GAGs, therefore their loss has profound consequences in the mechanical behaviour and in the cellular functions of successively repopulated scaffolds [31]. Associated to GAG content is also the hydrated state of the tissue: a reduction in hydration following decellularization can induce collapse of collagen fibres and introduces a less suitable environment for colonizing cells [32], 33].

While GAG and water preservation is pivotal, an opposite decellularizing effect is expected as far as DNA/RNA content. Similar to cell membrane residues, the phosphate groups of the nucleic acid backbone behave as powerful calcification triggers [34]. Aspecific endonucleases are often applied as efficient tools for the complete removal of nucleic acid debris [25-26].

Extracting processes should be hence developed ad hoc depending on the specific tissue to use as starter matrix, otherwise adversely affecting the original mechanical and bioactive properties of the natural ECM.

In addition, the realization of viable constructs must not be regardless of detergent scaffold retention. Incomplete washout of detergents could induce the creation of a toxic microenvironment for engrafting cells. *In vitro* evaluations should be critically performed in respect to each decellularization procedure currently applied [unpublished data, 35, 36].

2.2. Cells

Cells embody the second key-component of a TEHV: it is this element that provides viability to the ECM and consequently permits its remodelling and maturation towards a functional organ. Furthermore, the use of cell elements of allogeneic or autologous source can prevent from non-self reactions towards synthetic biomaterials or decellularized natural tissues.

2.2.1. Differentiated cells

For a similar selection principle operated by those researchers preferring the more committed animal-derived matrix, endothelial cells, fibroblasts, myofibroblasts and/or smooth muscle cells isolated from vascular or valve conduits have been extensively utilized to seed nude matrices and obtain both endothelial coverage with antithrombotic activity and tissue repopulation [24, 37].

Endothelial cells (ECs) were first applied in the '90s to test the feasibility of endothelialisation on Biomer and Mitrathane thromboresistant polyurethane ureas in response to physiological shear stress [38]. Commonly harvested from cardiovascular structures, as adult saphenous or more immature umbilical veins, endothelial cells were also seeded onto bioprosthetic heart valves to increase their low thrombogenic properties [39]. In an analogous fashion, a previous endothelial coverage on harshly decellularized native tissues can avert *in vivo* thromboembolic events, related to basal membrane damage/loss resulting in collagen fibres exposure.

More frequently, ECs were employed in combination to other cell elements, as for example myo/fibroblasts. A sequential seeding of fibroblasts and ECs was demonstrated effective in the *in vitro* creation of tissue-engineered valve constructs endowed with appropriate cell topography [40]. However, the district of fibroblast cell origin is able to significantly affect the degree of recellularization with better outcome associated to the usage of arterial myofibroblasts rather than of dermal fibroblasts [41, 42].

Valve fibroblasts, known as valve interstitial cells (VICs) for their cusp origin, have been successfully employed as sole repopulating cell population, exhibiting unmodified proliferative and synthetic abilities once engrafted in decellularized scaffolds [24].

While dissimilar to VICs, smooth muscle cells of vascular derivation (vSMCs) can be chemically manipulated with epidermal growth factor (EGF), platelet-derived growth factor (PDGF) and transforming growth factor beta-1 (TGF-beta1) for a phenotypic switch towards leaflet cells [43].

2.2.2. Stem cells and progenitors

Marrow stromal cells, umbilical cord myofibroblasts and progenitor cells, chorionic villi-derived cells and placenta or amniotic fluid progenitors share not only the potential to transdifferentiate in valve phenotypes after appropriate stimulation, but are also associated to several positive aspects, making them particularly attractive for bioengineering applications [25, 44-46].

Stem and progenitor cells are now of relatively safe isolation from foetal and neonatal tissues, such as amniotic fluid, chorionic villi or umbilical cord. Most of them demonstrate mesenchymal properties, potentiated by higher cell plasticity in relation to their immature state. The embryonic-like phenotype, possessed by these early precursors, can be 'frozen' in cell banks at its genuine isolation state without further differentiation/maturation and loss of stemness [45, 47-51].

While neonatal progenitor cells can be cryopreserved at birth in view of a future use, adult bone marrow-derived cells, and especially their mesenchymal compartment, can be easily harvested from the same cardiopathic patient for a fully autologous TEHV or even employed for the creation of allogeneic constructs [25], with no risk of cell rejection thanks to their beneficial immunomodulatory properties [52, 53]. MSCs reside virtually in all post-natal body departments, as for example adipose tissue or dermis [54, 55]. MSCs obtained from bone marrow (BM-MSCs) offer some advantages over other stem or progenitor cells in terms of their prospects for use in routine clinical practice, i.e. relatively simple protocols for their isolation, storage and *in vitro* expansion and a surprising phenotypic resemblance to valve cells [56, 57]. Indeed, their phenotypic convertibility into ECs, fibroblasts/myofibroblasts and SMCs might allow in a single step-seeding procedure to reconstruct the cell geographic distribution typical of valve cusps [25, 47, 58-60]. hBM-MSCs display a repertoire of molecules that may be relevant to their adhesion and penetration in synthetic or decellularized scaffolds, including b1-integrin (which plays a pivotal role by mediating cell–ECM interactions), CD54, CD105 and CD44 (which act cooperatively in cell homing via binding to hyaluronan, the major non-protein glycosaminoglycan of the ECM) [25].

Another cell type with attractive potential for heart valve tissue engineering is the equally rare, but more easily harvestable circulating fraction of endothelial progenitor cells (EPCs). Commonly isolated from the peripheral blood with a simple venous drawing (i.e. umbilical vein), these progenitors have a high proliferation activity and can commit to transform into a mesenchymal phenotype, reminiscent of the endothelial-mesenchyme transition during embryonic valve development [61-63].

2.2.3. Bioreactors

Scaffolds and cells do not represent alone sufficient components for a successful TEHV, but conditioning is indispensable to achieve a perfect maturation of the construct prior to implantation. This last step in manufacturing a viable valve can be guaranteed by the use of bioreactors able to submit it to physiological pressures and flow [64, 65]. Besides mechanical stimulation, the addition of specific chemicals can further train tissue-engineered valve constructs towards their proper functionality [66].

Firstly developed devices were very simple systems based on common or modified petri supports, in which TEHVs could be statically cultured.

The introduction of a dynamic conditioning was hence operated to improve cell engraftment and differentiation through the assemblage of two chambers: one for lodging the valvular construct, the other mimicking ventricular function. Connected to an air pump, the ventricle-like compartment can exert defined hydrodynamic settings in terms of flow and pressure. Diaphragms of different materials, as for example silicone, separate the two chambers and are displaced periodically by air influx [16].

The small size of the device has been primarily regarded for ensuring long-term culturing in defined temperature/gaseous environment. A compact system can, in fact, easily fit in an incubator, where CO_2 saturation, humidity and temperature are already set for cell culture [16]. To this aim, the implementation with gas sensors directly placed in the device can result in a superior chemical control of CO_2, N_2, O_2, glucose and lactate [67, 68].

Single specific mechanical stresses were successively applied to better induce tissue matura-tion and, furthermore, to activate endothelial-mesenchymal transformation. Laminar flow-, flexure- and cyclic strain-based stimulations could have profound effects on mechanical stiffness, collagen synthesis and alignment in the tissue-engineered valve [69-71].

A three-chamber bioreactor was developed by Sierad et al. in 2010 to respect previously indicated criteria and other important conditions, as easy valve mounting, physiological stimulation (transvalvular pressures, pulsatile forces, flow rate, frequency, stroke rate and shear stresses) and full control over parameters. Absence of toxic or degradable fabrication materials, maximum visibility, together to ease of sterilization and waste removal, further increase the yield of repeatable results. Compliance and reservoir tanks with sterile filters for gas exchange, one-way and resistance valves, pressure transducers, a web-cam and a ventilator pump complement this efficient system [72].

2.2.4. In Vitro applications

The reconstruction of a heart valve tissue in a plate dish was first endeavoured by the Bostonian teams of R. Langer, J.P. Vacanti and J.E. Jr Mayer, who published in 1995 the results of this pioneering work [12]. Vascular cells, outgrown from ovine neonatal femoral artery explants, were divided into two populations by LDL selection. LDL-negative SMCs/fibroblasts and LDL-positive ECs were sequentially seeded onto polyglycolic acid/polyglatin scaffolds in a 2-week-long procedure. Later, different cells and polymers were combined in the most efficient valve tissue combinations [41, 73, 74]. The introduction of PHAs, PH4B/PHAs and pulsatile flow conditioning in a bioreactor for heart valve construction allowed the attainment of more pliable scaffolds. After dynamic seeding, cells demonstrated to be actively involved in GAG and collagen synthesis, leading to an autologous replacement of the polymeric mesh [16, 75, 76]. PH4B/PHA became, in particular, the most promising scaffold for several successful TEHV approaches relying on diverse stem cells [44, 45, 49, 77-79].

Elastomeric poly(glycerol sebacate) scaffolds treated with multiple coating strategies based on ECM-derived proteins allowed adhesion and transdifferentiation of EPCs [61, 80].

In respect to the application of bioabsorbable polymers, the other TEHV modality, founded on natural ECMs, was experimented some years later. After the development of various decellularizing treatments, the combination with differentiated cells, as ECs and VICs, was able to generate directly *in vitro* by static conditioning surrogates of early heart valve tissues [24, 81]. As well as polymeric TEHVs, cell-repopulated decellularized ECMs were positively remodelled after dynamic stimulation with proper mechanical signals. In this case, actually, also elastin content was demonstrated to increase [82-84].

The usage of stem cells as cell source for the engineering of plain ECMs led to even better *in vitro* outcomes. Multipotent differentiation potential of human bone marrow MSCs can represent the ideal characteristic for complete repopulation of natural valve matrices. MSC engrafting ability was evaluated on decellularized porcine and human scaffolds. In both considered interactions, stem cells were able to adhere, spread within the ECM and transdifferentiate towards typical valve phenotypes (ECs, VICs). Collagen, GAG and elastin synthesis was indeed activated in engrafted cells, which tend to distribute similarly to the original valve cell topography. It was, however, the homotypic combination to better favour MSC-to-SMC conversion in the *ventricularis* layer [25].

3. Tissue regeneration

TEHV is not the sole approach investigated to obtain new viable valve devices: tissue-guided regeneration has been proposed as an alternative method for *in vivo* direct tissue reconstruction, by exploiting ECM instructive abilities. Once eliminated the allogeneic or xenogeneic cell component through decellularizing treatment, the fibre mesh still maintains biomechanical proficiency assuring in vivo prompt restoration of hydrodynamic performance. Furthermore, in the body, conceived as physiological bioreactor, naked natural scaffolds recruit recipient's cells thanks to their chemo-attractant properties. Positive aspects associated with this option should be identified in the possibility to construct autologous-like tissues, by skipping difficultly controllable procedures of cell seeding and chemo-mechanical stimulation *in vitro*.

Among the first experimental evidences, biomaterials, as patches of pure type I collagen, have been successfully introduced in the therapy of ischemic myocardium: once applied to the diseased tissue, the collagen sponge attracts progenitors and less undifferentiated cells, which in turn or alone are able to fully colonize it and start a cardiovascular transdifferentiation [85]. It is noteworthy to remember that these patches, either synthetic or cell-purified from biological tissues, have found FDA-approved applications as haemostatics or for skin reconstruction with excellent results [86].

A further surprising element for a positive consideration of this method has been given by Campbell and colleagues, who were able to obtain a tubular cell construct by implanting a polymeric tube in the animal peritoneal cavity. The newly formed tissue, pulled from the tube, had anatomical and histological resemblance to a quite mature blood vessel and it could be hence considered an optimal vascular substitute [87].

Also offering the opportunity to create tissue banks for ready-to-use devices at the moment of clinical need, the investigation on tissue-guided regenerated heart valves (TGRHVs) has particularly increased in recent years.

4. Preclinical and clinical applications of tissue engineering and tissue regeneration approaches

The preclinical proof-of-principle of TEHVs as valve substitutes has been demonstrated in the lamb model already with the polymeric bioconctructs firstly produced *in vitro* [12]. Vascular cell-repopulated polyglycolic acid/polyglactin matrices were implanted in the pulmonary position up to 21 days. Function assessment by Doppler echocardiography demonstrated no stenosis or regurgitation signs, even if a substantial leaflet thickness was reported.

Each subsequent modification in scaffold or cell types, as introduced by the same group, was generally tested *in vivo*, validating progressive functional improvements in transplanted lambs or sheep [41, 73, 74].

Further TEHVs applications in preclinical models were substantially based on the use of P4HB/ PHA with few exceptions, as electrospun polydioxanone [88]. In combination with stem cells of various stromal origins, P4HB/PHA-formulated engineered tissues were evaluated in a long-term animal model, showing replacement of the exogenous matrix after nearly 8 weeks *in vivo* [16].

A MSC-engineered mesh of polyglycolic and polylactic acids was evaluated as autologous pulmonary valve replacement in juvenile sheep. The good performance of this *in vitro* generated construct could be appreciated in a long follow-up of 4 months with restoration of a native-like pulmonary heart valve [59].

Despite biomechanical stimulation induced optimal results in term of cell viability and differentiation almost independently from the cytotype utilised, combined polymer/cell-based efforts to obtain a valve substitute have usually failed in recreating the fibre arrangement of a native ECM. In fact, trilaminate distribution of collagens, GAGs and elastin has been reported only in few cases [88].

A finely organized ECM already exists in native heart valves and can be conserved after cell removal. After decellularization with trypsin/EDTA, heart valve conduits were seeded with ECs and myofibroblasts. Allogenically implanted in orthotopic position, they performed adequately. Ex vivo tissue analyses revealed surface endothelium reconstitution, myofibro-blasts-mediated repopulation and ECM synthesis with no signs of inflammation and calcifi-cation [89].

Sole ECs were used to obtain *in vitro* endothelium coverage of ovine acellular scaffolds. After 6 months of *in vivo* evaluation, explanted tissues presented no calcifications as assessed by atomic absorption spectrometry [90].

Lutter et al. coated stented pulmonary valves with small interstinal submucosa, both pig-derived and decellularized. These scaffolds, dynamically seeded *in vitro* with ECs and myofibroblasts, were deployed in orthotopic position by means of transcatheter assistance. Valve performance and macroscopic appearance demonstrated to be normal during *in vivo* and post-mortem evaluation [91].

Despite rare reports of deleterious therapeutic effects associated to TEHVs' implantation in humans [92], clinical application of these substitutes, attained by combination of acellular scaffolds and ECs or EPCs, reached already more than 10 years of experience with proved function and absence of calcifications [93, 94].

Another modality of heart valve tissue engineering has been more recently proposed. It is realized by means of a one-phase intraoperative approach. The rational of such a strategy rises from the necessity of a ready-to-apply TEHV, when the surgical therapy has to be promptly adopted with no time for *in vitro* cell seeding and bioreactor conditioning. Weber and colleagues implanted such prepared TEHVs in the RVOT of non-human primates through minimally invasive, transapical procedures. These polymeric trileaflet heart valves have been just seeded with unselected autologous bone marrow cells before the crimping necessary for valve insertion. After one month, the completely remodelled valves were still functioning [95]. Similarly conceived TEHVs demonstrated patency also in the aortic position, being able to sustain the higher pressure regimen of the systemic circulation [96,97]. Another *in situ* TEHV delivery has been applied by Vincentelli et al, by injecting mesenchymal stem cells into a just deployed decellularized heart valve. As element of comparison, they used acellular scaffolds: these ones showed equal performance and reconstructed tissue [98]. However, these are no more TE-, but TGRHVs.

The first attempt of tissue-guided heart valve regeneration has been challenged by the extensive work of Konertz and colleagues, who, moving from the classical paradigm of tissue engineering, compared the two methods. Common for each approach is only the application of the same decellularizing detergent, deoxy-cholic acid. By using an allogeneic decellularized valve for the reconstruction of the right ventricular outflow tract in sheep, they ascertained there was no need to seed the scaffolds prior to implantation, after the good repopulation observed at six months [99]. Follow-up of the valve function revealed increase in the annulus diameter in response to animal growth [100]. As further step to the clinic, they developed a xenogeneic model again with substitution of the autologous pulmonary valve, transferred in aortic position during Ross intervention. They tested porcine decellularized valves, called Matrix P, in a pig-to-sheep interaction. By comparison to sheep cryopreserved allografts, decellularized porcine valves demonstrated better valvular performance, decreased calcific potential and feasible tissue regeneration [101]. Another group compared the haemodynamic function of valve allografts, either cryopreserved and/or decellularized, verifying a reduced calcification tendency in the sheep implanted with decellularized matrices [102].

Equivalently promising results have been reported for the implantation of Triton X100/sodium cholate-decellularized allogeneic valves in the longest preclinical follow-up ever realized for a TGRHV. Evaluated in Vietnamese minipigs as RVOT replacements in heterotopic position, these acellular, alpha-gal-free certified valve substitutes have demonstrated good haemodynamic performance with low transvalvular gradients in a 15-month-long *in vivo* observation.

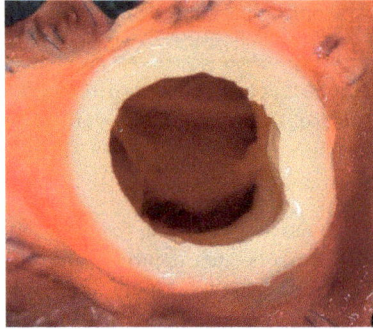

Figure 1. *In vivo* tissue-regenerated heart valve after 12 months of implantation in Vietnamese minipig

No calcification events could be appreciated within engrafted tissues by trans-thoracic echocardiography: these macroscopic observations found ex vivo confirmation by undetectable calcific foci after von Kossa staining. In addition, no inflammatory or immunogenic cells could be observed. A progressive repopulating process occurred in implanted valves: most tissues were endothelialised and engrafted by rare stem cells and numerous myo/fibroblasts, both highly proliferating and suggesting the onset of a smooth muscle cell conversion. Provision of oxygen and nutrients was again established by a dense capillary network and re-created vasa vasorum. Moreover, re-innervation aspects were also identified [26, 27].

Acellular allologous conduits were also favourably approved as aortic valve substitutes in a sheep model [103].

Few unfavourable outcomes with a TGRHV have been seldom disclosed. Two groups of heart valves, cryopreserved or decellularized and treated with an anticalcinosis devitalisation (digitonin and ethylenediaminetetraacetic acid), were tested in dogs by substituting an aorta fragment with the non-coronary sinus of the cusp allografts: albeit the lack of immune infiltrate in inserted decellularized specimens in contrast to cryopreserved ones, no engrafting of recipient 's cells was observed in both cases [104].

The reasons for such different findings should first be searched in the used decellularization procedure for TGRHV production.

Apart from animal studies, allollogeneic TGR approaches were also applied in humans with optimal outcomes. Decellularized allogeneic valves, as obtained with the deoxycholic acid procedure, were evaluated in 68 patients in the medium term for RVOT reconstruction in Ross aortic valve substitution. Up to 4 years, Costa et al. observed very low mortality (1, 4 %), a good valve function, both comparable with the cryopreserved allografts used as control, and a progressive engraftment – even if discontinuous [105].

TGR has been further practised as an alternative RVOT replacement strategy for human paediatric and young patients with confident results in a follow-up of more than 5 years. Freedom from re-intervention, lower transvalvular gradients and adaptive dimensional modifications in response to somatic growth have been reported from *in vivo* early-term comparison with pulmonary allografts [106]. In a just slighter observational window, allogeneic pulmonary valves were evaluated in a multicentre study with 342 patients undergoing RVOT reconstruction: improvement in haemodynamic function was registered for implanted valves and suggested to be related to decreased tissue antigenicity [107]. After a 5-year follow-up in 48 patients, Burch et al. put the accent on the relevance of the economic burden, related to the use of decellularized cryopreserved allografts in respect to their untreated counterparts [108].

Although good reported outcomes open the route for a promising treatment of heart valve failure, it will be imperative to reconsider therapeutic effects in a longer clinical evaluation, by taking into account also socio-economic considerations.

A debated note is, however, represented by the clinical application of unseeded decellularized xenogeneic tissues as valvular replacement solutions. *In vivo* infiltration of tissue-engineered Matrix P heart valves by human cells, not related to inflammatory or immune system, was observed in some explanted specimens [109]. These relevancies were at the basis of the pure Matrix P adoption in the clinical arena. Although favourable performance and lack of xenogeneic tissue-mediated immune reactions have been demonstrated by the same valve-manufacturing group in respect to current RVOT substitutes [110, 111], controversial issues were evidenced after implantation of the same Matrix P valves in other studies [112, 113].

These reports, together with the dramatic results of the early failed Synergraft decellularized valves [114], should lower the speed in the human application of xenogeneic tissues-derived devices, moving a step backward to more robust human-like preclinical trials, as non-human primate animal models.

5. New insights on heart valve regenerative medicine

5.1. Immunogenicity of xenogeneic tissues

Allotransplantation has been widely consolidated as valid therapy to rescue a failed vital function, but the shortage of human cells, tissues and organs dramatically increases the waiting lists for replacement: in 2006, Eurotransplant referred almost 16.000 patients were attending to receive a substitute, while in the United States these ones were reaching the number of 90.000 [115]. The numerical entity of these registers is expected to sensitively grow during the near future. Surely, the employ of unlimitedly supplied, animal-derived organs could allow an immediate intervention to recover the lost function and in combination with bioengineering methodologies, might favour the achievement of human-like organs throughout strictly controlled fabrication procedures. So far, animal tissues fixed in glutaraldehyde have been the reserve to exploit at the time of clinical need. However, this should be no longer considered as viable route in accordance to vitality maintenance, above all for those organs that cannot perform a correct function in absence of a proper cell physiology. The use of non-human sources is accompanied by a major raising concern for a broad clinical application, i.e. the immunological barrier. For a donor-receiver mismatched allocombination, the most serious medical issue is the inability of accommodation and therefore the onset of chronic rejection, whose main manifestation, in the case of heart transplant, is graft vascular disease. This allotransplantation drawback is characterized by an unchanged gravity and entity in respect to 40 years ago, when this research line started to be investigated as possible treatment of end-stage pathologies [116].

A peculiar atherosclerotic process interests the heart transplant with few calcifications, but increased cellularity and extracellular matrix deposition at the entire intimal level with a concentric distribution [117].

A similar event occurs in the xenotransplantation approach, where an even more severe expression is attended. Furthermore, in addition to a chronic response, antibody-mediated hyperacute rejection represents a dramatic hurdle to early-term xenograft survival, when a trans-species interaction has to be considered. By developing in a time period from minutes to hours in the pig-to-primate combination, hyperacute rejection, commonly defined as HAR, is a typical humoral immune response in vascularized organs with deposition of xenoreactive natural antibodies and complement activation [118]. Pig-to-primate xenotransplantation has properly enabled to discover the progression of delayed immunological answer to the cardiac graft (DXR): besides a strong humoral activity, acute cellular infiltrates and endothelium activation seriously compromise the function of newly transplanted organ [119].

5.1.1. Alpha-gal and other xenoantigens

Not well known - and in the last years very debated- is the real immunological trigger able to cause the complete loss of the xenograft during time. Probably the prompts of this phenomenon are not to be found in a unique opponent, but in more factors, which alone or in cooperation provoke it. One of the most powerful antigens is definitely Galα1-3Galβ1-4GlcNAc, commonly identified as α-Gal. This oligosaccharide is a component of the glycoproteins and glycolipids, displayed on the surface of vascular endothelial cells in all mammals except apes, Old World monkeys and humans, unable to metabolize it for evolutionary gene silencing of the related enzyme α1-3-Galactosyltransferase [120, 121]. Reaching an expression concentration of at least 10^7 epitopes per pig cell, alpha-gal is recognized by human cells in a highly specific pattern soon after birth similarly to ABO antibodies. In fact, microorganisms colonizing or transiting through the intestinal flora express it on their surface and due also to the dietary use of animal-derived nourishment, 1% of serum circulating IgGs are specifically directed against this epitope with a quite pure protective role against parasite and viral attacks [122, 123]. Already at the end of the previous century, a restricted but well developed body of evidence considered alpha-gal as an immunogenic suspect, but it was only more recent the full demonstration of its causative role in HAR, by studying the pig-to-primate interaction

[124]. Other important observations have been made available with this research about the amount of natural anti-pig antibodies in humans and their specific subclasses. At least 85% of humoral anti-pig players are specific for alpha-gal and belong to IgG and IgM classes: more recurrently, IgMs tend to deposit on the graft endothelium [124-126]. Anti-Gal antibodies have been shown to contribute both to HAR and lately DXR, if an initial tolerance regimen has been introduced [127].

Hence, the issue is unquestionably alarming for new therapeutic approaches of biomedicine using xenogeneic biological materials.

In order to face this problem, different strategies have been developed just from the observation of the glyco-composition differences between pig and human cells. In the endothelium of both species, N-acetyllactosamine and sialic acid are expressed, but the human one –as previously mentioned- lacks alpha-gal and is characterized by the presence of ABH-Galβ1-4GlcNAcβ1-R (ABO system) and a supplementary sugar, NeuGca2-3Galβ1-4GlcNAcβ1-R (N-glycolylilneur-aminic acid). Since the complete elimination of anti-Gal IgMs resulted in null complement-mediated cytotoxicity by human serum without side effects on the IgG counterpart, various methods to deplete the whole range of anti-alpha gal antibodies have been tested.

First xenotransplantation experiments have been started in the 1960s, when the existence of alpha-gal and its antibodies was still ignored, however a decrease in xenoreaction could be achieved by perfusing the recipient's blood in a donor-specific organ, such as the liver, possessing high immunoadsorbent ability. Analogously, other depletion procedures have ameliorated the survival of the xenogeneic tissue, even if still at the initial developmental phases: plasma exchange and plasma perfusion through column systems based on specific protein interaction or on immunoaffinity could extend implant durability, but rarely for more than one month due to failed establishment of accommodation.

A more direct method, independent from external devices, is the intravenous approach based on similar affinity principles. Infused antibodies precisely targeting idiotypes of anti-gal humoral effectors, immunoglobulin (IVIG) or even oligosaccharides behave as silencers, by blocking –at least quite completely- any possible immunological response against alpha-gal. In the case of IVIG, it has been postulated an indirect beneficial role through the acceleration of IgG physiological catabolism and inhibition of macrophage function [126].

A further procedure inducing an accommodation state can be identified in the suppression of anti-gal cell effectors, by full depletion of B-lymphocytes and plasma cells. Methods proposed for this purpose are irradiation, pharmacological therapy, anti-B cells specific antibodies (mAbs) and immunotoxins. The irradiation of the entire body with the clinically used dose of 300 cGy does not result in a lethal condition, but provokes a transient B-cell ablation, whose effects are therefore time-limited. The administration of mAbs underlies a more selective way of action and benefits from clinical experiences completed in the haemato-oncological field. Anti-CD20 mAbs, for instance, have been used to treat baboons for 4 weeks: at the end of this course, a complete deficiency in B cells could be maintained both in bone marrow and peripheral blood for at least 3 months. A combination of immunotoxins, such as ricin A and sapporin, and mAbs can promote better ablation results [126]. In the transplantation setting, a wide line of investigation has been directed to discover chemical agents able to perform immunosuppressive effects. Even in xenografting, this kind of therapy seems to have a supporting role for other strategies in order to induce accommodation.

Cyclophosphamide is one of the most common pharmacological agents with this task: in heart transplant, function prolongation induced by this drug is positive without doubt, but many risks are associated with its permanent use, as leukopenia [128].

Alkylating agents, as melphalan, or DNA polymerase blockers, as zidovudine, or even enzymatic inhibitors, as methotrexate, have been analogously experimented with different results. The first ones are particularly interesting because they are quite the unique to target plasma cells. Although reducing anti-alpha gal IgGs, suppressive effects of zidovudine are not so important in a prospective clinical use. Methotrexate, on the contrary, appears to be a valid agent if added to other B cell-destroying therapies. In new-born baboons, mycophenolate mofetil (MMF), an inhibitor of the purine synthesis, has allowed, as therapeutic adjuvant, to prolong the survival of transplanted porcine hearts of at least the double time in respect to non-treated animals [129]. These results in themselves could not seem particularly appealing if compared to the effects of other drugs, but MMF is able to offer a similar efficacy in the face of lack of side consequences and seems very promising for future uses on xenotransplanted patients.

A special mention should be addressed to a therapeutic approach based on a quite new soluble glycoconjugate, GAS914, in combination with different drugs (among which MMF too). GAS594 has demonstrated a constant proficiency in lowering the titres of anti-gal IgGs and IgMs, and hence prolonging durability of transgenic porcine hearts transplanted in cynomolgus monkeys [130].

All these methods search to abate the recipient's response to this carbohydrate, but generally a certain refractoriness does not allow a long permanence of the xenograft and consequently provokes the inability to maintain the organ function [126].

5.1.2. Animal humanization

Alpha-gal-induced rejection could be possibly avoided also throughout the modulation of the donor tissue, i.e. by bioengineering the animal donor for elimination of antigenicity sources. Gene engineering techniques enable to introduce human genes directly in the animal genome. So-generated porcine transgenic cell lines expressing human α1, 2-fucosyltransferase display in their cell membranes more universal donor O antigens than alpha-gal epitopes, therefore evoke decreased antibody reactivity [131]. Genetically induced human decay-accelerating factor (hDAF) expression in animal grafts plays an inhibitory role in the onset of HAR [132]. Nevertheless, more incisive approaches are gene knocking down or out of α1, 3-galactosyltransferase (Galt). When transplanted in heterotopic position into immunosuppressed baboons, Galt-KO porcine hearts could survive *in vivo* for at least 6 months with graft surviving at least HAR, but failing for later complications [133].

5.1.3. Decellularization strategies

Xenoantigens are commonly accepted to be cell-derived, so the removal of membranes, where these epitopes are displayed, should definitely circumvent xenoreactions. Such a perspective could particularly fit the case of engineered arterial vessels or heart valves, based on decellularized tissues. When the first human paediatric implantations of plain porcine heart valves, produced in an industrialized and controlled manner, were performed, a severe inflammatory/ immune response provoked premature graft failure [114]. These dramatic events could be attributed to an incomplete cell removal: the same Authors imputed in residual alpha-Gal the responsibility of observed HAR occurrences and later, suggested the use of the detergent IGEPAL CA-630 for total extraction and correctly wash-out from treated heart valves [134].

More recently, clinical evaluations by Bloch et al. have revealed no IgG-mediated, but minor IgM-related responses towards decellularized valves in respect to common bioprostheses [111].

It is undeniably important to improve decellularization strategies for alpha-gal removal. *Ex vivo* investigations on bovine and porcine valve tissues revealed that alpha-Gal is not only expressed at the endothelial level of the leaflet surface coverage, but also by ECs lining the arterioles' vascular lumen at the cusp base [25]. Also some stromal cells in the *interstitium* display this antigen on their cell membrane [134].

Particular attention should be addressed to validate techniques used for alpha-gal revelation. The isolectin BSI-B4, commonly suggested in the literature as detector, gives consistent results only for fresh specimens, but displays an aspecific affinity when applied to decellularized leaflets. The affinity binding of BSI-B4 towards glucidic molecules contained in alpha-Gal epitopes is less stable than the link achieved by immunodetection with the highly specific antibody M86 [25].

For future applications in this field, implantable valve substitutes should be certified for alpha-gal subtraction. Furthermost, for the good manufacture practice of therapeutic strategies based on decellularized extracellular matrices, it would be of paramount importance to rely on specific assays able to quantitatively detect the residual amount of alpha-gal xenoantigens (i.e. M86-based alpha-gal ELISA test) [25, 135, 136].

5.1.4. Decellularized scaffolds obtained from tissue-engineered constructs

A completely new approach to overcome xenograft/allograft-related immunogenicity has been recently proposed, by drastically bypassing the use of non-human tissues. Dijkam et al. decellularized a previously tissue-engineered heart valve and demonstrated the feasibility of an *in vitro* regeneration guided by the acellular ECM. First, TEHVs were obtained by seeding vascular cells on poly-4-hydroxybutyrate/polyglycolic acid scaffolds and by dynamic conditioning. Then, cell removal was operated using a detergent-based treatment (Triton X100, sodium deoxycholate and EDTA), followed by endonuclease digestion. Decellularized matrices were consequently repopulated with MSCs and tested for haemodynamic performance through a simulated transapical implantation. Mechanical characteristics of acellular scaffolds were also evaluated. Considerably, obtained scaffolds could be conserved for up to 18 months without modifying their bioactivity and biomechanical properties [137].

While representing an absolutely novel therapeutic concept to solve immunologic issues, it is associated to some significant drawbacks. The procedure to generate such a fully biocompatible scaffold is quite long, complicated and depending on multiple conditionings.

By the way, by exploiting a controlled large-scale industrial production, it would be possible to manufacture off-the-shelf valve substitutes. The major limitation is represented, indeed, by the immature nature of fabricated scaffolds. As in other tissue engineering-based solutions, the synthesized ECM, rich in collagen and GAGs, risks to be deficient in resilience following the absence of an elastin network.

5.2. Mimicking aortic valve formation

5.2.1. Valve cell progenitors: Possible surrogates and gene engineering for their generation

In the development of cardiac valves, the endocardial cushions appear to be the primordial of the valvular leaflets and the membranous septa: they derive from regionalized expansions of extracellular matrix between cardiomyocyte sheets and endocardial cells of the cardiac tube. A subset of endothelial cells acquires specific abilities of delamination and invasion of the cardiac jelly, by assuming a typical mesenchymal phenotype, with high proliferative activity and able to remodel the cushions in definitive cusps. The work of Markwald and Colleagues about Endothelial-Mesenchymal Transition (EMT) first evidenced the involvement of soluble factors in the extracellular matrix and nevertheless a close myocardium-endothelium relationship, likely to emphasize the unique responsive property of endocardial cells to cardiomyocytes' mechanical and paracrine stimuli [138].

At the end of the developmental process, at least four are the cellular contributions which constitute the different valvular phenotypes: the myocardium, whose involvement is immediate in the formation of the atrioventricular valves; the endocardium, which undergoes an endothelial-mesenchymal transdifferentiation; the epicardium, contributing to the atrioventricular valves; and the neural crest cells, which migrate from the brachial arches to the distal outflow tract, participating to the aorto-pulmonary septation [139-141].

Excluding embryonic cells for ethical concerns, cells with EMT potentiality should be endowed with a certain degree of plasticity: as seen before, EPCs and MSCs, isolable from several tissue sources of various donor ages, could possess among other cell phenotypes these requisites and find, in fact, broad application in tissue engineering practices.

Not yet followed in heart valve manufacturing are two other modalities to achieve more committed valve cell lines. On one hand, it would be possible to introduce genome modifications in cells already applied in TEHVs to induce paracrine mechanisms able to foster cell differentiation. On this basis, VEGF-overexpressing stem cells transplanted in the ischemic myocardium induced an improvement in vascularization [142]. Indeed, MSCs engineered to express Akt did not only participate to the repair of the infarcted heart, but also improved cardiac function [143].

The other more attracting frontier in advanced TEHV formulations is represented by the conversion of adult somatic cells to pluripotent stem cells (iPSCs) mediated by gene engineering. Cellular reprogramming to pluripotency is induced by the ectopic expression of 4 factors, i.e. Klf-4, c-Myc, Oct4 and Sox2 [144], rendering these cells phenotypically similar to embryonic stem cells but for an ethically acceptable use. iPSC cardiovascular applications range from the modelling of congenital cardiac diseases to the heart restoration after myocardial infarction [145, 146]. iPSC-based tissue-engineered heart valves could represent new powerful tools for the therapy of valvulopathies both as replacement solutions and as *in vitro* 3D valvular disease models.

5.2.2. Scaffold incorporation of growth factors

The close observation of the molecular events undergoing in heart valve formation would give specific indications on which signals bioengineered constructs could benefit for their maturation.

Endocardial cells undergo a profound phenotypic switch loosing the initial morphology, specific surface molecule expression and ability of acetylated-low density lipoprotein uptake in favour of a contractile, invasive profile. Transforming growth factor 1 and 2 (TGF-beta1 and 2), vascular endothelial growth factor (VEGF), bone morphogenetic protein 2 (BMP-2), mitogen-activated protein kinase 3 (MEKK3) and Notch1 are known to activate and strictly regulate EMT by direct control of Wnt/beta-catenin pathway. In addition, other molecular pathways are involved in heart valve development and the high complexity of regulation can be appreciated in the following chart (Figure 2):

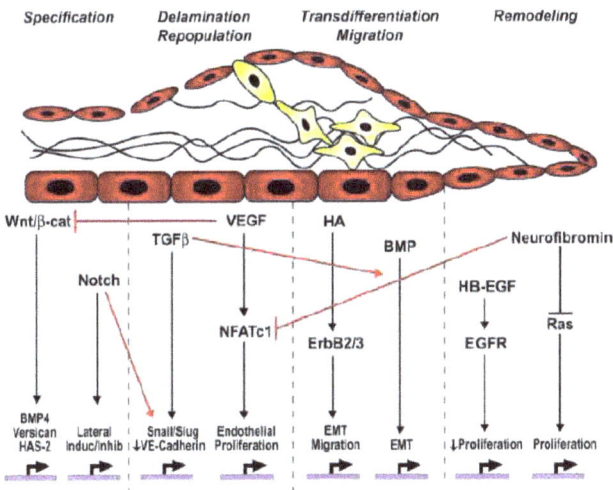

Figure 2. Valvulogenesis signalling complexity as proposed by Armstrong EJ and Bischoff J. From [147]

The pleiotropic factor VEGF is considered a specific mediator in EMT, favouring endothelial cell proliferation. Downstream of VEGF, the transcriptional factor NFATc1 has intranuclear expression: this is limited to the endocardium not activated in the EMT process during the temporal window of cushion development, while it is expressed by some valve endothelial cells in the post-natal life, leading to hypothesize their participation in the repopulation of the adult endothelium. Even RANKL (receptor activator of nuclear factor κB ligand) exercises a control role on NFATc1, by inhibiting VEGF-induced cell proliferation when the endocardial cushion is more mature [148]. Upstream of NFATc1, two elements, connexins and DSCR1 (Down Syndrome Critical Region 1) play their function via signalling pathways associated to calcium cellular gradients. In cardiomyocytes, DSCR1 seems to be overexpressed during the increase of the cytosolic calcium and acts as modulator of the calcineurin dephosphorilating activity on NFATc1, by preventing its translocation to the nucleus. Connexin 45-composed gap junctions might allow the calcium extracellular diffusion in the endocardial cushions after the VEGF-mediated activation of the calcium transients in endothelial subpopulations[147].

The transcriptional factor Notch1 rules osteogenic differentiation as well as valve development: its signalling in the endocardium might induce an increase of TGF-β2 expression in the myocardium, able to trigger EMT in endocardial cells through the cytosolic activation of Snail and Smad [149]. Activators of the TGF-β transduction pathway are even the bone morphogenetic proteins (BMPs), in particular BMP2, which causes powerful induction of Smad6 in the cusp endothelium [150, 151].

During EMT, PECAM down-regulation in endothelial cells is followed by smooth muscle actin hyper-regulation: Wnt/β-catenin pathway can be hence considered a link in between the mesenchymal activation and the populating process of the cardiac jelly with mesenchymal cells.

Beside these transduction pathways, it is equally important the integration of extracellular matrix signals, so called matrikines. ErbB proteins are involved in cell proliferation of cardiac cushions and their signalling is mediated by hyaluronic acid (HA), a highly hydrophilic glycosaminoglycan, which is able to extend the extracellular space and controls the ligand availability [147]. For both development and maintenance of mesenchymal cells in the valve leaflet, Sox9 is necessary by favouring cell proliferation and ECM correct alignment [152]. Recently, it has been recognized to the epicardium cell-secreted protein periostin a particular importance during the atrioventricular valve development in promoting differentiation of epicardial stem cells [153, 154].

New high-speed fluorescence microscopic technologies have allowed verifying the large interplay of different pathways in the development of the cusps and especially, they enabled a better understanding of the first events in valvulogenesis, arguing in favour of an invagination rather than a formation of endocardial cushions [155].

Recent gene expression studies revealed an up-regulation for α-SMA, Snail and β-catenin as well as acetyltransferase p300 (ATp300). Indeed, microRNA analysis identified a specific role for miR-125b in the down-regulation of p53 [156].

Growth factors involved in embryonic development have been incorporated as widely contemplated strategy in bone and joint regenerative medicine. In the heart valve field, this approach has not been frequently applied [157], until now preferring *in vitro* comparative investigations on cell stimulation with sole growth factors, as TGF-beta, VEGF and BMPs [158, 159].

5.2.3. EMT-inducing biomaterials

Heart valve development is a complex process where signalling molecules and specific extracellular matrix elements interact. In response to these several stimuli, endocardial and epicardial cells adhere to the surface of the cardiac cushions and start an endothelial-to-mesenchymal transition (EMT), leading to the formation of an elongated cusp structure [138].

The initial phase of valve formation depends on many extracellular matrix proteins [160]. The highly hydrophilic glycosaminoglycan HA is the major component of the endocardial cushions and its content is also elevated in the adult *spongiosa* layer, guaranteeing appeasement from the shocks provoked by the enormous pressure variations during the cardiac cycle. When seeded *in vitro* with VICs, hydrogels at various HA percentage have demonstrated to modulate ECM synthesis and induce also the production of elastin [161, 162].

Composite scaffolds of collagen and elastin have shown to reproduce the anisotropic spatial distribution of aortic ECM fibres and hence possess the potential to create heart valve replacements with a native-like microenvironment [163]. Mechanical strength properties of collagen have also been previously exploited in combination with HA, thus obtaining a cell-bioactive ECM milieu [164].

5.3. Biocompatibility indications

5.3.1. Biomimetic strategies

Functional endothelium together to resistant and flexible mechanical performance, mainly ensured by collagen and elastin, are critical components in the early clinical patency of a viable valve substitute. Starter matrices both for TEHV and TGRHV approaches should possess attractive properties towards cell elements facilitating their adhesion, penetration and further maturation. Most decellularized heart valves retain an intact basal membrane lamina, which represent the ideal microenvironment for endothelial cell attachment and spreading. This so-called contact guidance takes advantage of the specific nanotopography of the heart valve intimal ECM to increase cell bioaffinity. In order to recreate a valve-like microenvironment, surface functionalization with peptides, as laminin-extracted YIGSR (Tyr-Ile-Gly-Ser-Arg), selectively enhances endothelial cell adhesion and proliferation without thrombogenic effects [165]. Protein pre-coating of valve scaffolds with fibronectin or elastin-derived VAPG (Val-Ala-Pro-Gly) can enhance cell engrafting and differentiation [25, 80]. Self-assembling peptides containing YIGSR or VAPG create nanomatrix milieu mimicking the endothelium and resulting in increased endothelialisation and proliferation of vSMCs [166].

RGD and GRGDSP are both functional domains belonging to fibronectin. Stent biofunction-alisation with these cell adhesive ligands has been reported to result in controversial issues: while promoting endothelial cell adhesion and coverage, it favours platelet attachment [167-169]. Thus, the usage of these adhesive sequences should be cautious in perspective of thrombotic events.

Positive cell-affinity effects can be instead obtained by coating scaffold surfaces with fibrin, which however can be employed only as coating solution lacking of important mechanical assets [170, 171].

Particularly appealing is the application of peptides selected by phage display. This technology offers the possibility to create combinatorial peptide libraries, where still unknown cell recognition surface molecules can be discovered. A new peptide ligand, i.e. TPS, was identified through cell-SELEX system (Systematic Evolution of Ligands by EXponential enrichment) and covalently linked to methacrylic polymeric matrix to selectively capture endothelial cells [172].

In combination with natural materials, new matrices based on silk and chitosan, a polysac-charide found in Crustaceans, could consent the accomplishment of hybrid valve scaffolds, where endothelial cells can better adhere and proliferate [173].

5.3.2. Antimicrobial treatments

Although no infections have been recorded yet after implantation of porcine- or bovine-derived tissues, the risk of transmission of porcine retroviruses or Creutzfeldt-Jacob disease has not to be underestimated. In order to avoid new trans-species viral combinations, endo-nuclease treatments generally applied after decellularization could be therefore preventing in this sense. The use of foetal bovine serum in heart valve tissue engineering and cryopreser-vation is also controversial and its substitution with serum replacement should be introduced in good manufacture practice.

The first infective risk is primarily represented by bacterial/fungal contamination. Current antimicrobial treatments are based on cocktails of large spectrum antibiotics and antimycotics and are performed on decellularized scaffolds prior to further *in vitro* cell seeding or *in vivo* implantation. Synthetic biomaterials are mostly submitted to gaseous disinfection with plasma gas or ethylene oxide.

While UV rays have a low penetration power for disinfection, gamma-irradiation is effective in abrogating contaminations. However, even when combined with the radioprotective cryopreservant DMSO, it is able to induce deep damages on the ECM fibres with deleterious effects in the long-term performance of so-treated heart valve substitutes [174].

5.3.3. Cues for thrombosis and neointimal hyperplasia prevention

Scaffold modifications for antithrombogenicity have been developed using endothelial coverage, ECM peptides inducing endothelium formation or by engineering their surface with inhibitors of platelet function or anticoagulant agents [175].

As already discussed, a normal endothelium is protective from platelet adhesion and aggregation in the first phases after implantation. Achievable *in vitro* with endothelial cells and their circulating progenitors, endothelialisation has to occur on all surfaces contacting blood, otherwise uncovered regions can be platelet-attractive. The implementation of extracellular matrix with endothelial adhesive ligands, as YIGSR, can foster a complete endothelial coverage [165].

Other cell sources for non-thrombogenic surfaces are represented by MSCs, which offer high compatibility with blood cells and are lacking of the platelet selective surface ligand HSPG [176].

Besides its EC and SMC affinity, HA, similarly to other GAGs, is effective in the prevention of platelet adhesion [177].

Other molecules able to inhibit thrombotic formations are phosphorylcholine phospholipid and polyethylene glycol, which counteract the adsorption of serum proteins [178, 179].

Instead of its preventive blockage, protein adsorption can be opportunely manipulated with fibrinogen to circumvent further diffusion of other serum molecules: while some hydrophobic domains of the molecule are adsorbed, others are exposed creating fibrous conformations able to attract endothelial cells [180].

Nitric oxide (NO), a chemical compound normally produced by functional endothelial cells and owning antithrombogenic efficacy can be also derived from decomposition of diazenium-diolates. The incorporation of these molecules in scaffolds is able to drastically reduce *in vivo* thrombi formation [165, 181]. NO performs a second function in preventing valve complications. In fact, it is able to directly down-regulate proliferation pathways in vSMCs, thus precluding neointimal hyperplasia [182, 183]. Upon NO treatment, the activity of the protein synthesis machinery is reduced in these cells, observing a drastic reduction in the production of collagen [182]. Local delivery of stable S-nitrosothiol groups, incorporated in different compounds of serum albumin, has demonstrated to significantly reduce both platelet aggregation and neointimal proliferation in animal models of vascular injury [184]. Other NO formulations were identified to ensure a sustained and controlled release of the endothelial-derived molecule. When applied to VICs from the porcine aortic valve, combinations of poly(L-lactic acid) (PLLA) matrix systems incorporating NO-delivering poly(lactic-co-glycolic acid) (PLGA) nanoparticles reduced intercellular adhesion molecule 1 signalling and increased cyclic guanosine monophosphate levels, demonstrating therefore NO antiinflammatory and anticalcific potentialities [185].

Among anticoagulants, heparin is the most employed drug in the clinical activity. Resembling the glycosaminoglycan heparin sulphate in its chemical composition, it exerts blocking effect on the coagulation cascade also when immobilized into a scaffold. However, its pharmaceutical validity in this setting is not so good as in its soluble form [186].

Limited activity shown by immobilized heparin is surpassed by hyrudin scaffold incorporation. When conjugated to several biomaterials, this chemical agent is able both *in vitro* and *in vivo* to quench thrombin and prevent its further activity [187, 188].

Neointimal hyperplasia represents another complication in the *in vivo* performance of new viable valve substitutes. Besides NO, other chemical agents are currently used to counteract vSMC proliferation at the basis of neointima development. Local delivery of growth factors involved in the apoptotic pathways of vSMCs has been reported to attenuate the phenomenon with efficiency extents depending on the local concentration of the cytokine at the injury site [190, 191]. In lieu of locally delivering specific growth factors, the oral administration of drugs stimulating their cell production could represent a more compliant therapy for treated patients [192].

Other blocking strategies have been developed by directly targeting oligonucleotides or receptor molecules involved in vSMC proliferation. The use of antisense strategies or humanized monoclonal antibodies contributes to abolish the expression of proteins needed for cell cycling [193-195].

As for the administration of growth factors, these approaches rely on a non-functional endothelium and on the local vector availability.

Nevertheless, even if not yet tested in other formulations than soluble particles, growth factor- and antisense-based approaches could show promising potential when incorporated in scaffolds for cardiovascular applications.

More specifically tackling tactics can be exercised throughout the usage of viral particles with vascular tropism. Attenuated herpes simplex virus 1, obtained by removing only $\gamma_1 34.5$ genes, originally demonstrated its efficacy in malignant cancer therapies. Indeed, its ability to infect dividing cells can be used together with its tropism to vSMCs as efficient antiproliferative agent. In particular, while showing no systemic toxicity and a persistent activity for at least 4 weeks, its infective state can be electively blocked by antiviral drugs [196].

TGF-beta 1 and PDGF-BB pathways are up-regulated in the genesis of intimal hyperplasia. These growth factors contribute to the recruitment of adventitial cells by neighbouring medial SMCs through a paracrine mechanism and are, therefore, perfect targets in a blockade strategy. Cell-selective adenoviral gene transfer of Smad7 or PDGF-beta receptor reduced adventitial cell migration and vascular remodelling after balloon injury [197, 198].

Notwithstanding the efficiency and the possibility of control related to these systems, the use of viral agents is still accompanied by ethical and safety concerns, which argue in favour of other therapeutic strategies.

Already evaluated in combination to biomaterials is another drug class, which has been firstly applied in the immunotransplantation field. Limus derivatives are a large family of compounds preventing either allograft rejections or restenosis after angioplasty. Conversely, systemic toxic effects, unspecific antiproliferation activity on ECs and SMCs, and variable efficacy associated with their usage *in vitro* or *in vivo* are at the basis of the reported controversial results [199-203].

5.3.4. Functionalization of decellularized extracellular matrices

While decellularized ECMs have demonstrated the ability of *in vivo* self-regeneration, their structural and functional properties can be improved by conditioning with synthetic biomaterials. The advantage of such strategies resides in the combination of uniform and mouldable artificial products with bioactive natural scaffolds. Nanotechnology approaches are currently under investigation for the stable introduction of adhesive sequences or for the entrapment of structure-mouldable peptides (unpublished data).

5.3.5.. Anticalcification approaches

From the observation of the pathological events occurring in vessel/valve deterioration, different anticalcification strategies have been developed. In the bioprosthetic valves, mineralization is strictly related to the presence of phospholipids (phosphatidil serine and phosphaditil choline) and phosphate backbone of degraded nucleic acids in the extracellular milieu of a no more vital tissue [204, 205]. These extracellular phosphate groups are perfect nucleation sources for mineral deposition. The progression and entity of calcification is dependent on many factors and surely, the lack of a cell-favoured homeostatic pathway, provoked by glutaraldehyde (GA) cytotoxicity, can be useful to accelerate the phenomenon of diffuse mineralization on ECM fibres.

A reduction in the mineral deposition has been attempted through addition of several GA-detoxifying approaches. Challenged alone with valvular cells or cross-linked to GA-fixed bioprostheses in simulated body fluid, procyanidines have demonstrated cell biocompatibility, dose-dependent inhibition of alkaline phosphatase cellular activity and consequently, of matrix mineralization [206].

Lipid extraction for the removal of cell membrane phospholipids has been pursued by applying solvents or detergents with special attention to the preservation of ECM fibres. In an *in vivo* model, the long chain aliphatic alcohol octanediol in 40% concentration has proven to be an efficient anticalcification agent for GA-treated bovine pericardium [207].

A more diluted octanediol is in the organic solvent used as buffer for genypin/glutaraldehyde fixation of bovine pericardial tissues, previously submitted to sodium dodecyl sulphate decellularization and/or successively treated with several amino acids or sodium bisulphite. In respect to GA-fixed samples, all these different genypin-based variants turned out in in decreased calcium/phosphorus content and conserved tissue stability by resistance to pronase enzymatic degradation [208]. However, despite the concomitant evaluation of decellularization, which could have partaken in the removal of alpha-gal epitopes, the levels of these xenoantigens were valuated only between genipin/GA- versus sole GA-fixations particularly [208].

Ethanol cross-linked to triglycidyl amine is also able to reduce GA-associated calcification both in rat subdermal and sheep models, however it is responsible of structural instability in treated tissues [209]. In another study by Sacks et al, triglycidyl epoxy-crosslinking without GA addition demonstrated improved biomechanics in respect to GA alone [210].

Amino acids, as glycine, phenylalanine or aspartic acid, are largely employed in anticalcification processes to potentiate the action of alcohols and metallocene dichlorides [211].

Detergent application, at the basis of most decellularizing techniques, exploits tensioactivity to eliminate membrane lipids, indistinctly from the presence of phosphate groups. Treatments with Triton X100 and sodium cholate, deoxycholic acid, N-lauroyl sarcosinate or sodium dodecyl sulphate, especially if combined with DNA/RNA nucleases, resulted in no calcific events both *in vitro*, in preclinical animal models and/or in the clinical stage [25-28, 102, 212].

Calcium and phosphorus signalling has been tackled via calcimimetics and biphoshonates by directly acting on calcifying cells. So far evaluated mainly in the renal district, calcimimetics, as R-568 and AMG 641, could in the future be incorporated in synthetic and natural matrices to selectively block parathyroid hormone pathway responsible for renal artery calcification [213]. Interestingly, another calcimimetic, cinacalcet, has been reported to reduce vascular calcification in the renal aorta of uremic rats in association with further encouraging outcomes on vascular remodelling and myocardial fibrosis [214].

Testified as possible medical therapy for calcific aortic stenosis, bisphosphonate molecules incorporated into polyurethane scaffolds induced resistance from calcification in 60 day-long rat subdermal tests and in 90 day-long evaluation in the circulation as pulmonary valve cusp [215].

5.4. *In vitro* and *in vivo* novel tissue technologies

5.4.1. Bio-electrospray

Further advances in cardiovascular regenerative medicine have recently been introduced to ease the achievement of intraoperative tissue-engineered organ units: bioelectrospray is emerging as a powerful tool both for the creation of specific nanotopographic surface and for homogeneous/spatial cell seeding or coating of valve scaffolds [216, 217].

5.4.2. Monoclonal antibodies and DNA aptamers

Monoclonal antibodies can be applied to selectively capture cell populations expressing specific cluster differentiation molecules: an increase in the attachment of endothelial or mesenchymal stem cells was achieved by coating scaffold surface with anti-CD34, anti-CD90 or anti-CD133 [218-220].

Aptamers, 70-90 nucleotide-long single strand oligos, can bind to specific molecules with high selectivity and affinity. Identified through combinatorial phage display technology, they were immobilized on the surface of polydimethylsiloxan or polytetrafluoroethylene patches precoated with the antithrombogenic PEG. The scaffold formulation was able to block serum protein adsorption and selectively recruit EPCs from the bloodstream [221]. EPC-attracting aptamer technology has also been applied with similar results in valve scaffolds [222].

5.4.3. Organ printing

Extremely fascinating in bioengineering is the possibility to fabricate complex living structures by organ printing. This approach contemplates different sequential steps for the realization of biological tissue and organ substitutes: computer-aided design (CAD), image processing, modelling with solids, free-form fabrication, designing, simulation and finally manufacturing [223]. Several applications of this technology have been proposed since 2001 [224] and are currently focusing also in the preparation of cardiovascular tissues [225, 226]. Until now, organ printing has been rendered useful in the heart valve field not for biofabrication, but for pre-operative planning and valve replacement simulation in complex interventions [227].

5.4.4. In body tissue architecture

Actually, the concept of in body tissue architecture finds limited exploitation in the development of heart valves substitutes. Interestingly, the Japanese group of Nakayama et al. has produced a trileaflet valved-shaped construct based on this technology. As in the case of Campbell et al. [87], the approach takes advantage of the normal biological response to a foreign material developed by the body, implanting silicon rods in the subcutaneous tissues. In a period of 4 weeks, these grafts are first 'embedded' by granulation-like tissue, then removed and fused each other for correct valvular shaping and reinserted to complete the cell covering. At the end of the process, the particular arrangement given by the researchers allows eliminating supporting artificial materials to attain a trileaflet valve conduit [228].

5.5. Implantation techniques: Classical cardio-surgical implant versus transapical and TAVI access

Open chest interventions have represented the main surgical modality for diseased heart valve treatment. The classic cardio-surgical implant generally implies median sternotomy and cardio-pulmonary bypass with cannulation of both venae cavae and aorta in hypothermic conditions. This technique is largely used for the implantation of bioengineered valves in animal model testing or in clinical valve substitutions [93].

Classic cardio-surgical valve substitution is for sure a life-saving procedure. However, its invasiveness results in infective risk and pain in the immediate post-intervention period. Additionally, in children the current lack for valve substitutes with somatic adaptation ability submits these paediatric patients to several re-do procedures until their adulthood.

Owing to the improvement in life expectancy, the elderly represent another cardiopathic population in need for re-intervention.

Catheter-assisted techniques are minimally invasive implantation approaches, experimented in animal models in 1965 and in humans in 2000 [229, 230]. The percutaneous trans-catheter implantation of an aortic valve prosthesis (TAVI) was firstly performed by Cribier et al. some years later [231]. In a TAVI device, a bioprosthetic aortic valve is mounted on an expandable stainless steel stent. It is then compressed to nearly one-third of its diameter through a crimping procedure and introduced in a catheter before its implantation in the patient. Once the correct position has been assessed by fluoroscopy imaging, the crimped valve is balloon- or self-expanded and tightly juxtaposed to the insufficient aortic valve. The procedure of trans-catheter aortic valve insertion in degenerated surgically implanted bioprostheses is particularly indicated for high surgical risk patients, since a minimal thoracotomy access is required instead of sternotomy and cardio-pulmonary bypass.

Through a catheter-assisted system, tissue-engineered heart valves were transapically implanted in sheep and non-human primates as pulmonary valve replacements following a minithoracotomy [95, 232]. Although performing during 2 month-long experimental evaluation, cusp thickening was reported in these poly-4-hydroxybutyrate coated nonwoven polyglycolic acid-based TEHVs [233].

A similar transapical approach was adopted by the same group for TEHV implantation in sheep systemic circulation. Haemodinamically evaluated up to 2 weeks, these tissue-engineered aortic replacements were found post-mortem in active remodelling, with merely collagen/GAG ECM synthesis and freedom from thrombotic formations or structural degenerations [97].

These intriguing experimental evidences demonstrate the feasibility of such an approach also for bioengineered valve substitutes. In addition, a transapically-delivered bioengineered TAVI could be a particularly beneficial option for patients with severe aortic valve calcification.

However, crimping/re-opening effects on cell survival, ECM microstructure and valve function should be further examined both *in vitro* and *in vivo* within a longer observational time. Decellularized scaffold-relying approaches could be especially influenced by this mounting-related shock with immediate and significant consequences on tissue hydration, GAG content and collagen/elastin fibre interplay.

5.6. Imaging tools

5.6.1. Two Photon-laser scanning confocal microscopy

More and more advanced optical visualization systems are offering sophisticated functions for non-invasive deeper penetration and dynamic evaluation of developing organs and bioengineered constructs. Cell adhesion and spreading in thick 3D structures can now be analysed until almost millimetre depth by means of 2 photon-laser scanning confocal microscopy (2P-LSCM). Differently from more common linear-based imaging, 2P-LSCM exploits the simultaneous adsorption of two near IR-photons to excite endogenous fluorophores, as tricarboxylic triamipiridinium elastin-derivates, without previous sectioning or staining. Besides elastin networks, it is possible to study collagen fibres through second harmonic generation in an adsorption-free process [234]. This unique imaging modality offers the unquestionable possibility to dynamically monitor relatively small living tissues without manipulation artefacts [235].

5.6.2. MRI

Another non-invasive imaging modality is magnetic resonance: widely applied in the clinical setting, it surpasses ionizing radiation-based echocardiography for the optimal spatio-temporal resolution [236]. *In vivo* performance of bioengineered heart valves can be constantly monitored by MRI with the feasibility of precise dimensional measurements [229, 237]. Cell passive loading of magnetic resonance nanoparticles *in vitro* allows for their dynamic tracing in implanted tissue-engineered constructs. Formulated in different diameter size (10-1.000 nm), most used MR nanoparticles, i.e. 50 nm-diameter superparamagnetic iron oxide (SPIO) ones, are cell-incorporated by endocytotic loading or up-taken in enhanced way by combination with protamine sulphate. Cell survival, motility and differentiation abilities have been reported to be not strongly influenced by SPIOs, thus perturbing mainly the magnetic field in the populated tissue [238].

5.6.3. μOCT, PET and SPECT

While MR technology allows qualitative and quantitative dynamic functional studies, detailed information on valve degeneration can be attained by means of tomography-based imaging [239]. With its 1-μm-axial resolution, micro-optical coherence tomography (μOCT) would be a particularly interesting tool in in bioengineering to elucidate cellular and subcellular events in the early tissue engraftment as well as in the initial onset of valve disease [240].

Positron emission and single photon emission computed tomography (respectively PET and SPECT) possess an inferior spatial resolution. As SPIOs, radionuclide-labelled cells can be obtained by means of passive loading. Cell tracking, however, will be strictly limited by the radioisotope half-life: among the commonly used radionuclides, the SPECT probe ^{111}In-Oxine has the longest detectable radioactivity of 2.8 days. Another limitation associated with SPECT is the necessity to load a relatively high amount of radioisotopes for quantitative evaluations, at the expense of cell viability. The more sensitive PET suffers instead of the shorter half-life of used probes [241]. On this account, PET and SPECT are not ideal to evaluate *in vivo* mid/long-term dynamic remodelling of bioengineered valves, but necessary to identify calcific degenerations [28].

5.7. Heart valve tissue banks

After the production of new valve substitutes, their storage and further capillary distribution are essential steps to the prompt realization of interventional therapies.

Off-the-shelf solutions must rely on appropriate conservation procedures, avoiding the use of cytotoxic fixatives able to compromise further *in vivo* remodelling/regeneration of TEHVs and TGRHVs.

Cryopreservation has been established as alternative storage technique to GA-fixation, when allografts started to be employed in clinic 50 years ago. Initially called homografts, pulmonary valves from cadaveric donors found large usage in the Ross procedure instead of the patient's own valve, eterotopically transposed for the replacement of the degenerated aortic root [242]. After isolation, donor tissues are examined to exclude lacerations and/or unsuitability sources and graded following macroscopic qualitative evaluation. Antimicrobial procedures are then performed to eliminate bacterial and fungal infective risks with constant control for effective microbe removal [243, 244]. Decontaminated tissues are immersed in cryopreserving solutions, usually based on cell culture medium added with a low percentage of the cryoprotectant dimethyl sulfoxide (DMSO). DMSO contributes to reduce hyperosmolarity shocks and ice crystal formation, which would induce deleterious effects on heart valve structure and mechanics. Tissues, introduced in highly resistant package, are then submitted to time- and condition-controlled cryofreezing and stored in vapour-phase nitrogen tanks for a maximum 5 years long period if unused.

On a constantly updated survey of the European Homograft Bank, nearly 4.500 cryopreserved valves on about 5.200 selected tissues were employed for complex valve malformations in children, women of child-bearing age with diseased cardiac valves, patients with anticoagulation contra-indication or patients with severe endocarditis [245].

While undoubtedly more immunotolerable than xenogeneic bioprostheses, their performance in the patients has a comparable endurance. Causes for this restricted durability have been firstly searched in the survival of populating cell elements. Strips of aortic valve cusps and walls were stimulated with vasoactive concentrations of potassium, 5-hydroxytryptamine, noradrenaline, endothelin-1 and prostaglandin F-(2alpha) to test cell contractility after cryopreservation: no significant differences were observed in comparison to fresh tissues [246]. Apoptotic studies revealed cell necrosis, related to ischemia rather than a cryopreservation-dependent activation of death program [247]. Indeed, albeit its cryoprotective action, DMSO is cytotoxic at physiologic temperature and could be responsible for cell death in unwell washed out thawed valves [248]. In addition, ultrastructural damage was reported as major source of scarce ECM stability.

Cryopreservation technique has already been tested as possible storage modality of tissue-engineered or *in vivo* regenerating decellularized valve substitutes: independent deep imaging analyses revealed however contrasting observations upon this treatment. Evaluations with transmission electron microscopy of cryopreserved/decellularized specimens found typical ECM pattern with no collagen swelling/shrinkage or clearly distorted/disrupted elastin fibres [25]. Two photon-laser scanning confocal microscopy on decellularized/cryopreserved valves demonstrated structural integrity of ECM fibres [249]. Cryopreservation detrimental effects were instead reported with the application of the same imaging technology by Schenke-Layland et al. [250]. The same group proposed vitrification as ECM preserving alternative to cryopreservation. Vitrification, defined by the Authors as 'ice-free cryopreservation', mainly differs from the standard method for the additional use of formamide and 1,2-propanediol. Vitrified porcine pulmonary valves showed better haemodynamic and biologic performance in comparison to cryopreserved tissues [251]. However, chemical compounds added to the cryopreserving medium could negatively affect cell viability.

5.8. Inflammation in heart valve regenerative medicine

5.8.1. Adverse effects of inflammation on cardiovascular tissue engineering/regeneration

The natural response of a body to an implanted tissue develops similarly to the healing process of a wound and analogously resolves at the graft acceptance. The implant is initially surrounded and infiltrated by a granulation tissue rich in inflammatory mononucleated cells, as monocytes and neutrophils acquiring *in situ* a mature, active phenotype. Debris removal and cytokine release, operated by macrophages, contribute to activate the last remodelling phases, depending on recruited fibroblasts and smooth muscle cells. A delicate balancing is involved in this rejecting/engrafting process. An intensification in the pro-inflammatory macrophage function, related to a not fully biocompatible synthetic or natural scaffold, provokes the onset of immunologic responses by enrolling further cells, as lymphocytes.

A related aspect is also the genesis of firstly cell calcification and hence extended ECM mineralization. Remained into incompletely decellularized tissues (especially of xenogeneic origin) or fruit of cell death activation (necrosis or apoptosis) in tissue-engineered constructs, cellular debris can, in fact, trigger inflammatory and/or immunologic response activation. Comparably to foam cells in atherosclerotic lesions, cell death of foreign body giant cells, i.e. fused collections of macrophages, generates apoptotic bodies. These latter, together to the similar ones or to the debris both released by dying construct cells, further propagate inflammation and generate a suitable microenvironment for calcium nucleation [252-254].

As previously mentioned, retention of xenoantigens and detergents could further increase the *in vivo* pro-inflammatory potential of decellularized matrix-based approaches [255]. Nevertheless, some unsuccessful results described for both TEHVs and TGRHVs, trusting on decellularized tissues, could hypothetically reside in the decellularization-induced exposure of previously masked epitopes or even in ECM micro-modifications, recognized as non-self by the immune system. A recent paper by Zhou and coll. discussed upon the effects of different decellularizing treatments on ECM preservation, thrombogenicity and immunogenicity, by *in vitro* direct human blood contact. While sodium deoxycholate-based decellularization induced no ECM disruption and complete decellularization, for all proposed methods, including sodium dodecyl sulphate, trypsin/EDTA or trypsin-detergent-nuclease, thrombotic and immunological responses were surely higher than those in glutaraldehyde-fixed specimens [256]. A confirmation about these findings is supported by another work published in the same year: through a quantitative approach based on immunoblotting technique, Arai and Orton were able to demonstrate the detection of soluble protein antigens still maintained in bovine pericardium and porcine heart valves after decellularization with sodium dodecyl sulphate and sodium deoxycholate [257].

The treatment based on Triton X100, sodium cholate and endonucleases, not evaluated in the previously cited studies, demonstrated to produce acellular heart valve substitutes, evoking *in vivo* null thrombogenic or inflammatory/immunogenic responses thanks to the complete alpha-gal elimination [26, 27, 135, 136].

So far, endothelialisation strategies represent - also in the clinical setting - the almost unique modalities to prevent thrombogenicity-related excessive inflammation in tissue-engineered heart valves approaches, especially when autologous endothelial cells are employed [93].

5.8.2. Favourable inflammatory events on cardiovascular tissue engineering/regeneration

Differently from any other cardiovascular tissue, as the adjacent myocardium and arterial wall, adult heart valve atrioventricular and semilunar leaflets possess a highly represented CD34-

positive interstitial population (Figure 3), as also evidenced in the work of Barth and colleagues [258]. The presence of CD34-expressing cells in these tissues reminds on almost two possible and equally valuable hypotheses on the role of these cytotypes in these districts. CD34 is a glycoprotein expressed on endothelial cells and on their circulating progenitors (EPCs). It is also identifiable on the surface of bone marrow-residing haematopoietic stem cells, which are known to be myeloid cell precursors of EPCs and of other cells, among which monocytes and macrophages (their tissue-activated form) [259]. Other inflammatory cell markers have been found positive even in uncompromised cusps of young donor's valve allografts (Figure 3) [260]. In particular, CD68-expressing macrophages are widespread both in semilunar and atrioventricular valve tissues, without the intensely site-concentrated cell distribution usually observed in pathological specimens.

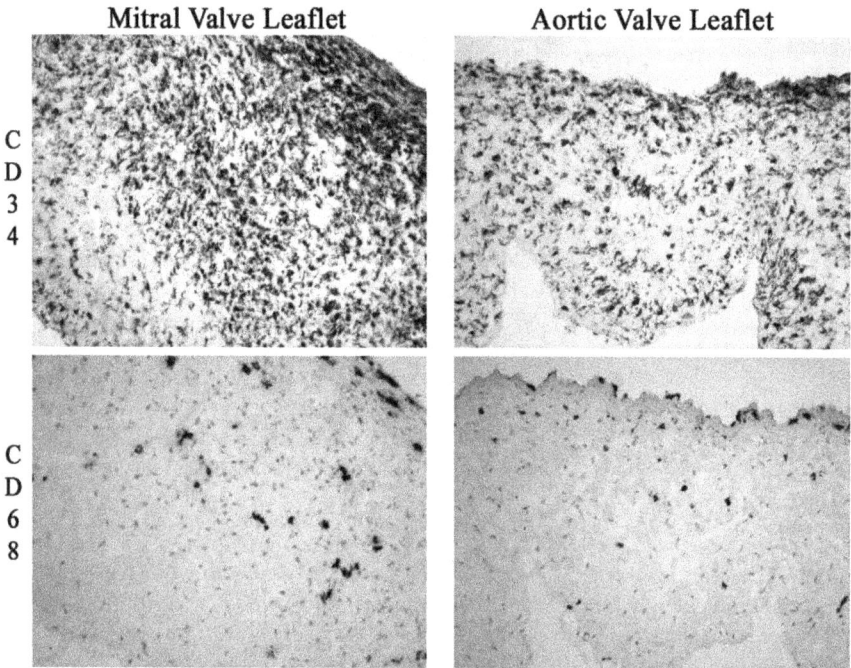

Figure 3. Hematopoietic cell markers expressed in the mitral and aortic valve leaflets of a 26 year-old donor allograft. CD34 is widely positive in all cusps tissues. CD68 expression is scattered and homogenously distributed in all leaflets, likely to identify a protective function, as that observable in the healthy myocardium. Magnification: 70x

The meaning of this presence in healthy tissues is not known, but it could be likely that the continuous mechanical stress imposed to the thin leaflets, together with the direct exposure to blood, needs a sentinel function exerted by macrophages and other cells.

Another interesting hypothesis rises from the observation of the double nature of the macro-phage cell. In effect, a phenotype committed to tissue regeneration has been discovered besides the typical protective tasks played by these cells. For the similarity to T2 helper lymphocytes, these macrophages have been named M2 and can be characterized by the expression of interleukin-10 (IL-10) and mannose receptor (MR) [261]. In the analysed valve specimens, the immunodetection of CD68, a broad macrophage marker, is associated to the expression of MR and IL-10, as visible in Figure 4.

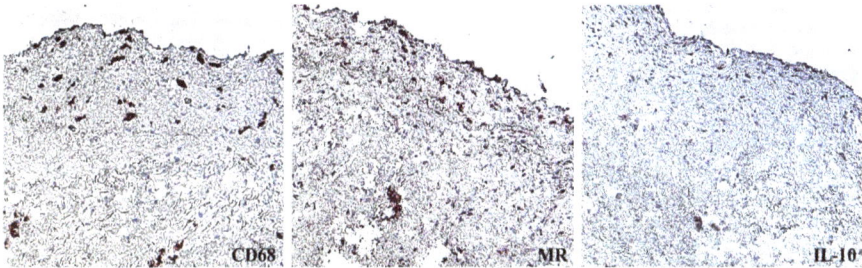

Figure 4. Evaluation of M2 macrophages in the mitral valve leaflet of a 26 year-old donor allograft. MR and IL-10 are likely to be expressed by the same CD68-positive cells. Magnification: 100x

This expression pattern of M2 macrophage typical markers is also preserved interspecies in mammals, further corroborating the notion of an evolutionarily conserved, constantly undergoing protection/regeneration process in the heart valve tissue. Porcine, bovine, sheep and non-human primate heart valves share, in fact, a similar cell distribution and localisation of CD68, MR and IL-10 markers (Figure 5).

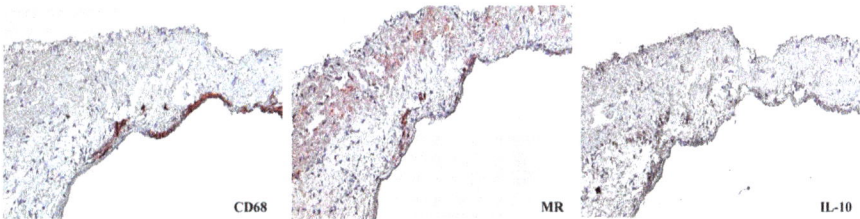

Figure 5. M2 macrophage pattern in the aortic valve leaflet of a Macaca fascicularis subject. Magnification: 50x

As further supportive remark, the extensive identification of stem cells with diverse lineages in heart valves evidences the unique regenerative properties endowed by these tissues [260].

Type 2 macrophages have been additionally found in the early post-implantation phases of bioengineered valve replacements and reported to remain in the implanted tissues until the construct scaffold has been completely replaced by an autologous matrix [262].

The engraftment of differently attainable biocompatible TEHVs and TGRHVs could be facilitated with the modulation of the M1/M2 ratio in favour of the second player: as often verified for other cardiovascular tissues [263], inflammatory responses could be mitigated through specific pharmaceutical treatments. While still at the sunrise of a possible clinical application in cardiovascular disease treatments, RNA interference (RNAi) technology could be an attenuator of inflammation, thanks to the selective silencing of targeted genes. Scaffold-mediated therapeutic delivery of RNAi could enable localize treatment of inflammation without secondary systemic effects [264].

Author details

Laura Iop* and Gino Gerosa

*Address all correspondence to: laura.iop@unipd.it

Department of Cardiac, Thoracic and Vascular Sciences School of Medicine, University of Padua, Padua, Italy

References

[1] Wells FC and Crowe T. Leonardo da Vinci as a paradigm for modern clinical research. J Thorac Cardiovasc Surg 2004;127(4): 929-4

[2] Hufnagel CA. Surgery of acquired diseases of the cardiac valves. GP. 1953;7(2):69-81

[3] Starr A, Edwards ML. Mitral replacement: clinical experience with a ball-valve prosthesis. Ann Surg 1961;154: 726-40

[4] Langer R, Vacanti JP. Tissue engineering. Science 1993;260: 920–6

[5] Agrawal CM, Ray RB. Biodegradable polymeric scaffolds for musculoskeletal tissue engineering. J Biomed Mater Res 2001;55: 141–150

[6] Braunwald NS. Performance of materials in vascular prosthetic devices: heart valves. Bull N Y Acad Med 1972;48(2): 357-61

[7] Wisman CB, Pierce WS, Donachy JH, Pae WE, Myers JL, Prophet GA. A polyurethane trileaflet cardiac valve prosthesis: in vitro and in vivo studies. Trans Am Soc Artif Intern Organs 1982;28: 164-8

[8] Bernacca GM, O'Connor B, Williams DF, Wheatley DJ. Hydrodynamic function of polyurethane prosthetic heart valves: influences of Young's modulus and leaflet thickness.Biomaterials2002;23(1): 45-50

[9] Kolff WJ, Yu LS. The return of elastomer valves. Ann Thorac Surg 1989;48(3 Suppl): S98-9

[10] Joshi RR, Frautschi JR, Phillips RE Jr, Levy RJ. Phosphonated polyurethanes that resist calcification.J Appl Biomater 1994;5(1): 65-77

[11] Rahmani B, Tzamtzis S, Ghanbari H, Burriesci G, Seifalian AM. Manufacturing and hydrodynamic assessment of a novel aortic valve made of a new nanocomposite polymer. J Biomech2012;45(7): 1205-11

[12] Shinoka T, Breuer CK, Tanel RE, Zund G, Miura T, Ma PX, Langer R, Vacanti JP, Mayer JE. Tissue engineering heart valves: valve leaflet replacement study in a lamb model. Ann Thorac Surg 1995;60(Suppl. 3): S513–6

[13] Shinoka T, Ma PX, Shum-Tim D, Breuer CK, Cusick RA, Zund G, Langer R, Vacanti JP, Mayer JE. Tissue engineered heart valves. Autologous valve leaflet replacement study in a lamb model. Circulation 1996;94(Suppl.): II164–8

[14] Shinoka T, Shum-Tim D, Ma PX, Tanel RE, Isogai N, Langer R, Vacanti JP, Mayer JE. Creation of viable pulmonary artery autografts through tissue engineering. J Thorac Cardiovasc Surg 1998;115: 536–546

[15] Schmidt D, Stock UA, Hoerstrup SP. Tissue engineering of heart valves using decellularized xenogeneic or polymeric starter matrices. Philos Trans R Soc Lond B Biol Sci 2007;362(1484): 1505-12

[16] Hoerstrup SP, Sodian R, Daebritz S, Wang J, Bacha EA, Martin DP, Moran AM, Guleserian KJ, Sperling JS, Kaushal S, Vacanti JP, Schoen FJ, Mayer JE Jr. Functional living trileaflet heart valves grown *in vitro*. Circulation 2000;102: III44–49

[17] Hoerstrup SP, Cummings Mrcs I, Lachat M, Schoen FJ, Jenni R, Leschka S, Neuenschwander S, Schmidt D, Mol A, Günter C, Gössi M, Genoni M, Zund G. Functional growth in tissue-engineered living, vascular grafts: follow-up at 100 weeks in a large animal model. Circulation 2006;114(1 Suppl): I159-66

[18] Yin W, Gallocher S, Pinchuk L, Schoephoerster RT, Jesty J, Bluestein D. Flow-induced platelet activation in a St. Jude mechanical heart valve, a trileaflet polymeric heart valve, and a St. Jude tissue valve.Artif Organs 2005;29(10): 826-31

[19] Mohammadi H. Nanocomposite biomaterial mimicking aortic heart valve leaflet mechanical behaviour. Proc Inst Mech Eng H 2011;225(7): 718-22

[20] Koroleva A, Gittard S, Schlie S, Deiwick A, Jockenhoevel S, Chichkov B. Fabrication of fibrin scaffolds with controlled microscale architecture by a two-photon polymerization-micromolding technique.Biofabrication 2012;4(1): 015001

[21] Ghanbari H, Viatge H, Kidane AG, Burriesci G, Tavakoli M, Seifalian AM. Polymeric heart valves: new materials, emerging hopes.Trends Biotechnol 2009;27(6): 359-67

[22] Grauss RW, Hazekamp MG, Oppenhuizen F, van Munsteren CJ, Gittenberger-de Groot AC, De Ruiter MC. Histological evaluation of decellularised porcine aortic

valves: matrix changes due to different decellularisation methods. Eur J Cardiothorac Surg 2005;27(4): 566-71

[23] Rieder E, Kasimir MT, Silberhumer G, Seebacher G, Wolner E, Simon P, Weigel G. Decellularization protocols of porcine heart valves differ importantly in efficiency of cell removal and susceptibility of the matrix to recellularization with human vascular cells. J Thorac Cardiovasc Surg 2004;127(2): 399-405

[24] Bertipaglia B, Ortolani F, Petrelli L, Gerosa G, Spina M, Pauletto P, Casarotto D, Marchini M, Sartore S. Cell characterization of porcine aortic valve and decellularized leaflets repopulated with aortic valve interstitial cells: the VESALIO Project (Vitalitate Exornatum Succedaneum Aorticum Labore Ingenioso Obtenibitur). Ann Thorac Surg 2003;75: 1274-1282

[25] Iop L, Renier V, Naso F, Piccoli M, Bonetti A, Gandaglia A, Pozzobon M, Paolin A, Ortolani F, Marchini M, Spina M, De Coppi P, Sartore S, Gerosa G. The influence of heart valve leaflet matrix characteristics on the interaction between human mesenchymal stem cells and decellularized scaffolds. Biomaterials 2009;30(25): 4104-16

[26] L, Gandaglia A, Bonetti A, Marchini M, Spina M, Basso C, Thiene G, Gerosa G. *In vivo* Spontaneous Tissue Regeneration Of Allogeneic Decellularized Aortic Valves. Conference Proceedings *5th Biennial Meeting of the Society for Heart Valve Disease (Joint meeting with Heart Valve Society of America)* – Berlin, Germany, 27-30 June 2009

[27] Gallo M, Naso F, Poser H, Rossi A, Franci P, Bianco R, Micciolo M, Zanella F, Cucchini U, Aresu L, Buratto E, Busetto R, Spina M, Gandaglia A, Gerosa G. Physiological performance of a detergent decellularized heart valve implanted for 15 months in Vietnamese pigs: surgical procedure, follow-up, and explant inspection. Artif Organs 2012;36(6): E138-50

[28] Dohmen PM, Lembcke A, Holinski S, Kivelitz D, Braun JP, Pruss A, Konertz W. Midterm clinical results using a tissue-engineered pulmonary valve to reconstruct the right ventricular outflow tract during the Ross procedure. Ann Thorac Surg 2007;84(3): 729-36

[29] Yang M, Chen CZ, Wang XN, Zhu YB, Gu YJ. Favourable effects of the detergent and enzyme extraction method for preparing decellularized bovinepericardium scaffold for tissue engineered heart valves.J Biomed Mater Res B Appl Biomater 2009;91(1): 354-61

[30] Cigliano A, Gandaglia A, Lepedda AJ, Zinellu E, Naso F, Gastaldello A, Aguiari P, De Muro P, Gerosa G, Spina M, Formato M. Fine structure of glycosaminoglycans from fresh and decellularized porcine cardiac valves and pericardium.Biochem Res Int 2012;2012: 979351

[31] Kuschert GS, Coulin F, Power CA, Proudfoot AE, Hubbard RE, Hoogewerf AJ, Wells TN. Glycosaminoglycans interact selectively with chemokines and modulate receptor binding and cellular responses.Biochemistry 1999;38(39): 12959-68

[32] Badylak SF, Freytes DO, Gilbert TW. Extracellular matrix as a biological scaffold material: Structure and function. Acta Biomater2009;5(1): 1-13

[33] Naso F, Gandaglia A, Formato M, Cigliano A, Lepedda AJ, Gerosa G, Spina M. Differential distribution of structural components and hydration in aortic and pulmonary heart valve conduits: Impact of detergent-based cell removal. Acta Biomater 2010;6(12): 4675-88

[34] Lau WL, Festing MH, Giachelli CM. Phosphate and vascular calcification: Emerging role of the sodium-dependent phosphate co-transporter PiT-1.Thromb Haemost 2010;104(3): 464-70

[35] Cebotari S, Tudorache I, Jaekel T, Hilfiker A, Dorfman S, Ternes W, Haverich A, Lichtenberg A. Detergent decellularization of heart valves for tissue engineering: toxicological effects of residual detergents on human endothelial cells.Artif Organs 2010;34(3): 206-10

[36] Bayrak A, Tyralla M, Ladhoff J, Schleicher M, Stock UA, Volk HD, Seifert M. Human immune responses to porcine xenogeneic matrices and their extracellular matrix constituents in vitro.Biomaterials 2010;31(14): 3793-803

[37] Schnell AM, Hoerstrup SP, Zund G, Kolb S, Sodian R, Visjager JF, Grunenfelder J, Suter A, Turina M. Optimal cell source for cardiovascular tissue engineering: venous vs. aortic human myofibroblasts. Thorac Cardiovasc Surg 2001;49(4): 221-5

[38] Zhu L, Williams WG, Bellhouse B, Pugh S, Rabinovitch M. Effective endothelialization of polyurethane surfaces. Response to shear stress and platelet adhesion. ASAIO Trans 1990;36(4): 811-6

[39] Bengtsson LA, Phillips R, Haegerstrand AN. In vitro endothelialization of photooxidatively stabilized xenogeneic pericardium. Ann Thorac Surg 1995;60(2 Suppl): S365-8

[40] Kim WG, Park JK, Park YN, Hwang CM, Jo YH, Min BG, Yoon CJ, Lee TY. Tissue-engineered heart valve leaflets: an effective method for seeding autologous cells on scaffolds.Int J Artif Organs 2000;23(9): 624-8

[41] Shinoka T, Shum-Tim D, Ma PX, Tanel RE, Langer R, Vacanti JP, Mayer JE Jr. Tissue-engineered heart valve leaflets: does cell origin affect outcome?Circulation 1997;96(9 Suppl): II-102-7

[42] Hoffman-Kim D, Maish MS, Krueger PM, Lukoff H, Bert A, Hong T, Hopkins RA. Comparison of three myofibroblast cell sources for the tissue engineering of cardiac valves.Tissue Eng 2005;11(1-2): 288-301

[43] Appleton AJ, Appleton CT, Boughner DR, Rogers KA. Vascular smooth muscle cells as a valvular interstitial cell surrogate in heart valve tissue engineering. Tissue Eng Part A 2009;15(12): 3889-97

[44] Hoerstrup SP, Kadner A, Melnitchouk S, Trojan A, Eid K, Tracy J, Sodian R, Visjager JF, Kolb SA, Grunenfelder J, Zund G, Turina MI. Tissue engineering of functional tri-leaflet heart valves from human marrow stromal cells. Circulation 2002;106(12 Suppl 1): I143-50

[45] Schmidt D, Achermann J, Odermatt B, Breymann C, Mol A, Genoni M, Zund G, Hoerstrup SP. Prenatally fabricated autologous human living heart valves based on amniotic fluid derived progenitor cells as single cell source. Circulation 2007;116(11 Suppl): I64-70

[46] Castrechini NM, Murthi P, Gude NM, Erwich JJ, Gronthos S, Zannettino A, Brennecke SP, Kalionis B. Mesenchymal stem cells in human placental chorionic villi reside in a vascular Niche. Placenta 2010;31(3): 203-12

[47] Iop L, Chiavegato A, Callegari A, Bollini S, Piccoli M, Pozzobon M, Rossi CA, Calamelli S, Chiavegato D, Gerosa G, De Coppi P and Sartore S. Different cardiovascular potential of adult and fetal-type mesenchymal stem cells in a rat model of heart cryoinjury. *Cell Transplantation* 2008;17: 679-694

[48] Schmidt D, Achermann J, Odermatt B, Genoni M, Zund G, Hoerstrup SP. Cryopreserved amniotic fluid-derived cells: a lifelong autologous fetal stem cell source for heart valve tissue engineering. J Heart Valve Dis 2008;17(4): 446–55

[49] Schmidt D, Mol A, Breymann C, Achermann J, Odermatt B, Gössi M, et al. Living autologous heart valves engineered from human prenatally harvested progenitors. Circulation 2006;114(1 Suppl): I125–31

[50] Sodian R, Schaefermeier P, Abegg-Zips S, Kuebler WM, Shakibaei M, Daebritz S, et al. Use of human umbilical cord blood-derived progenitor cells for tissue-engineered heart valves. Ann Thorac Surg 2010;89(3): 819–28

[51] Schmidt D, Mol A, Odermatt B, Neuenschwander S, Breymann C, Gössi M et al. Engineering of biologically active living heart valve leaflets using human umbilical cord-derived progenitor cells. Tissue Eng 2006;12(11): 3223–32

[52] Haniffa MA, Wang XN, Holtick U, Rae M, Isaacs JD, Dickinson AM, Hilkens CM, Collin MP. Adult human fibroblasts are potent immunoregulatory cells and functionally equivalent to mesenchymal stem cells. J Immunol 2007 1;179(3): 1595-604

[53] Batten P, Sarathchandra P, Antoniw JW, Tay SS, Lowdell MW, Taylor PM, et al. Human mesenchymal stem cells induce T cell anergy and downregulate T cell allo-responses via the TH2 pathway: relevance to tissue engineering human heart valves. Tissue Eng 2006;12: 2263–73

[54] Colazzo F, Sarathchandra P, Smolenski RT, Chester AH, Tseng YT, Czernuszka JT, Yacoub MH, Taylor PM. Extracellular matrix production by adipose-derived stem cells: implications for heart valve tissue engineering.Biomaterials 2011;32(1): 119-27

[55] Vaculik C, Schuster C, Bauer W, Iram N, Pfisterer K, Kramer G, Reinisch A, Strunk D, Elbe-Bürger A. Human dermis harbors distinct mesenchymal stromal cell subsets.J Invest Dermatol 2012;132(3 Pt 1): 563-74

[56] Pittenger MF, Mackay AM, Beck S, Jaiswal RK, Douglas R, Mosca JD, et al. Multilineage potential of adult human mesenchymal stem cells. Science 1999;284: 143–7

[57] Latif N, Sarathchandra P, Thomas PS, Antoniw J, Batten P, Chester AH, et al. Characterization of structural and signaling molecules by human valve interstitial cells and comparison to human mesenchymal stem cells. J Heart Valve Dis 2007; 16:56

[58] Della Rocca F, Sartore S, Guidolin D, Bertipaglia B, Gerosa G, Casarotto D, et al. Cell composition of the human pulmonary valve: a comparative study with the aortic valve – the VESALIO Project. Vitalitate Exornatum Succedaneum Aorticum Labore Ingenioso Obtenibitur. Ann Thorac Surg 2000;70: 1594–600

[59] Sutherland FW, Perry TE, Yu Y, Sherwood MC, Rabkin E, Masuda Y, et al. From stem cells to viable autologous semilunar heart valve. Circulation 2005; 111: 2783–91

[60] Bin F, Yinglong L, Nin X, Kai F, Laifeng S, Xiaodong Z. Construction of tissue engineered homograft bioprosthetic heart valves *in vitro*. ASAIO J 2006;52: 303–9

[61] Sales VL, Mettler BA, Engelmayr GC Jr, Aikawa E, Bischoff J, Martin DP, Exarhopoulos A, Moses MA, Schoen FJ, Sacks MS, Mayer JE Jr. Endothelial progenitor cells as a sole source for ex vivo seeding of tissue-engineered heart valves.Tissue Eng Part A 2010;16(1): 257-67

[62] Dvorin EL, Wylie-Sears J, Kaushal S, Martin DP, Bischoff J. Quantitative evaluation of endothelial progenitors and cardiac valve endothelial cells: proliferation and differentiation on poly-glycolic acid/poly-4-hydroxybutyrate scaffold in response to vascular endothelial growth factor and transforming growth factor beta1.Tissue Eng 2003;9(3): 487-93

[63] Fang NT, Xie SZ, Wang SM, Gao HY, Wu CG, Pan LF. Construction of tissue-engineered heart valves by using decellularized scaffolds and endothelial progenitor cells.Chin Med J (Engl) 2007;120(8): 696-702

[64] Hoerstrup SP, Sodian R, Sperling JS, Vacanti JP, Mayer JE. New pulsatile bioreactor for *in vitro* formation of tissue engineered heart valves. Tissue engineering 2000; 6: 75–79

[65] Ramaswamy S, Gottlieb D, Engelmayr GC Jr, Aikawa E, Schmidt DE, Gaitan-Leon DM, Sales VL, Mayer JE Jr, Sacks MS. The role of organ level conditioning on the promotion of engineered heart valve tissue development in-vitro using mesenchymal stem cells. Biomaterials 2010;31(6): 1114-25

[66] Wang L, Wilshaw SP, Korossis S, Fisher J, Jin Z, Ingham E. Factors influencing the oxygen consumption rate of aortic valve interstitial cells: application to tissue engineering. Tissue Eng Part C Methods 2009;15(3): 355-63

[67]   Warnock JN, Konduri S, He Z, Yoganathan AP.Design of a sterile organ culture sys-
       tem for the ex vivo study of aortic heart valves. J Biomech Eng2005;127(5): 857-61

[68]   Lichtenberg A, Tudorache I, Cebotari S, Suprunov M, Tudorache G, Goerler H, Park
       JK, Hilfiker-Kleiner D, Ringes-Lichtenberg S, Karck M, Brandes G, Hilfiker A, Haver-
       ich A. Preclinical testing of tissue-engineered heart valves re-endothelialized under
       simulated physiological conditions.Circulation2006;114(1 Suppl): I559-65

[69]   Jockenhoevel S, Zund G, Hoerstrup SP, Schnell A, Turina M. Cardiovascular tissue
       engineering: a new laminar flow chamber for in vitro improvement of mechanical tis-
       sue properties.ASAIO J2002;48(1): 8-11

[70]   Engelmayr GC Jr, Sales VL, Mayer JE Jr, Sacks MS. Cyclic flexure and laminar flow
       synergistically accelerate mesenchymal stem cell-mediated engineered tissue forma-
       tion: Implications for engineered heart valve tissues.Biomaterials 2006;27(36): 6083-95

[71]   Balachandran K, Alford PW, Wylie-Sears J, Goss JA, Grosberg A, Bischoff J, Aikawa
       E, Levine RA, Parker KK. Cyclic strain induces dual-mode endothelial-mesenchymal
       transformation of the cardiac valve.Proc Natl Acad Sci USA 2011;108(50): 19943-8

[72]   Sierad LN, Simionescu A, Albers C, Chen J, Maivelett J, Tedder ME, Liao J, Simiones-
       cu DT. Design and Testing of a Pulsatile Conditioning System for Dynamic Endothe-
       lialization of Polyphenol-Stabilized Tissue Engineered Heart Valves.Cardiovasc Eng
       Technol 2010;1(2): 138-153

[73]   Breuer CK, Shin'oka T, Tanel RE, Zund G, Mooney DJ, Ma PX, Miura T, Colan S,
       Langer R, Mayer JE, Vacanti JP.Tissue engineering lamb heart valve leaflets.Biotech-
       nol Bioeng 1996;50(5): 562-7

[74]   Zund G, Breuer CK, Shinoka T, Ma PX, Langer R, Mayer JE, Vacanti JP. The in vitro
       construction of a tissue engineered bioprosthetic heart valve.Eur J Cardiothorac Surg
       1997;11(3): 493-7

[75]   Sodian R, Hoerstrup SP, Sperling JS, Martin DP, Daebritz S, Mayer JE Jr, Vacanti JP.
       Evaluation of biodegradable, three-dimensional matrices for tissue engineering of
       heart valves.ASAIO J 2000;46(1): 107-10

[76]   Sodian R, Hoerstrup SP, Sperling JS, Daebritz SH, Martin DP, Schoen FJ, Vacanti JP,
       Mayer JE Jr. Tissue engineering of heart valves: in vitro experiences.Ann Thorac
       Surg. 2000 Jul;70(1):140-4

[77]   Kadner A, Hoerstrup SP, Tracy J, Breymann C, Maurus CF, Melnitchouk S, Kadner
       G, Zund G, Turina M. Human umbilical cord cells: a new cell source for cardiovascu-
       lar tissue engineering.Ann Thorac Surg 2002;74(4): S1422-8

[78]   Kadner A, Zund G, Maurus C, Breymann C, Yakarisik S, Kadner G, Turina M,
       Hoerstrup SP. Human umbilical cord cells for cardiovascular tissue engineering: a
       comparative study.Eur J Cardiothorac Surg 2004;25(4): 635-41

[79] Schmidt D, Breymann C, Weber A, Guenter CI, Neuenschwander S, Zund G, Turina M, Hoerstrup SP. Umbilical cord blood derived endothelial progenitor cells for tissue engineering of vascular grafts.Ann Thorac Surg 2004;78(6): 2094-8

[80] Sales VL, Engelmayr GC Jr, Johnson JA Jr, Gao J, Wang Y, Sacks MS, Mayer JE Jr. Protein precoating of elastomeric tissue-engineeringscaffolds increased cellularity, enhanced extracellular matrix protein production, and differentially regulated the phenotypes of circulating endothelial progenitor cells.Circulation 2007;116(11 Suppl): I55-63

[81] Bader A, Schilling T, Teebken OE, Brandes G, Herden T, Steinhoff G, Haverich A. Tissue engineering of heart valves--human endothelial cell seeding of detergent acellularized porcine valves. Eur J Cardiothorac Surg. 1998 Sep;14(3):279-84

[82] Cebotari S, Mertsching H, Kallenbach K, Kostin S, Repin O, Batrinac A, Kleczka C, Ciubotaru A, Haverich A. Construction of autologous human heart valves based on an acellular allograft matrix.Circulation 2002;106(12 Suppl 1): I63-I68

[83] Schenke-Layland K, Opitz F, Gross M, Döring C, Halbhuber KJ, Schirrmeister F, Wahlers T, Stock UA. Complete dynamic repopulation of decellularized heart valves by application of defined physical signals-an in vitro study.Cardiovasc Res 2003;60(3): 497-509

[84] Lichtenberg A, Tudorache I, Cebotari S, Ringes-Lichtenberg S, Sturz G, Hoeffler K, Hurscheler C, Brandes G, Hilfiker A, Haverich A. In vitro re-endothelialization of detergent decellularized heart valves under simulated physiological dynamic conditions.Biomaterials 2006;27(23): 4221-9

[85] Callegari A, Bollini S, Iop L, Chiavegato A, Torregrossa G, Pozzobon M, Gerosa G, De Coppi P, Elvassore N, Sartore S. Neovascularization induced by porous collagen scaffold implanted on intact and cryoinjured rat hearts. Biomaterials 2007;28(36): 5449-61

[86] Menon NG, Rodriguez ED, Byrnes CK, Girotto JA, Goldberg NH, Silverman RP. Revascularization of human acellular dermis in full-thickness abdominal wall reconstruction in the rabbit model. Ann Plast Surg 2003;50(5): 523-7

[87] Chue WL, Campbell GR, Caplice N, Muhammed A, Berry CL, Thomas AC, Bennett MB, Campbell JH. Dog peritoneal and pleural cavities as bioreactors to grow autologous vascular grafts. J Vasc Surg 2004;39(4): 859-67

[88] Kalfa D, Bel A, Chen-Tournoux A, Della Martina A, Rochereau P, Coz C, Bellamy V, Bensalah M, Vanneaux V, Lecourt S, Mousseaux E, Bruneval P, Larghero J, Menasché P. A polydioxanone electrospun valved patch to replace the right ventricular outflow tract in a growing lamb model.Biomaterials 2010;31(14): 4056-63

[89] Steinhoff G, Stock U, Karim N, Mertsching H, Timke A, Meliss RR, Pethig K, Haverich A, Bader A. Tissue engineering of pulmonary heart valves on allogenic acellular

matrix conduits: in vivo restoration of valve tissue.Circulation 2000;102(19 Suppl 3): III50-5

[90] Dohmen PM, Ozaki S, Yperman J, Flameng W, Konertz W. Lack of calcification of tissue engineered heart valves in juvenile sheep.Semin Thorac Cardiovasc Surg 2001;13(4 Suppl 1): 93-8

[91] Lutter G, Metzner A, Jahnke T, Bombien R, Boldt J, Iino K, Cremer J, Stock UA. Percutaneous tissue-engineered pulmonary valved stent implantation.Ann Thorac Surg 2010;89(1): 259-63

[92] Perri G, Polito A, Esposito C, Albanese SB, Francalanci P, Pongiglione G, Carotti A. Early and late failure of tissue-engineered pulmonary valve conduits used for right ventricular outflow tract reconstruction in patients with congenital heart disease. Eur J Cardiothorac Surg 2012;41(6): 1320-5

[93] Cebotari S, Lichtenberg A, Tudorache I, Hilfiker A, Mertsching H, Leyh R, Breymann T, Kallenbach K, Maniuc L, Batrinac A, Repin O, Maliga O, Ciubotaru A, Haverich A. Clinical application of tissue engineered human heart valves using autologous progenitor cells. Circulation 2006;114(1 Suppl): I132-7

[94] Dohmen PM, Lembcke A, Holinski S, Pruss A, Konertz W. Ten years of clinical results with a tissue-engineered pulmonary valve. Ann Thorac Surg 2011;92(4): 1308-14

[95] Weber B, Scherman J, Emmert MY, Gruenenfelder J, Verbeek R, Bracher M, Black M, Kortsmit J, Franz T, Schoenauer R, Baumgartner L, Brokopp C, Agarkova I, Wolint P, Zund G, Falk V, Zilla P, Hoerstrup SP. Injectable living marrow stromal cell-based autologous tissue engineered heart valves: first experiences with a one-step intervention in primates.Eur Heart J 2011;32(22): 2830-40

[96] Emmert MY, Weber B, Behr L, Frauenfelder T, Brokopp CE, Grünenfelder J, Falk V, Hoerstrup SP. Transapical aortic implantation of autologous marrow stromal cell-based tissue-engineered heart valves: first experiences in the systemic circulation.JACC Cardiovasc Interv 2011;4(7): 822-3

[97] Emmert MY, Weber B, Wolint P, Behr L, Sammut S, Frauenfelder T, Frese L, Scherman J, Brokopp CE, Templin C, Grünenfelder J, Zünd G, Falk V, Hoerstrup SP. Stem cell-based transcatheter aortic valve implantation: first experiences in a pre-clinical model.JACC Cardiovasc Interv 2012;5(8): 874-83

[98] Vincentelli A, Wautot F, Juthier F, Fouquet O, Corseaux D, Marechaux S, Le Tourneau T, Fabre O, Susen S, Van Belle E, Mouquet F, Decoene C, Prat A, Jude B. In vivo autologous recellularization of a tissue-engineered heart valve: are bone marrow mesenchymal stem cells the best candidates? J Thorac Cardiovasc Surg 2007;134(2): 424-32

[99] Dohmen PM, da Costa F, Yoshi S, Lopes SV, da Souza FP, Vilani R, Wouk AF, da Costa M, Konertz W. Histological evaluation of tissue-engineered heart valves im-

planted in the juvenile sheep model: is there a need for in-vitro seeding? J Heart Valve Dis 2006;15(6): 823-9

[100] Dohmen PM, da Costa F, Holinski S, Lopes SV, Yoshi S, Reichert LH, Villani R, Posner S, Konertz W. Is there a possibility for a glutaraldehyde-free porcine heart valve to grow? Eur Surg Res 2006;38(1): 54-61

[101] Affonso da Costa FD, Dohmen PM, Lopes SV, Lacerda G, Pohl F, Vilani R, Affonso Da Costa MB, Vieira ED, Yoschi S, Konertz W, Affonso da Costa I. Comparison of cryopreserved homografts and decellularized porcine heterografts implanted in sheep.Artif Organs 2004;28(4): 366-70

[102] Hopkins RA, Jones AL, Wolfinbarger L, Moore MA, Bert AA, Lofland GK. Decellularization reduces calcification while improving both durability and 1-year functional results of pulmonary homograft valves in juvenile sheep. J Thorac Cardiovasc Surg 2009;137(4):907-13, 913e1-4

[103] Baraki H, Tudorache I, Braun M, Höffler K, Görler A, Lichtenberg A, Bara C, Calistru A, Brandes G, Hewicker-Trautwein M, Hilfiker A, Haverich A, Cebotari S. Orthotopic replacement of the aortic valve with decellularized allograft in a sheep model.Biomaterials 2009;30(31): 6240-6

[104] Muratov R, Britikov D, Sachkov A, Akatov V, Soloviev V, Fadeeva I, Bockeria L. New approach to reduce allograft tissue immunogenicity. Experimental data. Interact Cardiovasc Thorac Surg 2010;10(3): 408-12

[105] Costa F, Dohmen P, Vieira E, Lopes SV, Colatusso C, Pereira EW, Matsuda CN, Cauduro S. Ross Operation with decellularized pulmonary allografts: medium-term results. Rev Bras Cir Cardiovasc 2007;22(4): 454-62

[106] CebotariS, Tudorache I, Ciubotaru A, Boethig D, Sarikouch S, Goerler A, Lichtenberg A, Cheptanaru E, Barnaciuc S, Cazacu A, Maliga O, Repin O, Maniuc L, Breymann T, Haverich A. Use of freshdecellularizedallografts for pulmonary valve replacement may reduce the reoperation rate in children and young adults: early report. Circulation 2011;124(11 Suppl): S115–23

[107] Brown JW, Elkins RC, Clarke DR, Tweddell JS, Huddleston CB, Doty JR, Fehrenbacher JW, Takkenberg JJ. Performance of the CryoValve SG human decellularized pulmonary valve in 342 patients relative to the conventional CryoValve at a mean follow-up of four years. J Thorac Cardiovasc Surg 2010;139(2): 339-48

[108] Burch PT, Kaza AK, Lambert LM, Holubkov R, Shaddy RE, Hawkins JA. Clinical performance of decellularized cryopreserved valved allografts compared with standard allografts in the right ventricular outflow tract. Ann Thorac Surg 2010;90(4): 1301-5

[109] Erdbrugger W, Konertz W, Dohmen PM, Posner S, Ellerbrok H, Brodde OE, Robenek H, Modersohn D, Pruss A, Holinski S, Stein-Konertz M, Pauli G. Decellularized xen-

ogeneic heart valves reveal remodeling and growth potential *in vivo*. Tissue Eng 2006;12(8): 2059-68

[110] Konertz W, Angeli E, Tarusinov G, Christ T, Kroll J, Dohmen PM, Krogmann O, Franzbach B, Pace Napoleone C, Gargiulo G. Right ventricular outflow tract reconstruction with decellularized porcine xenografts in patients with congenital heart disease. J Heart Valve Dis 2011;20(3): 341-7

[111] Bloch O, Golde P, Dohmen PM, Posner S, Konertz W, Erdbrügger W.Immune response in patients receiving a bioprosthetic heart valve: lack of response with decellularized valves. Tissue Eng Part A 2011;17(19-20): 2399-405

[112] Rüffer A, Purbojo A, Cicha I, Glöckler M, Potapov S, Dittrich S, Cesnjevar RA. Early failure of xenogenous de-cellularised pulmonary valve conduits--a word of caution! Eur J Cardiothorac Surg2010;38(1): 78-85

[113] Cicha I, Rüffer A, Cesnjevar R, Glöckler M, Agaimy A, Daniel WG, Garlichs CD, Dittrich S. Early obstruction of decellularized xenogenic valves in pediatric patients: involvement of inflammatory and fibroproliferative processes.Cardiovasc Pathol 2011;20(4): 222-31

[114] Simon P, Kasimir MT, Seebacher G, Weigel G, Ulrich R, Salzer U, Rieder E and Wolner E. Early failure of the tissue engineered porcine heart valve Synergraft™ in paediatric patients. Eur J Cardiothorac Surg 2003;23: 1002-6

[115] Sprangers B, Waer M, Billiau AD. Xenograft rejection-all that glitters is not Gal. Nephrol Dial Transplant 2006;21: 1486-8

[116] Terasaki PI, Cecka JM, Gjertson DW, Takemoto S, Cho YW, Yuge J. Risk rate and long-term kidney transplant survival. Clin Transpl 1996: 443-58

[117] Billingham ME, Cary NR, Hammond ME, Kemnitz J, Marboe C, McCallister HA, Snovar DC, Winters GL, Zerbe A. A working formulation for the standardization of nomenclature in the diagnosis of heart and lung rejection: Heart Rejection Study Group. The International Society for Heart Transplantation. J Heart Transplant 1990;9(6): 587-93

[118] Edge ASB, Gosse ME and Dinsmore J. Xenogeneic cell therapy: current progress and future developments in porcine cell transplantation. Cell Transplant 1998;7: 525-539

[119] Kobayashi T, Taniguchi S, Neethling FA, Rose A, Hancock WW, Ye Y, Niekrasz M , Kosanke S, Wright JL,White DJG and Cooper DKC. Delayed xenograft rejection of pig-to-baboon cardiac transplants after cobra venom factor therapy. Transplantation 1997; 64: 1255-1261

[120] Galili U, Clark MR, Shohet SB, Buehler J, Macher BA. Evolutionary relationship between the natural anti-Gal antibody and the Gal alpha 1-3Gal epitope in primates. Proc Natl Acad Sci USA 1987;84: 1369-1373

[121] Galili U, Shohet SB, Kobrin E, Stults CL, Macher BA. Man, apes, and Old World monkeys differ from other mammals in the expression of alpha-galactosyl epitopes on nucleated cells. J Biol Chem 1988;263(33): 17755-62

[122] Galili U, Rachmilewitz EA, Peleg A, Flechner I. A unique natural human IgG antibody with anti-alphagalactosyl specificity. J Exp Med 1984;160(5): 1519-31

[123] Galili U, Mandrell RE, Hamadeh RM, Shohet SB, Griffiss JM. Interaction between human natural anti-alphagalactosyl immunoglobulin G and bacteria of the human flora. Infect Immun 1988;56(7):1730

[124] Cooper DK, Good AH, Koren E, Oriol R, Malcolm AJ, Ippolito RM, Neethling FA, Ye Y, Romano E, Zuhdi N. Identification of alpha-galactosyl and other carbohydrate epitopes that are bound by human anti-pig antibodies: relevance to discordant xenografting in man. Transpl Immunol 1993;1(3): 198-205

[125] Koren E, Kujundzic M, Koscec M, Neethling FA, Richards SV, Ye Y, Zuhdi N, Cooper DK. Cytotoxic effects of human preformed anti-Gal IgG and complement on cultured pig cells. Transplant Proc 1994;26(3): 1336-9

[126] Alwayn IPJ, Basker M, Buhler L and Cooper DKC. The problem of anti-pig antibodies in pig-to-primate xenografting: current and novel methods of depletion and/or suppression of production of anti-pig antibodies. Xenotransplantation 1999; 6: 157-168

[127] Kozlowski T, Shimizu A, Lambrigts D, Yamada K, Fuchimoto Y, Glaser R, Monroy R, Xu Y, Awwad M, Colvin RB, Cosimi AB, Robson SC, Fishman J, Spitzer TR, Cooper DKC, Sachs DH. Porcine kidney and heart transplantations in baboons undergoing a tolerance induction regimen and antibody adsorption. Transplantation 1999;67: 18-30

[128] Schmoeckel M, Bhatti FN, Zaidi A, Cozzi E, Waterworth PD, Tolan MJ, Pino-Chavez G, Goddard M, Warner RG, Langford GA, Dunning JJ, Wallwork J, White DJ. Orthotopic heart transplantation in a transgenic pig-to-primate model. Transplantation 1998;65: 1570-7

[129] Minanov OP, Artrip JH, Szabolcs M, Kwiatkowski PA, Galili U, Itescu S, Michler RE. Triple immunosuppresion reduces mononuclear cell infiltration and prolongs graft life in pig-to-newborn baboon cardiac xenotransplantation. J Thorac Cardiovasc Surg 1998;115: 998-1006

[130] Lam TT, Paniagua R, Shivaram G, Schuurman HJ, Borie DC, Morris RE. Anti-non-Gal porcine endothelial cell antibodies in acute humoral xenograft rejection of hDAF-transgenic porcine hearts in cynomolgus monkeys. Xenotransplantation 2004;11: 531-535

[131] Costa C, Zhao L, Burton WV, Bondioli KR, Williams BL, Hoagland TA, Di Tullio PA, Ebert KM and Fodor WL. Expression of α1-2-fucosyltransferase in transgenic pigs

modifies the surface carbohydrate phenotype and confers resistance to human se-rum-mediated cytolysis. FASEB J 1999;6: 6-11

[132] Cozzi E, Yannoutsous N, Langford GA, Pino-Chavez G, Wallwork B and White DJG. Effect of transgenic expression of human decay-accelerating factor on the inhibition of hyperacute rejection of pig organs. In Xenotransplantation by Cooper DKC and Kemp E, pp. 665-682, Springer-Verlag, Berlin

[133] Kuwaki K, Tseng YL, Dor FJMF, et al. Heart transplantation in baboons using α1,3-galactosyltransferase gene-knockout pigs as donors: initial experience. Nat Med 2005;11: 29–31

[134] Kasimir MT, Rieder E, Seebacher G, Wolner E, Weigel G and Simon P. Presence and elimination of the xenoantigen Gal (α1-3) Gal in tissue-engineered heart valves. Tissue Engineering 2005;11: 1274-1280

[135] Naso F, Gandaglia A, Iop L, Spina M, Gerosa G. Alpha-Gal detectors in xenotransplantation research: a word of caution.Xenotransplantation 2012;19(4): 215-20

[136] Naso F, Gandaglia A, Iop L, Spina M, Gerosa G. First quantitative assay of alpha-Gal in soft tissues: presence and distribution of the epitope before and after cell removal from xenogeneic heart valves.Acta Biomater 2011;7(4): 1728-34

[137] Dijkman PE, Driessen-Mol A, Frese L, Hoerstrup SP, Baaijens FP. Decellularized homologous tissue-engineered heart valves as off-the-shelf alternatives to xeno- and homografts. Biomaterials 2012;33(18): 4545-54

[138] Krug EL, Markwald RR. Extracellular cardiac proteins activate chick endothelial transition to prevalvular mesenchyme. Prog Clin Biol Res1986;217B: 195-8

[139] de Lange FJ, Moorman AFM, Anderson H, Maenner J,. Soufan AT, de Gier-de Vries C, Schneider MD, Webb S, van den Hoff MJB, Christoffels VM. Lineage and Morphogenetic Analysis of the Cardiac Valves. Circ Res 2004;95; 645-654

[140] Snider P, Olaopa M, Firulli AB, Conway SJ. Cardiovascular Development and the Colonizing Cardiac Neural Crest Lineage. The Scientific World Journal 2007;7: 1090–1113

[141] Eisenberg LM, Markwald RR. Molecular Regulation of Atrioventricular Valvulo-septal Morphogenesis. Circulation Research 1995; 77:1-6

[142] von Wattenwyl R, Blumenthal B, Heilmann C, Golsong P, Poppe A, Beyersdorf F, Siepe M.Scaffold-based transplantation of vascular endothelial growth factor-overexpressing stem cells leads to neovascularization in ischemic myocardium but did not show a functional regenerative effect.ASAIO J 2012;58(3): 268-74

[143] Noiseux N, Gnecchi M, Lopez-Ilasaca M, Zhang L, Solomon SD, Deb A, Dzau VJ, Pratt RE. Mesenchymal stem cells overexpressing Akt dramatically repair infarcted

myocardium and improve cardiac function despite infrequent cellular fusion or differentiation.Mol Ther 2006;14(6): 840-50

[144] Takahashi K, Tanabe K, Ohnuki M, Narita M, Ichisaka T, Tomoda K, Yamanaka S.Induction of pluripotent stem cells from adult human fibroblasts by defined factors.Cell 2007;131(5): 861-72

[145] Jung CB, Moretti A, Mederos y Schnitzler M, Iop L, Storch U, Bellin M, Dorn T, Ruppenthal S, Pfeiffer S, Goedel A, Dirschinger RJ, Seyfarth M, Lam JT, Sinnecker D, Gudermann T, Lipp P, Laugwitz KL. Dantrolene rescues arrhythmogenic RYR2 defect in a patient-specific stem cell model of catecholaminergic polymorphic ventricular tachycardia.EMBO Mol Med 2012;4(3): 180-91

[146] Templin C, Zweigerdt R, Schwanke K, Olmer R, Ghadri JR, Emmert MY, Müller E, Küest SM, Cohrs S, Schibli R, Kronen P, Hilbe M, Reinisch A, Strunk D, Haverich A, Hoerstrup S, Lüscher TF, Kaufmann PA, Landmesser U, Martin U. Transplantation and tracking of human-induced pluripotent stem cells in a pig model of myocardial infarction: assessment of cell survival, engraftment, and distribution by hybrid single photon emission computed tomography/computed tomography of sodium iodide symporter transgene expression. Circulation 2012;126(4): 430-9

[147] Armstrong EJ and Bischoff J. Heart Valve Development: Endothelial Cell Signaling and Differentiation. Circ Res 2004;95; 459-470

[148] Combs MD and Yutzey KE. VEGF and RANKL Regulation of NFATc1 in Heart Valve Development. Circ Res 2009;105; 565-574

[149] de la Pompa JL. Notch Signaling in Cardiac Development and Disease. Pediatr Cardiol 2009;30: 643–650

[150] Rivera-Feliciano J, Tabin CJ. Bmp2 instructs cardiac progenitors to form the heart-valve-inducing field. Developmental Biology 2006;295:580–588

[151] MCCulley DJ, Kang J, Martin JF, Black BL. BMP4 is required in the anterior heart field and its derivatives for endocardial cushion remodeling, outflow tract septation, and semilunar valve development. Developmental Dynamics 2008;237: 3200–3209

[152] Lincoln J, Kist R, Scherer G, Yutzey KE. Sox9 is required for precursor cell expansion and extracellular matrix organization during mouse heart valve development. Developmental Biology 2007;305: 120–132

[153] Lie-Venema H, Eralp I, Markwald RR, van den Akker NM, Wijffels MC, Kolditz DP, van der Laarse A, Schalij MJ, Poelmann RE, Bogers AJ, Gittenberger-de Groot AC. Periostin expression by epicardium-derived cells is involved in the development of the atrioventricular valves and fibrous heart skeleton. Differentiation 2008;76(7): 809-19

[154] Norris RA, Potts JD, Yost MJ, Junor L, Brooks T, Tan H, Hoffman S, Hart MM,. Kern MJ, Damon B, Markwald RR, Goodwin RL. Periostin Promotes a Fibroblastic Lineage

Pathway in Atrioventricular Valve Progenitor Cells. Developmental Dynamics 2009;238: 1052–1063

[155] Scherz PJ, Huisken J, Sahai-Hernandez P, Stainier DYR. High-speed imaging of developing heart valves reveals interplay of morphogenesis and function. Development 2008;135: 1179-1187

[156] Ghosh AK, Nagpal V, Covington JW, Michaels MA, Vaughan DE. Molecular basis of cardiac endothelial-to-mesenchymaltransition (EndMT): differential expression of microRNAs during EndMT. Cell Signal 2012;24(5): 1031-6

[157] Hong H, Dong N, Shi J, Chen S, Guo C, Hu P, Qi H. Fabrication of a novel hybrid heart valve leaflet for tissue engineering: an in vitro study.Artif Organs2009;33(7): 554-8

[158] Paruchuri S, Yang JH, Aikawa E, Melero-Martin JM, Khan ZA, Loukogeorgakis S, Schoen FJ, Bischoff J. Human pulmonary valve progenitor cells exhibit endothelial/mesenchymal plasticity in response to vascular endothelial growth factor-A and transforming growth factor-beta2. Circ Res 2006;99(8): 861-9

[159] Chiu YN, Norris RA, Mahler G, Recknagel A, Butcher JT. Transforming growth factor β, bone morphogenetic protein, and vascular endothelial growth factor mediate phenotype maturation and tissue remodeling by embryonic valve progenitor cells: relevance for heart valve tissue engineering. Tissue Eng Part A 2010;16(11): 3375-83

[160] Sewell-Loftin MK, Chun YW, Khademhosseini A, Merryman WD. EMT-inducing biomaterials for heart valve engineering: taking cues from developmental biology.J Cardiovasc Transl Res 2011;4(5): 658-71

[161] Ramamurthi A, Vesely I. Evaluation of the matrix-synthesis potential of crosslinked hyaluronan gels for tissue engineering of aortic heart valves.Biomaterials2005;26(9): 999-1010

[162] Camci-Unal G, Nichol JW, Bae H, Tekin H, Bischoff J, Khademhosseini A. Hydrogel surfaces to promote attachment and spreading of endothelial progenitor cells.J Tissue Eng Regen Med 2012; doi: 10.1002/term.517

[163] Koens MJ, Faraj KA, Wismans RG, van der Vliet JA, Krasznai AG, Cuijpers VM, Jansen JA, Daamen WF, van Kuppevelt TH. Controlled fabrication of triple layered and molecularly defined collagen/elastin vascular grafts resembling the native blood vessel.Acta Biomater 2010;6(12): 4666-74

[164] Smith MD, Shearer MG, Srivastava S, Scott R, Courtney JM. Quantitative evaluation of the growth of established cell lines on the surface of collagen, collagen composite and reconstituted basement membrane.Urol Res 1992;20(4): 285-8

[165] Taite LJ, Yang P, Jun HW, West JL. Nitric oxide-releasing polyurethane-PEG copolymer containing the YIGSR peptide promotes endothelialization with decreased platelet adhesion.J Biomed Mater Res B Appl Biomater 2008;84(1): 108-16

[166] Andukuri A, Minor WP, Kushwaha M, Anderson JM, Jun HW. Effect of endothelium mimicking self-assembled nanomatrices on cell adhesion and spreading of human endothelial cells and smooth muscle cells.Nanomedicine 2010;6(2): 289-97

[167] Blindt R, Vogt F, Astafieva I, Fach C, Hristov M, Krott N, Seitz B, Kapurniotu A, Kwok C, Dewor M, Bosserhoff AK, Bernhagen J, Hanrath P, Hoffmann R, Weber C. A novel drug-eluting stent coated with an integrin-binding cyclic Arg-Gly-Asp peptide inhibits neointimal hyperplasia by recruiting endothelial progenitor cells.J Am Coll Cardiol2006;47(9): 1786-95

[168] einhart JG, Schense JC, Schima H, Gorlitzer M, Hubbell JA, Deutsch M, Zilla P. Enhanced endothelial cell retention on shear-stressed synthetic vascular grafts precoated with RGD-cross-linked fibrin.Tissue Eng2005;11(5-6): 887-95

[169] Andrieux A, Rabiet MJ, Chapel A, Concord E, Marguerie G. A highly conserved sequence of the Arg-Gly-Asp-binding domain of the integrin beta 3 subunit is sensitive to stimulation.J Biol Chem1991;266(22): 14202-7

[170] Hasegawa T, Okada K, Takano Y, Hiraishi Y, Okita Y. Autologous fibrin-coated small-caliber vascular prostheses improve antithrombogenicity by reducing immunologic response.J Thorac Cardiovasc Surg2007;133(5): 1268-76

[171] Flanagan TC, Cornelissen C, Koch S, Tschoeke B, Sachweh JS, Schmitz-Rode T, Jockenhoevel S. The in vitro development of autologous fibrin-based tissue-engineered heart valves through optimised dynamic conditioning.Biomaterials 2007;28(23): 3388-97

[172] Veleva AN, Heath DE, Cooper SL, Patterson C. Selective endothelial cell attachment to peptide-modified terpolymers.Biomaterials2008;29(27): 3656-61

[173] Rodas AC, Polak R, Hara PH, Lee EI, Pitombo RN, Higa OZ. Cytotoxicity and endothelial cell adhesion of lyophilized and irradiated bovine pericardium modified with silk fibroin and chitosan.Artif Organs 2011;35(5): 502-7

[174] Sarathchandra P, Smolenski RT, Yuen AH, Chester AH, Goldstein S, Heacox AE, Yacoub MH, Taylor PM. Impact of γ-Irradiation on Extracellular Matrix of Porcine Pulmonary Valves.J Surg Res 2012;176(2): 376-85

[175] Li S, Henry JJ. Nonthrombogenic approaches to cardiovascular bioengineering.Annu Rev Biomed Eng 2011;13: 451-75

[176] Hashi CK, Zhu Y, Yang GY, Young WL, Hsiao BS, Wang K, Chu B, Li S. Antithrombogenic property of bone marrow mesenchymal stem cells in nanofibrous vascular grafts. Proc Natl Acad Sci USA 2007;104(29): 11915-20

[177] Kito H, Matsuda T. Biocompatible coatings for luminal and outer surfaces of small-caliber artificial grafts.J Biomed Mater Res 1996;30(3): 321-30

[178] Gombotz WR, Wang GH, Horbett TA, Hoffman AS. Protein adsorption to poly(ethyl-ene oxide) surfaces.J Biomed Mater Res 1991;25(12): 1547-62

[179] Jordan SW, Faucher KM, Caves JM, Apkarian RP, Rele SS, Sun XL, Hanson SR, Chai-kof EL. Fabrication of a phospholipid membrane-mimetic film on the luminal surface of an ePTFE vascular graft. Biomaterials 2006;27(18): 3473-81

[180] Koo J, Galanakis D, Liu Y, Ramek A, Fields A, Ba X, Simon M, Rafailovich MH. Con-trol of anti-thrombogenic properties: surface-induced self-assembly of fibrinogen fi-bers. Biomacromolecules 2012;13(5): 1259-68

[181] Smith DJ, Chakravarthy D, Pulfer S, Simmons ML, Hrabie JA, Citro ML, Saavedra JE, Davies KM, Hutsell TC, Mooradian DL, Hanson SR, Keefer LK. Nitric oxide-releas-ing polymers containing the [N(O)NO]- group.J Med Chem 1996;39(5): 1148-56

[182] Kolpakov V, Gordon D, Kulik TJ. Nitric oxide-generating compounds inhibit total protein and collagen synthesis in cultured vascular smooth muscle cells.Circ Res 1995;76(2): 305-9

[183] Yu J, Zhang Y, Zhang X, Rudic RD, Bauer PM, Altieri DC, Sessa WC. Endothelium derived nitric oxide synthase negatively regulates the PDGF-survivin pathway dur-ing flow-dependent vascular remodeling. PLoS One 2012;7(2): e31495

[184] Marks DS, Vita JA, Folts JD, Keaney JF Jr, Welch GN, Loscalzo J. Inhibition of neoin-timal proliferation in rabbits after vascular injury by a single treatment with a protein adduct of nitric oxide.J Clin Invest 1995;96(6): 2630-8

[185] Acharya G, Hopkins RA, Lee CH. Advanced polymeric matrix for valvular complica-tions.J Biomed Mater Res A 2012;100(5): 1151-9

[186] De Scheerder I, Wang K, Wilczek K, Meuleman D, Van Amsterdam R, Vogel G, Pies-sens J, Van de Werf F. Experimental study of thrombogenicity and foreign body reac-tion induced by heparin-coated coronary stents.Circulation 1997;95(6): 1549-53

[187] Lahann J, Plüster W, Klee D, Gattner HG, Höcker H. Immobilization of the thrombin inhibitor r-hirudin conserving its biological activity.J Mater Sci Mater Med 2001;12(9): 807-10

[188] Hashi CK, Derugin N, Janairo RR, Lee R, Schultz D, Lotz J, Li S. Antithrombogenic modification of small-diameter microfibrous vascular grafts.Arterioscler Thromb Vasc Biol 2010;30(8): 1621-7

[189] Pastore CJ, Isner JM, Bacha PA, Kearney M, Pickering JG. Epidermal growth factor receptor-targeted cytotoxin inhibits neointimalhyperplasia in vivo. Results of local versus systemic administration.Circ Res 1995;77(3): 519-29

[190] Asahara T, Bauters C, Pastore C, Kearney M, Rossow S, Bunting S, Ferrara N, Symes JF, Isner JM. Local delivery of vascular endothelial growth factor accelerates reendo-

thelialization and attenuates intimal hyperplasia in balloon-injured rat carotid artery.Circulation 1995;91(11): 2793-801

[191] Leppänen O, Rutanen J, Hiltunen MO, Rissanen TT, Turunen MP, Sjöblom T, Brüggen J, Bäckström G, Carlsson M, Buchdunger E, Bergqvist D, Alitalo K, Heldin CH, Ostman A, Ylä-Herttuala S. Oral imatinib mesylate (STI571/gleevec) improves the efficacy of local intravascular vascular endothelial growth factor-C gene transfer in reducing neointimal growth in hypercholesterolemic rabbits.Circulation 2004;109(9): 1140-6

[192] Sirois MG, Simons M, Edelman ER. Antisense oligonucleotide inhibition of PDGFR-beta receptor subunit expression directs suppression of intimal thickening.Circulation 1997;95(3): 669-76

[193] Coleman KR, Braden GA, Willingham MC, Sane DC. Vitaxin, a humanized monoclonal antibody to the vitronectin receptor (alphavbeta3), reduces neointimalhyperplasia and total vessel area after balloon injury in hypercholesterolemic rabbits.Circ Res 1999;84(11): 1268-76

[194] Miniati DN, Hoyt EG, Feeley BT, Poston RS, Robbins RC.Circulation 2000;102(19 Suppl 3): III237-42

[195] Skelly CL, Curi MA, Meyerson SL, Woo DH, Hari D, Vosicky JE, Advani SJ, Mauceri HJ, Glagov S, Roizman B, Weichselbaum RR, Schwartz LB. Prevention of restenosis by a herpes simplex virus mutant capable of controlled long-term expression in vascular tissue in vivo.Gene Ther 2001;8(24): 1840-6

[196] Mallawaarachchi CM, Weissberg PL, Siow RC. Smad7 gene transfer attenuates adventitial cell migration and vascular remodeling after balloon injury.Arterioscler Thromb Vasc Biol2005;25(7): 1383-7

[197] Mallawaarachchi CM, Weissberg PL, Siow RC. Antagonism of platelet-derived growth factor by perivascular gene transfer attenuates adventitial cell migration after vascular injury: new tricks for old dogs?FASEB J2006;20(10): 1686–1688

[198] Garcia-Touchard A, Burke SE, Toner JL, Cromack K, Schwartz RS. Zotarolimus-eluting stents reduce experimental coronary artery neointimal hyperplasia after 4 weeks. Eur Heart J 2006;27(8): 988-93

[199] Chen YW, Smith ML, Sheets M, Ballaron S, Trevillyan JM, Burke SE, Rosenberg T, Henry C, Wagner R, Bauch J, Marsh K, Fey TA, Hsieh G, Gauvin D, Mollison KW, Carter GW, Djuric SW. Zotarolimus, a novel sirolimus analogue with potent antiproliferative activity on coronary smooth muscle cells and reduced potential for systemic immunosuppression.J Cardiovasc Pharmacol 2007;49(4): 228-35

[200] Zhao L, Ding T, Cyrus T, Cheng Y, Tian H, Ma M, Falotico R, Praticò D. Low-dose oral sirolimus reduces atherogenesis, vascular inflammation and modulates plaque composition in mice lacking the LDL receptor.Br J Pharmacol 2009;156(5): 774-85

[201] Patel JK, Kobashigawa JA. Everolimus for cardiac allograft vasculopathy--every patient, at any time?Transplantation. 2011 Jul 27;92(2):127-8

[202] Baek I, Bai CZ, Hwang J, Park J, Park JS, Kim DJ. Suppression of neointimalhyperplasia by sirolimus-eluting expanded polytetrafluoroethylene (ePTFE) haemodialysis grafts in comparison with paclitaxel-coated grafts.Nephrol Dial Transplant 2012;27(5): 1997-2004

[203] Thiene G, Valente M. Calcification of valve bioprosthesis: the cardiac surgeon's nightmare. Eur J Cardiothorac Surg 1994;8(9): 476-8

[204] Pettenazzo E, Deiwick M, Thiene G, Molin G, Glasmacher B, Martignago F, Bottio T, Reul H, Valente M. Dynamic *in vitro* calcification of bioprosthetic porcine valves: evidence of apatite crystallization. J Thorac Cardiovasc Surg 2001;121(3): 500-9

[205] Zhai W, Chang J, Lü X, Wang Z. Procyanidins-crosslinked heart valve matrix: anticalcification effect.J Biomed Mater Res B Appl Biomater 2009;90(2): 913-21

[206] Pettenazzo E, Valente M, Thiene G. Octanediol treatment of glutaraldehyde fixed bovine pericardium: evidence of anticalcification efficacy in the subcutaneous rat model.Eur J Cardiothorac Surg 2008;34(2): 418-22

[207] Lim HG, Kim SH, Choi SY, Kim YJ. Anticalcification effects of decellularization, solvent, and detoxification treatment for genipin and glutaraldehyde fixation of bovine pericardium.Eur J Cardiothorac Surg 2012;41(2): 383-90

[208] Connolly JM, Bakay MA, Alferiev IS, Gorman RC, Gorman JH 3rd, Kruth HS, Ashworth PE, Kutty JK, Schoen FJ, Bianco RW, Levy RJ. Triglycidyl amine crosslinking combined with ethanol inhibits bioprosthetic heart valve calcification.Ann Thorac Surg 2011;92(3): 858-65

[209] Sacks MS, Hamamoto H, Connolly JM, Gorman RC, Gorman JH 3rd, Levy RJ. In vivo biomechanical assessment of triglycidylamine crosslinked pericardium. Biomaterials 2007;28(35): 5390-8

[210] Koutsopoulos S, Kontogeorgou A, Dalas E, Petroheilos J. Calcification of porcine and human cardiac valves: testing of various inhibitors for antimineralization. J Mater Sci Mater Med 1998;9(7): 421-4

[211] da Costa FD, Costa AC, Prestes R, Domanski AC, Balbi EM, Ferreira AD, Lopes SV. The early and midterm function of decellularized aortic valve allografts.Ann Thorac Surg 2010;90(6): 1854-60

[212] Rodríguez M, Aguilera-Tejero E, Mendoza FJ, Guerrero F, López I. Effects of calcimimetics on extraskeletal calcifications in chronic kidney disease. Kidney Int Suppl 2008;(111): S50-4

[213] Jung S, Querfeld U, Müller D, Rudolph B, Peters H, Krämer S. Submaximal suppression of parathyroid hormone ameliorates calcitriol-induced aortic calcification and remodeling and myocardial fibrosis in uremic rats. J Hypertens 2012;30(11): 2182-91

[214] Alferiev I, Vyavahare N, Song C, Connolly J, Hinson JT, Lu Z, Tallapragada S, Bianco R, Levy R. Bisphosphonate derivatized polyurethanes resist calcification.biomaterials 2001;22(19): 2683-93

[215] Ng KE, Joly P, Jayasinghe SN, Vernay B, Knight R, Barry SP, McComick J, Latchman D, Stephanou A. Bio-electrospraying primary cardiac cells: in vitro tissue creation and functional study.Biotechnol J 2011;6(1): 86-95

[216] Kaminski A, Klopsch C, Mark P, Yerebakan C, Donndorf P, Gäbel R, Eisert F, Hasken S, Kreitz S, Glass A, Jockenhövel S, Ma N, Kundt G, Liebold A, Steinhoff G. Autologous valve replacement-CD133+ stem cell-plus-fibrin composite-based sprayed cell seeding for intraoperative heart valvetissue engineering.Tissue Eng Part C Methods 2011;17(3): 299-309

[217] Lin Q, Ding X, Qiu F, Song X, Fu G, Ji J. In situ endothelialization of intravascular stents coated with an anti-CD34 antibody functionalized heparin-collagen multilayer.Biomaterials 2010;31(14): 4017-25

[218] Ye X, Zhao Q, Sun X, Li H. Enhancement of mesenchymal stem cell attachment to decellularized porcine aortic valve scaffold by in vitro coating with antibody against CD90: a preliminary study on antibody-modified tissue-engineered heart valve. Tissue Eng Part A 2009;15(1): 1-11

[219] Jordan JE, Williams JK, Lee SJ, Raghavan D, Atala A, Yoo JJ. Bioengineered self-seeding heart valves.J Thorac Cardiovasc Surg 2012;143(1): 201-8

[220] Hoffmann J, Paul A, Harwardt M, Groll J, Reeswinkel T, Klee D, Moeller M, Fischer H, Walker T, Greiner T, Ziemer G, Wendel HP. Immobilized DNA aptamers used as potent attractors for porcine endothelial precursor cells.J Biomed Mater Res A 2008;84(3): 614-21

[221] Schleicher M, Wendel HP, Fritze O, Stock UA. In vivo tissue engineering of heart valves: evolution of a novel concept.Regen Med 2009;4(4): 613-9

[222] Sun W, Darling A, Starly B, Nam J. Computer-aided tissue engineering: overview, scope and challenges. Biotechnol Appl Biochem 2004;39(Pt 1): 29-47

[223] Lalan S, Pomerantseva I, Vacanti JP. Tissue engineering and its potential impact on surgery.World J Surg 2001;25(11): 1458-66

[224] Norotte C, Marga FS, Niklason LE, Forgacs G. Scaffold-free vascular tissue engineering using bioprinting.Biomaterials 2009;30(30): 5910-7

[225] Masoumi N, Jean A, Zugates JT, Johnson KL, Engelmayr GC Jr. Laser microfabricated poly(glycerol sebacate) scaffolds for heart valve tissue engineering.J Biomed Mater Res A 2012. doi: 10.1002/jbm.a.34305

[226] Schmauss D, Schmitz C, Bigdeli AK, Weber S, Gerber N, Beiras-Fernandez A, Schwarz F, Becker C, Kupatt C, Sodian R. Three-dimensional printing of models for preoperative planning and simulation of transcatheter valve replacement. Ann Thorac Surg2012;93(2): e31-3

[227] Nakayama Y, Yamanami M, Yahata Y, Tajikawa T, Ohba K, Watanabe T, Kanda K, Yaku H. Preparation of a completely autologous trileaflet valve-shaped construct by in-body tissue architecture technology. J Biomed Mater Res B Appl Biomater 2009;91(2): 813-8

[228] Davies H. Catheter mounted valve for temporary relief of aortic insufficiency Lancet 1965;1: 250

[229] Bonhoeffer P, Boudjemline Y, Saliba Z, Merckx J, Aggoun Y, Bonnet D, Acar P, Le Bidois J, Sidi D, Kachaner J. Percutaneous replacement of pulmonary valve in a right-ventricle to pulmonary-artery prosthetic conduit with valve dysfunction.Lancet2000;356(9239): 1403-5

[230] Cribier A, Eltchaninoff H, Bash A, Borenstein N, Tron C, Bauer F, Derumeaux G, Anselme F, Laborde F, Leon MB. Percutaneous transcatheter implantation of an aortic valve prosthesis for calcific aortic stenosis: first human case description.Circulation2002;106(24): 3006-8

[231] Schmidt D, Dijkman PE, Driessen-Mol A, Stenger R, Mariani C, Puolakka A, Rissanen M, Deichmann T, Odermatt B, Weber B, Emmert MY, Zund G, Baaijens FP, Hoerstrup SP. Minimally-invasive implantation of living tissue engineered heart valves: a comprehensive approach from autologous vascular cells to stem cells.J Am Coll Cardiol2010;56(6): 510-20

[232] Schmidt D, Dijkman PE, Driessen-Mol A, Stenger R, Mariani C, Puolakka A, Rissanen M, Deichmann T, Odermatt B, Weber B, Emmert MY, Zund G, Baaijens FP, Hoerstrup SP. Minimally-invasive implantation of living tissue engineered heart valves: a comprehensive approach from autologous vascular cells to stem cells.J Am Coll Cardiol2010;56(6): 510-20

[233] Helmchen F, Denk W. Deep tissue two-photon microscopy. Helmchen F, Denk W. Nat Methods 2005;2(12): 932-40

[234] Schenke-Layland K, Riemann I, Opitz F, König K, Halbhuber KJ, Stock UA. Comparative study of cellular and extracellular matrix composition of native and tissue engineered heart valves.Matrix Biol 2004;23(2): 113-25

[235] Karamitsos TD, Myerson SG. The role of cardiovascular magnetic resonance in the evaluation of valve disease.Prog Cardiovasc Dis 2011;54(3): 276-86

[236] Dohmen PM, Lembcke A, Hotz H, Kivelitz D, Konertz WF. Ross operation with a tissue-engineeredheart valve.Ann Thorac Surg 2002;74(5):1438-42

[237] Ramaswamy S, Schornack PA, Smelko AG, Boronyak SM, Ivanova J, Mayer JE Jr, Sacks MS. Superparamagnetic iron oxide (SPIO) labeling efficiency and subsequent MRI tracking of native cell populations pertinent to pulmonary heart valve tissue engineering studies.NMR Biomed 2012;25(3): 410-7

[238] Aikawa E, Otto CM. Look more closely at the valve: imaging calcific aortic valve disease.Circulation2012;125(1): 9-11

[239] Liu L, Gardecki JA, Nadkarni SK, Toussaint JD, Yagi Y, Bouma BE, Tearney GJ. Imaging the subcellular structure of human coronary atherosclerosis using micro-opticalcoherencetomography.Nat Med 2011;17(8): 1010-4

[240] Ruggiero A, Thorek DL, Guenoun J, Krestin GP, Bernsen MR. Cell tracking in cardiac repair: what to image and how to image. Eur Radiol 2012;22(1): 189-204

[241] Ross DN. Homograft replacement of the aortic valve. Lancet 1962;2(7254): 487

[242] Jashari R, Tabaku M, Van Hoeck B, Cochéz C, Callant M, Vanderkelen A. Decontamination of heart valve and arterial allografts in the European Homograft Bank (EHB): comparison of two different antibiotic cocktails in low temperature conditions.Cell Tissue Bank 2007;8(4): 247-55

[243] Soo A, Healy DG, El-Bashier H, Shaw S, Wood AE. Quality control in homograft valve processing: when to screen for microbiological contamination?Cell Tissue Bank 2011;12(3): 185-90

[244] Jashari R, Goffin Y, Van Hoeck B, Vanderkelen A, du Verger A, Fan Y, Holovska V, Fagu A, Brahy O. Belgian and European experience with the European Homograft Bank (EHB) cryopreserved allograft valves.--assessment of a 20 year activity.Acta Chir Belg 2010;110(3): 280-90

[245] Wassenaar C, Bax WA, van Suylen RJ, Vuzevski VD, Bos E. Effects of cryopreservation on contractile properties of porcine isolated aortic valve leaflets and aortic wall.J Thorac Cardiovasc Surg 1997;113(1): 165-72

[246] Rendal Vázquez ME, Díaz Román TM, Rodríguez Cabarcos M, Zavanella Botta C, Domenech García N, González Cuesta M, Sánchez Dopico MJ, Pértega Díaz S, Andión Núñez C. Apoptosis in fresh and cryopreserved cardiac valves of pig samples.Cell Tissue Bank 2008;9(2): 101-7

[247] Gatto C, Dainese L, Buzzi M, Terzi A, Guarino A, Pagliaro PP, Polvani G, D'Amato Tothova J. Establishing a procedure for dimethyl sulfoxide removal from cardiovascular allografts: a quantitative study.Cell Tissue Bank 2012 Jul 27 [Epub ahead of print]

[248] Gerson CJ, Elkins RC, Goldstein S, Heacox AE. Structural integrity of collagen and elastin in SynerGraft® decellularized-cryopreserved human heart valves.Cryobiology. 2012 Feb;64(1):33-42

[249] Schenke-Layland K, Madershahian N, Riemann I, Starcher B, Halbhuber KJ, König K, Stock UA. Impact of cryopreservation on extracellular matrix structures of heart valve leaflets.Ann Thorac Surg 2006;81(3): 918-26

[250] Lisy M, Pennecke J, Brockbank KG, Fritze O, Schleicher M, Schenke-Layland K, Kaulitz R, Riemann I, Weber CN, Braun J, Mueller KE, Fend F, Scheunert T, Gruber AD, Albes JM, Huber AJ, Stock UA. The performance of ice-free cryopreserved heart valve allografts in an orthotopic pulmonary sheep model.Biomaterials 2010;31(20): 5306-11

[251] Rattazzi M, Iop L, Faggin E, Bertacco E, Zoppellaro G, Baesso I, Puato M, Torregrossa G, Fadini GP, Agostini C, Gerosa G, Sartore S, Pauletto P. Clones of interstitial cells from bovine aortic valve exhibit different calcifying potential when exposed to endotoxin and phosphate.Arterioscler Thromb Vasc Biol 2008;28(12): 2165-72

[252] Bertacco E, Millioni R, Arrigoni G, Faggin E, Iop L, Puato M, Pinna LA, Tessari P, Pauletto P, Rattazzi M. Proteomic analysis of clonal interstitial aortic valve cells acquiring a pro-calcific profile.J Proteome Res 2010;9(11): 5913-21

[253] New SE, Aikawa E. Cardiovascular calcification: an inflammatory disease.Circ J 2011;75(6): 1305-13

[254] Mathapati S, Verma RS, Cherian KM, Guhathakurta S.Inflammatory responses of tissue-engineered xenografts in a clinical scenario.Interact Cardiovasc Thorac Surg2011;12(3): 360-5

[255] Zhou J, Fritze O, Schleicher M, Wendel HP, Schenke-Layland K, Harasztosi C, Hu S, Stock UA. Impact of heart valve decellularization on 3-D ultrastructure, immunogenicity and thrombogenicity. Biomaterials 2010;31(9): 2549-54

[256] Arai S, Orton EC. Immunoblot detection of soluble protein antigens from sodium dodecyl sulphate- and sodium deoxycholate-treated candidate bioscaffold tissues. J Heart Valve Dis 2009;18(4): 439-43

[257] Barth PJ, KoÅNster H, Moosdorf R. CD34+ fibrocytes in normal mitral valves and myxomatous mitral valve degeneration. Pathol Res Pract 2005;201(4): 301-4

[258] Orkin SH. Diversification of haematopoietic stem cells to specific lineages. Nat Rev Genet 2000;1(1): 57-64

[259] Iop L, Basso C, Rizzo S, Piccoli M, Callegari M, Paolin A, De Coppi P, Thiene G, Sartore S, Gerosa G. Stem Cell Populations in Human Heart Valves: Identification, Isolation and Characterization in Valve Homografts and Surgical Specimens. Conference proceedings. World Conference on Regenerative Medicine– Leipzig, Germany, 29-31 October 2009

[260] Martinez FO, Sica A, Mantovani A, Locati M. Macrophage activation and polarization. Front Biosci 2008;13: 453-61

[261] Brown BN, Valentin JE, Stewart-Akers AM, McCabe GP, Badylak SF. Macrophage phenotype and remodeling outcomes in response to biologic scaffolds with and without a cellular component.Biomaterials 2009;30(8):1482-91

[262] Zheng C, Azcutia V, Aikawa E, Figueiredo JL, Croce K, Sonoki H, Sacks FM, Luscinskas FW, Aikawa M. Statins suppress apolipoprotein CIII-induced vascular endothelial cell activation and monocyte adhesion.Eur Heart J 2012 Aug 26 [Epub ahead of print]

[263] Monaghan M, Pandit A. RNA interference therapy via functionalized scaffolds. Adv Drug Deliv Rev 2011;63(4-5):197-208

Chapter 9

The Immune Response in *In Situ* Tissue Engineering of Aortic Heart Valves

S. L. M. van Loon, A. I. P. M. Smits, A. Driessen-Mol,
F. P. T. Baaijens and C. V. C. Bouten

Additional information is available at the end of the chapter

1. Introduction

The gold standard for treatment of advanced heart valve disease is surgical heart valve replacement. None of the currently available mechanical and bioprosthetic heart valve substitutes resembles normal heart valve function. While mechanical heart valves offer excellent durability, they require life-long anticoagulation to control thromboembolism, which inherently leads to an increased risk of hemorrhage complications. Bioprosthetic valves on the other hand, retain a more physiological blood flow pattern, but these valves are prone to calcification and structural deterioration, limiting their lifespan. For both types of replacement valves, the main limitation is that they are non-living prostheses, incapable of adapting to changes in the hemodynamic environment. It was shown that a living autograft implanted in the aortic position (the Ross procedure) improves long-term clinical outcome compared to a non-living homograft [1]. This illustrates the importance of the regulatory and adaptive properties of a living valve substitute. Tissue engineered aortic valves can provide such an autologous, viable valve with the potential to grow, adapt, and regenerate within the hemodynamic environment. Evidently, the pediatric and young adult population would benefit most from such a tissue engineered aortic valve. The valve's ability to grow as the recipient grows and matures, eliminates the need for repetitive surgeries. [2-7].

Foundational principle of regenerative medicine is restoring the native tissue structure and function by providing a microenvironment necessary to promote tissue regeneration. Tissue engineering scaffolds are biomaterials designed to create this microenvironment and to promote tissue regeneration [8]. The traditional tissue engineering paradigm for creating trileaflet heart valves consists of harvesting autologous cells from the patient, expanding the cells *in vitro*, and subsequently seeding the cells into a biodegradable scaffold. The cell-scaffold constructs are conditioned in a bioreactor to promote extracellular matrix formation (ECM), while the scaffold is degraded [9]. Although this approach leads to an autologous, living heart valve, the *in vitro* process is a very costly and time consuming procedure. Therefore, a novel approach emerged from this, in which the *in vitro* phase is completely omitted, the so-called *in situ* tissue engineering, or 'guided tissue regeneration' (figure 1). This approach relies on the body's natural regenerative potential and uses the human body as a bioreactor [4]. Key to this process is the use of a functional scaffold, capable of host cell repopulation and subsequent *in situ* tissue remodeling. After implantation, cells will colonize the scaffold to form tissue, while the scaffold withstands physiological stresses and strains from its hemodynamic environment and may gradually degrade [2,4]. Clearly, these characteristics put more stringent demands on the biomaterial used, as it should provide both mechanical strength and the cellular niche, balancing between material degradation and tissue formation. The scaffold can be biological or synthetic or a combination of both (a hybrid scaffold), loaded with bioactive components and/or cells to provide stimuli for favorable host cell repopulation, differentiation and tissue formation. The *in situ* approach allows for the minimization of risks and costs associated with cell and tissue culture, while providing off-the-shelf availability.

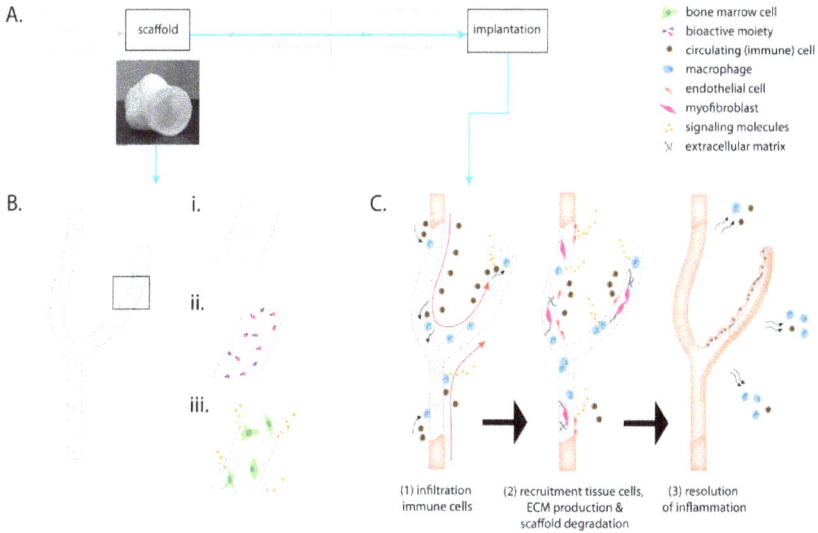

Figure 1. (A) The *in situ* tissue engineering paradigm in which the scaffold is directly implanted, omitting lengthy *in vitro* conditioning phases. (B) The scaffold consists of the bare biomaterial (*i*), which may harbor incorporated bioactive moieties (*ii*) and/or cells (e.g. bone marrow stromal cells) seeded directly prior to implantation (*iii*). (C) Hypothesized mechanism of *in situ* heart valve tissue engineering: after implantation, the scaffold will trigger the host immune response, leading to recruitment of various immune cells and macrophage infiltration. The infiltrated cells secrete cytokines and growth factors to attract additional immune cells, as well as tissue cells, originating from surrounding tissue and/or circulating (progenitor) cells. Endothelial cells cover the blood-scaffold interface and activated myofibroblasts migrate into the scaffold to produce extracellular matrix. Scaffold degradation correlates to a decrease in pro-inflammatory stimuli, eventually leading to resolution of inflammation. Ideally, the valve remodels into the physiological three-layered structure with endothelial cells covering the blood-contact area and quiescent myofibroblasts as valve interstitial-like cells populating the spongiosa layer. Illustration by Anthal Smits.

The *in situ* tissue engineering approach is heavily reliable on the wound healing response. Both the injury incurred during the implantation process and the host inflammatory response to the implanted biomaterial and its degradation products, influence the local microenvironment created by the scaffold. The biomaterial intensifies the inflammatory response by inducing a foreign body response (FBR), propagated by infiltrating immune cells [10,11]. This response is characterized by the presence of macrophages and their fusion into multinucleated giant cells associated with chronic inflammation arising from the persistent presence of a foreign body. The FBR, especially inflammation, may drive valve calcification. However, inflammation is not merely a detrimental response to biomaterial scaffolds. Rather, it can be considered as a natural agent of tissue remodeling, orchestrated by various cell types and potent signaling molecules. By unraveling the inflammatory response towards the foreign biomaterial and the triggers for pathological outcome, targets may be identified to control the inflammatory response through modifications of the biomaterial. The goal is to develop strategies that harness the beneficial aspects of the inflammatory response, while limiting its potential deleterious effects by modulating the inflammatory response towards regeneration.

This chapter deals with the use of biomaterials for *in situ* heart valve tissue engineering and the immune response to the implanted biomaterial. The FBR to biomaterials is discussed, leading to biomaterial design approaches directed to immunomodulation towards tissue regeneration, identifying pitfalls as well as current research challenges for this innovative technology.

2. Biomaterial scaffolds

Biomaterials are materials that interact with the body and its cells. As such, they are central to many strategies for regenerative medicine. They are employed as vehicles for transplanting (progenitor) cells, timed and localized delivery of bioactive moieties, and/or as 3D scaffolds for tissue engineering. Scaffolds are biomaterials designed to create a microenvironment that promotes regeneration. Besides creating and maintaining a defined space for tissue growth, biomaterial scaffolds also provide mechanical stability, and support cell adhesion and migration. Ideally, a scaffold for tissue engineering should be bioresorbable, biocompatible and have a highly porous macrostructure necessary for cell growth, nutrient supply, and waste removal [2,3,6,8,12]. By engineering the proper cellular niche, such scaffolds can provide an environment suitable to modify host responses and direct cell survival, migration, proliferation, differentiation, as well as matrix formation and remodeling. The premise is that in order to unlock the full potential of the cells, at least some aspects of the native 3D tissue environment associated with their renewal, differentiation and organization needs to be mimicked in the applied scaffold materials [3].

2.1. Biomaterial scaffold use in *in situ* heart valve tissue engineering

Trileaflet heart valves are sophisticated tissues with an anisotropic three-layered structure, optimized to withstand the repetitive hemodynamic loads it is subjected to. A human heart valve opens and closes approximately 100.000 times per day, resulting in cyclic changes in the shape, dimensions, and stress of its leaflets and supporting structures. Furthermore, rather than being a purely passive structure, heart valves consist of active components that allow them to adapt to changes in the hemodynamic environment to a certain degree. This puts stringent demands on biomaterial scaffolds used for heart valve tissue engineering, in particular on the mechanical properties. The hemodynamic environment requires a strong biomaterial bearing the repetitive and substantial mechanical stresses applied, especially in the aortic position. This calls for excellent elastic and fatigue properties of the scaffold. A successful tissue engineered heart valve must not only accommodate the resulting deformations, but also have ongoing strength, flexibility, and durability, beginning at the instant of implantation and continuing throughout the lifetime of the recipient [2]. For the *in situ* tissue engineering approach, this means the scaffold has to maintain valve functionality while ECM is formed and remodeled and the biomaterial is degraded *in situ*. In contrast, for the traditional *in vitro* tissue engineering approach the load-bearing function of the biomaterial is overtaken by ECM *in vitro*, prior to implantation. This balance between scaffold resorption and synthesis of new matrix by the host's cells is one of the main challenges in designing scaffolds for *in situ* tissue engineering [4].

2.1.1. Biological scaffolds

The ECM is the natural scaffold for tissue and organ morphogenesis, maintenance, and reconstruction following injury, and is associated with constructive tissue remodeling [12]. The ECM proteins are potent regulators of cell adhesion and activation, and provide a 3D scaffold for cellular organization and migration. They provide mechanical support and store and mobilize signaling molecules. The fibrous ECM structure is provided by collagen, elastin, and fibrin, while non-fibrous proteins as fibronectin and laminin are domains for cell-matrix interactions. This protein scaffold is embedded in a gelatinous matrix composed of glycosaminoglycans (GAGs) and proteoglycans. It serves as a lubricant and as a reservoir for signaling molecules, regulating their distribution and mode of action serving cell-matrix interactions, and activation of enzymes and mediators [11]. Hence, ECM serves as a native modulator of cell activity, also in immune responses and tissue repair. The 3D organization of its components and the complexity of the composition distinguish the native ECM from synthetic scaffolds [4,12,13]. Consequently, the use of a decellularized valve is currently the predominant choice as scaffold material for application in *in situ* engineering of heart valves.

In contrast to cross-linked bioprostheses, decellularized xenografts or homografts allow for infiltration of host cells and matrix remodeling, which may render an autologous, living replacement valve in time. Upon decellularization, the xenograft or homograft is depleted of cells and cellular components. The decellularized matrix possesses a native-like geometry and structure with mechanical properties and physiological hemodynamics similar to its native counterpart [3,4,14]. Signaling components present in the matrix provide natural cues to dictate cell adhesion, proliferation, and growth. With respect to biocompatibility, it is crucial to remove all cellular components, without harming or altering the matrix properties by the decellularization treatment [15]. The method of decellularization strongly determines the degree of preservation of matrix integrity, as well as the efficiency of cell removal. Various decellularization techniques are being studied in an effort to suppress the immunogenic potential of such biological matrices while retaining matrix integrity [2,4,5,7,14]. Results from studies on recellularization of decellularized homografts and xenografts in animal models are controversial, as reviewed elsewhere [2-4,7,16]. In decellularized aortic valves, residual devitalized cells and their epitopes are primary initiators of valve calcification leading to failure of this bioprosthetic valve [7,17]. It is suggested that inflammation inhibitory factors, naturally present in the ECM, are lost due to the decellularization treatment, accounting for the activation of granulocytes and the initiation of the immune response [4]. Furthermore, xenografts are associated with the risk of immunogenic reactions or disease transmission and availability of homografts is limited. To overcome these issues, recent studies have suggested the use of homologous decellularized tissue engineered heart valves. For this, heart valves were engineered *in vitro* using adult saphenous vein cells seeded onto a synthetic polyglycolic acid (PGA)/poly-4-hydroxybutyrate (P4HB) scaffold. After conditioning the cell-scaffold construct in an *in vitro* bioreactor, the tissue engineered valve was decellularized and used as a starter matrix for subsequent recellularization and remodeling *in situ* [18].

An alternative, natural resorbable scaffold material suitable for *in situ* tissue engineering and studied extensively is small intestine submucosa (SIS) [2,3,13]. SIS consists almost entirely of acellular collagen so there is no need for these substrates to undergo extensive decellularization procedures, making it an attractive alternative to decellularized matrices [3]. The success of SIS has been attributed to its intrinsic ECM proteins, cytokines, and growth factors, showing rapid remodeling by the host tissue and exhibiting good vascularization and tissue growth without excessive inflammation and FBR [2]. With respect to heart valve tissue engineering, complete valvular replacements from SIS have been produced demonstrating remodeling potential *in vivo* [19]. As for all animal derived materials, a disadvantage of using SIS is the risk of transferring zoonoses and its availability may be a limiting factor when homograft material is used [3,14]. Further studies should clarify the underlying mechanisms involved before translating the use of decellularized matrices as heart valve scaffolds to human clinic.

2.1.2. Synthetic scaffolds

Synthetic scaffolds have the advantage that they can be tailored to demands, offering precise control of various aspects, such as mechanical properties, chemical properties, degradation rate, as well as the immunogenic potential [7,8]. However, this level of control comes at a price in the sense that multi-disciplinary in-depth knowledge is required to engineer a scaffold appropriate for *in situ* tissue engineering. Engineering of synthetic scaffolds is a discipline that spans multiple length-scales. On the macroscale, a scaffold should exhibit mechanical properties appropriate to fulfill its function. The 3D architecture affects the global mechanical properties of the scaffold, but additionally, on the microscale, it influences cell infiltration and organization (e.g. by contact guidance). Apart from the global mechanical properties of a scaffold, the local mechanical properties, such as material surface stiffness, determine the stimuli experienced by the cells. Surface chemistry (e.g. hydrophobicity/hydrophilicity) has a major effect on cell- and protein-biomaterial interactions and with state-of-the art incorporation of bioactive or even bioresponsive molecules, scaffold engineering has advanced down to the nanoscale [3]. This emphasizes that not only the choice of biomaterial but also the method of processing is of key importance in scaffold development.

Synthetic biodegradable materials, such as PGA, P4HB, polylactic acid (PLA), polycaprolactone (PCL) and copolymers, are the main biocompatible materials of choice, varying in their rates of degradation and manufacturing possibilities [2-4,6,7,14]. Their degradation rate can be tailored by varying their copolymer ratio [3]. Fast-degrading scaffolds such as PGA/P4HB have been used extensively as scaffolds for *in vitro* tissue engineering procedures of heart valves [9,20,21]. Whereas the use of synthetic scaffolds in traditional *in vitro* tissue engineering is abundant, experience with the use of synthetic scaffolds for *in situ* tissue engineering of heart valves is rather limited. However, recent studies applying synthetic scaffolds for small-caliber blood vessels demonstrate the ground-breaking potential of such scaffolds for endogenous regeneration. Small-diameter nanofibrous PCL grafts showed fast endothelialization and ECM formation in the systemic circulation of a rat model [22]. Vascular grafts composed of a nonwoven PGA mesh with a PCL/Poly-L-lactic acid (PLLA) copolymer, seeded with bone marrow stromal cells, demonstrated regeneration of mature blood vessels *in situ* via an inflammation-mediated response in a mouse model [23], as well as in clinical trials [24]. To improve mechanotransduction from the biomaterial to the cells, Wu *et al.* employed a fast degrading elastomeric graft, consisting of poly(glycerol sebacate) (PGS), resulting in fast *in situ* regeneration of neoarteries with mechanical properties and functionality similar to the native vascular tissue [25]. Alternatively, Yokota *et al.* developed a hybrid scaffold consisting of a collagen sponge with layered PGA and PLLA, resulting in regeneration of the canine carotid artery [26]. Although these results demonstrate the great potential of synthetic or hybrid scaffolds for *in situ* tissue engineering, translating these results to heart valves is not trivial due to the complexity of mechanical loads and high-demanding function of the heart valve. Furthermore, slow and/or incomplete polymer degradation may result in excessive chronic inflammation, possibly leading to fibrosis and hampered valve function.

Despite these challenges to overcome, synthetic scaffolds have the potential to offer a strong cost-effective off-the-shelf alternative for heart valve replacements, yielding them very interesting for future clinical application.

2.2. Modulating the immune response

Independent of the biomaterial, the injury incurred during the implantation process will trigger an immune response, due to the disruption of host tissue and induction of cell damage. However, the extent of the inflammatory response evoked is dependent on location, implantation procedure, and biocompatibility of the biomaterial [14,27]. The natural human host response to the scaffold is an excellent target to modulate and control cell and tissue fate. Valvular regeneration is hypothesized to start with a rapid infiltration of the scaffold by monocytes. These monocytes differentiate into macrophages and attract progenitor cells that differentiate into tissue-producing cells. In addition, the macrophages themselves may differentiate into tissue-producing cells. Next, clearance of the macrophages occurs and extracellular matrix is formed and remodeled toward the natural heart valve matrix architecture with quiescent cells. Detailed understanding of this response will provide guidelines to achieve cell and tissue homeostasis, while preventing adverse tissue development (e.g. fibrosis) by mitigating early cellular responses. As the nature of the infiltrating cells in the scaffold and their differentiation is believed to tune the balance of later stage tissue formation towards regeneration or fibrosis, controlling the endogenous production or presentation to the cells of key regulating cytokines in these early processes is essential. Thus, insights in the sequential cell influx and cytokine production and their role in cell differentiation/polarization and tissue formation, will allow the development of optimized scaffolds for *in situ* heart valve tissue engineering applications.

3. The immune response to biomaterials

The defensive response of the human body to invasion by disease-causing entities is referred to as the immune response. In general, its main function is to resolve the infection, restore the tissue damage and reestablish a state of homeostasis. The ideal response is rapid and destructive when necessary, yet specific and self limiting [28]. The immune response consists of two stages: the innate response and the adaptive response (figure 2). The innate immune response refers to the antigen-nonspecific defense mechanism that a host uses immediately or within several hours after exposure to a pathogen or other foreign entity, e.g. a biomaterial. The response is aimed at the recognition and removal of the entity, inhibiting infection and inducing a state of inflammation. When the innate immune response is outrun by a continuing infection and antigen is drained to regional lymph nodes, the adaptive immune response is triggered. Adaptive immunity is antigen-specific, generating responses that are tailored to maximally eliminate pathogens and cells displaying non-self antigens. A key feature of adaptive immunity is the development of immunological memory, in which specific antibodies are generated [29,30]. Synthetic biomaterials are thought not to initiate an adaptive response because they are typically not immunogenic. However, cells and mechanisms involved in the initiation of an adaptive immune response have been found at sites of synthetic implants, suggesting the involvement of an adaptive response in the immune response to biomaterials [11]. In *in situ* tissue engineering, an immune response is inevitable and its beneficial aspects, i.e. dead cell removal and initiation of wound healing, must be harnessed while the potential deleterious effects, i.e. excessive inflammation and fibrosis, must be limited.

3.1. The acute and chronic inflammatory response

The classification 'acute' or 'chronic' is primarily defined by the duration of the inflammatory response and the type of cells infiltrating in response to pro-inflammatory signals [27]. As part of the innate immune response, the acute inflammatory response occurs in the first days after implantation and is characterized by the presence of blood-derived polymorphonuclear leukocytes (PMNs, or granulocytes), predominantly neutrophils. The infiltrating cells cause a state of inflammation to develop within the tissue, generally described by the local accumulation of fluid accompanied by warming (*calor*), pain (*dolor*), reddening (*rubor*), swelling (*tumor*), and functional changes (*functio laesa*). These cells secrete reactive oxygen intermediates (ROIs) and inflammatory cytokines, including interleukin-1β (IL-1β), tumor necrosis factor-α (TNF-α), and interferon-γ (IFN-γ), which orchestrate the character and degree of the subsequent immune response [31]. Their actions can, besides eliminating the pathogen or other foreign entity, also cause secondary damage to the surrounding tissue. Controlling the numbers and types of immune cells at the implant site has the potential to reduce secondary tissue damage and promote regeneration [8].

The inflammatory response prolonging within subsequent weeks, months or even years after implantation is referred to as the chronic inflammatory response. Ideally, the chronic phase of the inflammatory response is avoided through adequate and quick elimination of the disease-causing entity during the acute phase. Chronic inflammation develops as inflammatory stimuli persist at the implant site, with macrophages representing the driving force in continuing the inflammatory response, mediating prolonged expression of cytokines, i.e. IL-1β and TNF-α [11]. Implantation of a biomaterial can intensify the inflammatory response by inducing a FBR, propagated by the infiltrating macrophages, which influences subsequent wound healing.

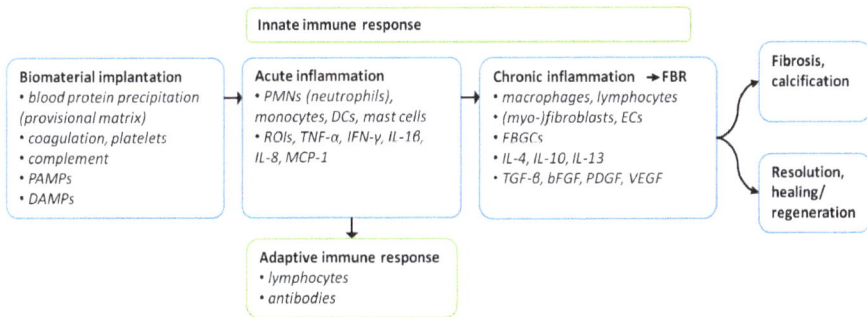

Figure 2. Overview of the immune response to a biomaterial; pathogen-associated molecular patterns (PAMPs), damage-associated molecular patterns (DAMPs), polymorphonuclear leukocytes (PMNs), dendritic cells (DCs), reactive oxygen intermediates (ROIs), tumor necrosis factor-α (TNF-α), interferon-γ (IFN-γ), interleukin-1β (IL-1β), monocyte chemotactic protein-1 (MCP-1], foreign body response (FBR), endothelial cells (ECs), foreign body giant cells (FBGCs), transforming growth factor-β (TGF-β), basic fibroblast growth factor (bFGF), platelet-derived growth factor (PDGF), vascular endothelial growth factor (VEGF).

3.2. Mediators of the immune response

The complete process from innate immune response to wound healing is tuned by a broad spectrum of cytokines and growth factors. Cytokines are a large family of proteins, peptides and glycoproteins, recognized as intercellular signaling immunomodulators [27]. Cytokines are produced by cells and affect the behavior of other cells by binding to specific receptors on their target cells. The term chemokine refers to a specific class of cytokines that is involved in guiding leukocytes to sites where their functions are needed, and as such, have a central role in inflammatory processes. This migration of cells to the site of interest via unidirectional movement towards an increasing gradient of a chemical signal is called chemotaxis [27,30].

Chemokines are not only involved in orchestrating cellular migration in inflammation and wound healing, but also play roles in hematopoiesis, angiogenesis, and tumor metastasis [10].

The secreted chemical mediators usually have a very short half-life due to their high susceptibility to proteolytic degradation. Local linkage to the ECM protects them from enzymatic cleavage, while others may become inactive when bound and can only act when released by matrix proteolysis [11]. Hereby, chemical mediators and ECM proteins collaborate in creating a distinct cellular niche that regulates tissue regeneration.

3.3. Initiation of the innate immune response

Implantation of a biomaterial scaffold typically leads to thrombus formation and initiation of an acute immune response by activation of the coagulation system, complement system, fibrinolytic system, and platelets. Interaction of the biomaterial with blood leads to protein deposition on the biomaterial surface forming a provisional matrix, which affects subsequent leukocyte adhesion interactions [8]. Synthetic polymers, their degradation products and/or the associated provisional matrix activate the complement cascade, marking the biomaterial as being foreign. Phagocytic cells are recruited to the implant by the chemokines released from the provisional matrix and surrounding cells. These phagocytic cells adhere to the matrix surface and further enhance secretion of inflammatory products.

3.3.1. Blood protein precipitation

Upon contact with blood, the blood-biomaterial interaction leads to adsorption of blood proteins, dependent on the biomaterial surface properties [10,11,29,31,32]. The adsorption of endogenous proteins from blood or interstitial fluid onto the surface of the biomaterial, rather than the biomaterial itself, dictates the immune cell response to implanted biomaterials [27]. All other host components, including leukocytes, encounter and/or interact with this surface as an adhesion substrate. It serves as a provisional matrix, which may also contain a milieu of cytokines, chemokines, or other bioactive agents. This provisional matrix furnishes structural, biochemical, and cellular components to the processes of wound healing and FBR. It can be seen as a naturally derived, biodegradable sustained release system in which bioactive moieties are released to control subsequent phases of wound healing [10].

The precipitation of proteins from blood and tissue occurring immediately after implantation determines the activation of the coagulation cascade, the complement system, platelets and immune cells. The proteins guide their interplay, leading to the formation of the provisional matrix and to the onset of the immune response [11,29]. The adsorbed protein layer includes complement activation fragments, immunoglobulin G (IgG), fibrinogen, fibronectin, and vitronectin. Fibrinogen and fibronectin bind a large number of extracellular macromolecules as well as cell surface proteins, providing a matrix for cell proliferation and organization [33]. Whereas complement and fibrinogen mainly contribute to the activation of inflammatory cells, fibronectin and vitronectin are critical in regulating the inflammatory response to biomaterials [11]. The composition of the protein layer changes over time, described as the Vroman effect [10,29]. Adsorbed proteins may desorb rapidly and, therefore, present time-dependent variations in the type and level of proteins which cells encounter. The highest mobility proteins of the blood serum generally arrive first, e.g. albumin and globulin, and are later replaced by less motile proteins that have a higher affinity for the biomaterial surface, e.g. fibronectin and factor XII.

Complement receptors function as a non-specific aid in detection and removal of foreign materials. Activation of the complement system leads to subsequent reactions in host defense and functions as one of the players in the tight cross-talk between the different cascade systems, platelets, and leukocytes, inducing clotting and inflammation. The complement system is activated by the coating of the implant with complement activation fragments within the provisional matrix, and through release of anaphylatoxins, i.e. C3a and C5a, which are chemo-attractants for leukocyte infiltration and cause leukocyte activation [32,34]. Upon complement activation, proteases in the system cleave specific proteins to release cytokines, e.g. TNF-α, IL-1β, IL-6, and IL-8, and initiate an amplifying cascade of further cleavages. Furthermore, it contributes to the onset of the inflammatory response by triggering degranulation of mast cells, attraction and activation of PMNs and monocytes, induction of ROI-release by PMNs, supporting platelet adhesion and activation, and promotion of tissue factor expression by monocytes and PMNs on biomaterial surfaces [11]. Destruction of host cells is prevented by the presence of membrane-bound complement regulatory proteins, e.g. CD46, CD55, and CD59 [29].

Blood coagulation on biomaterials requires the combination of contact activation by factor XII, platelet adhesion and their activation by thrombin. This leads to the cleavage of fibrinogen to fibrin and subsequent clot formation. Platelet adhesion and activation, through adsorbed IgG and fibrinogen, mediates neutrophil reactive oxygen generation and monocyte tissue factor expression, leading to neutrophil and monocyte adhesion [29]. Platelets trapped in the fibrin clot, as well as fibroblasts and leukocytes themselves are major resources of chemo-attractants at the site of implantation, initiating and modulating inflammatory reactions and immune responses [35,36].

Cell adhesion and activation on biomaterials primarily occurs through interaction of adhesion receptors with the adsorbed proteins. The major adhesion receptors of leukocytes are represented by integrins, which regulate aggregation, immune functions, cell migration, matrix deposition, and wound contraction [33]. Surface integrin molecules allow cells to migrate through the ECM and mediate signal transduction between the cell and its environment, enabling the cell to respond to its environment. Integrin molecule engagement on leukocytes promotes leukocyte survival, activation, and differentiation [29]. Ligands for integrin receptor binding and cellular adhesion are provided by the adsorbed proteins, including fibrinogen, IgG, iC3b, fibronectin, and vitronectin [10].

3.3.2. Pattern recognition

Besides recognition of biomaterials through adhesion receptors, i.e. integrins, immune cells are activated by another type of receptor-ligand interaction that is based on pattern recognition. A class of molecules classically defined as pathogen-associated molecular pattern (PAMP) molecules, alerts the innate immune system and triggers defensive immune responses. PAMPs include lipopolysaccharide (LPS), viral RNA and bacterial peptidoglycans, which interact with dedicated receptors on immune cells, the pattern recognition receptors (PRRs) [8,11,28,29,35,37,38]. These receptors are specialized in the recognition of microbial components that are chemically distinct from the host's endogenous molecules [39]. PRRs include transmembrane Toll-like receptors (TLRs), cytoplasmic NOD-like receptors (NLRs), and cytoplasmic C-type lectin receptors (CLRs) [28,37]. The TLR family is a well-known family of PRRs, in which each member recognizes a specific set of molecular patterns. For example, TLR2 and TLR4 recognize damaged ECM by binding breakdown products of hyaluronan cleaved in tissue damage, while TLR7, TLR8, and TLR9 recognize host RNA and DNA [28]. TLRs are expressed on e.g. platelets, macrophages, dendritic cells (DCs), neutrophils, and endothelial cells [36,37]. Tissue-resident macrophages and DCs, both functioning as antigen-presenting cells (APCs), are most influential in early PRR-signaling and are the primary inducers of an inflammatory reaction [28,39].

An inflammatory response can, besides initiation by PAMPs, also be initiated by several endogenous molecules interacting with signaling receptors. These innate danger signals are described as endokines or alarmins, but are also known as damage-associated molecular patterns (DAMPs) [11,35,38,40]. These signals have immunostimulatory effects and include an array of structurally diverse, multifunctional host proteins that are rapidly released during infection or tissue damage, e.g. after biomaterial implantation. The resulting necrotic cell death leads to the release of cytoplasmic and nuclear components that contain DAMPs, recognized by PRRs expressed by leukocytes. In addition, proteases and hydrolases released from dead cells modify extracellular components to generate mediators (e.g. complement fragments) or other DAMPs (e.g. ECM fragments), which can activate leukocytes [39]. DAMPs have intranuclear, intracellular and/or extracellular functions in mobilizing and activating receptor-expressing cells engaged in host defense and tissue repair, e.g. macrophages and DCs. One of the members of the DAMP family is the group of high-mobility-group box (HMGB) proteins, which are chromosomal proteins helping in transcription, replication, recombination, and DNA repair. HMGB-1 is one of the best known proteins within this family and is released by necrotic cells, cytolytic cells, and cells stimulated by pro-inflammatory stimuli. It was shown to have extracellular activity as a chemokine, attracting neutrophils and mononuclear inflammatory cells [28,39,40]. Other members of the DAMP family include interleukins, heat-shock proteins, defensins, eosinophil-derived neurotoxin, macrophage-/PMN-derived cathelicidins, and nucleosomes. Injury-related TLR-ligands are small hyaluronan fragments, fibrinogen, and fibronectin, of which the latter two are present in the adsorbed protein layer on a biomaterial surface [28].

Induction of inflammation through pattern recognition leads to activation of the receptor expressing cell. When a ligand has bound to a PRR, activation signals are sent out, which initiate signaling pathways leading to the activation of transcription factors, notably nuclear factor κB (NF-κB). This factor migrates into the nucleus and mediates gene transcription and production of inflammatory mediators, such as chemokines, adhesion molecules, growth factors, and pro-inflammatory cytokines, especially TNF-α, and IL-1, which themselves also mediate activation of NF-κB [37]. Many molecules with important functions in immunity and repair mediate their effects through activation of the NF-κB pathway. Transcriptional control of inflammation by NF-κB during the immune response has emerged as one of the most important signaling cascades in the regulation of the inflammatory response [35].

3.4. Cell recruitment in the acute inflammatory response

The acute inflammatory response is driven by fast acting leukocytes, mostly neutrophils and macrophages, as the primary defense against nonspecific infecting entities [11,27]. After implantation of a biomaterial, inherently causing cell damage, these immune cells are activated through the engagement of their integrins and PRRs with the protein-coated biomaterial surface. The activation of immune cells leads to the initiation of inflammatory cytokine production and subsequent chemokine recruitment of more immune cells, i.e. PMNs, monocytes, and macrophages, but also endothelial cells and fibroblasts to the site of implantation [28,35]. Activation of PMNs includes a phagocytic response and degranulation, which subsequently leads to biomaterial degradation and potential damaging of the surrounding tissue, prolonging the inflammatory response [11].

During the inflammatory response, macrophages and lymphocytes predominantly synthesize and release immunoregulatory cytokines, e.g. IL-1β, IL-6, and TNF-α, and chemokines, e.g. IL-8, monocyte chemotactic protein-1 (MCP-1), and macrophage inflammatory protein-1β (MIP-1β). These are potent chemo-attractants and activation factors for inflammatory effector cells such as PMNs, monocytes, macrophages, immature DCs, natural killer (NK) cells, and lymphocytes. Changes in cellularly released chemical factors mediate additional cell recruitment and activity [27]. The increasing influx of mononuclear cells over time is balanced by a decreased infiltration of PMNs, leading to a decrease in PMN activation signals followed by their apoptosis and engulfment by macrophages. Within two days after implantation PMNs typically disappear from the site [11].

3.4.1. Neutrophils

Neutrophils are the most dominant cell type among the PMNs present in the acute inflammatory response. They are phagocytic leukocytes containing granules and are activated by pro-inflammatory cytokines, such as IL-1β, TNF-α, and IFN-γ [35]. The life span of a neutrophil inside the blood stream is 12 hours, but increases to 24-48 hours upon activation outside the vasculature [27,39]. Crucial mediators for neutrophil recruitment in acute inflammation are chemokines and their receptors, e.g. IL-8 [35]. The primary function of IL-8 is induction of the chemotaxis of neutrophils, with their arrival at the site within hours after injury, followed by a later influx of monocytes [38].

Neutrophils eradicate foreign entities by immediate phagocytosis, a process by which solid particles are uptaken by the cell. After phagocytosis of the biomaterial, neutrophils die, and are, together with other material debris, cleared by resident macrophages [27]. This uptake promotes anti-inflammatory lipoxin production by the macrophage, which down-regulates further neutrophil recruitment and activity, while promoting monocyte migration [39]. When neutrophils detect TNF-α, but do not directly encounter any exogeneous particles, they mobilize and release their granules into the extracellular space, a process called degranulation, to create an inhospitable environment for nearby foreign entities [28]. The granules of neutrophils are loaded with proteases, which, together with the production of ROIs and reactive nitrogen intermediates (RNIs), leads to the denaturation of proteins, disruption of lipids, and damaging of DNA [28,39]. Upon degranulation, the neutrophil reorganizes its surrounding microenvironment and promotes the recruitment of additional immune responsive cells, mainly monocytes, but also generates secondary damage to the host tissue and cells [8,28]. Therefore, neutrophil activation has to be tightly controlled to avoid excessive tissue damage while enabling the rapid recruitment of monocytes [39].

3.4.2. Monocytes

After neutrophils, monocytes enter the site of implantation and subsequently mature into tissue macrophages or DCs. Bone marrow precursors give rise to the monocytes in the blood, which circulate for a few days before they migrate into the tissue and mature [41]. Monocytes are recruited by cytokines and chemotactic factors, released by resident macrophages and neutrophils [27]. In general, monocytes reach maximum numbers 24-36 hours after injury [37]. There is a guided movement of monocytes in response to chemokines and other chemo-attractants [10]. MCP-1, also known as C-C chemokine ligand 2 (CCL2), binds to C-C chemokine receptor 2 (CCR2) and mediates monocyte recruitment [42]. Although expression of CCR2 is restricted to only a few cell types including monocytes, most (if not all) nucleated cells express MCP-1 in response to activation by pro-inflammatory cytokines or stimulation of innate immune receptors. A hypothesis on the mechanism of action of MCP-1 in monocyte recruitment from the bone marrow is that MCP-1 dimerizes and associates with tissue GAGs, creating a gradient which guides monocytes toward the site of infection or inflammation [42].

In the blood, monocytes are not a homogeneous population of cells. Human monocytes are divided into subsets according to their surface expression of CD14 and CD16 [39,42]. CD14 is a PRR that can recognize and bind various structures from invading microbes (e.g. LPS), while CD16 is a receptor binding IgG antibodies [41]. CD14^{++}CD16^{-} monocytes are the most prevalent monocyte subset present in the blood (~85% of total monocytes) and express CCR2 [43]. The CD16^{+} monocyte population comprises two subsets, CD14^{++}CD16^{+} and CD14^{+}CD16^{++} monocytes [41,42]. There appears to be a developmental relationship between these different subtypes in that, during the course of an inflammatory reaction, the CD14^{++}CD16^{-} monocytes first develop into CD14^{++}CD16^{+} monocytes to then become CD14^{+}CD16^{++} monocytes. Hence, CD14^{+}CD16^{++} monocytes may represent a more mature subset [41]. The precise role of the different monocyte subsets in initiating immune responses remains unclear, although CD14^{++}CD16^{-} monocytes are believed to contribute more effectively to pathogen clearance while CD14^{+}CD16^{++} monocytes show a patrolling role and account for more vigorous production of pro-inflammatory cytokines [39,42].

At the site of implantation, monocytes become activated and develop into DCs or mature tissue macrophages, undergoing a phenotypic change. This process is directed by mediators present in the microenvironment, such as cytokine receptors, TLRs, and complement receptors, which are crucial for the proper adaptation of cell function to the specific requirements at the site.

[11,35]. For example, TLR-activated monocytes produce IL-10, which has a central role in preventing excessive inflammation [38]. Additionally, there is substantial debate about whether specific monocyte populations give rise to specific tissue macrophages [39,44]. It has been suggested that monocytes continue maturing in the blood and can be recruited to the tissue at various points during this maturation continuum. The point at which they leave the blood may define their function [42].

3.4.3. Dendritic cells

Dendritic cells (DCs), monocytes, and macrophages are closely related, as blood monocytes can differentiate into macrophages and DCs and, in their turn, DCs can differentiate into macrophages [41]. The main function of DCs is to function as APCs, processing foreign material and presenting it on its surface to other immune cells, e.g. T-lymphocytes (T cells) [45]. They act as messengers between the innate and adaptive immune response, initiating the T-cell response [29]. Besides their presence as resident cells in tissues, they are also found in the blood, circulating in an immature state. Upon activation, DCs migrate to the lymph nodes and interact with lymphocytes to initiate and modulate the adaptive immune response [30].

By triggering receptors and signaling cascades of the pathogen recognition system, biomaterials activate DCs through the adherent protein layer [11,29]. DC maturation is promoted or inhibited depending on which PRR is engaged, leading to immunity or tolerance, respectively. Immunogenic DCs may prolong the immune response to biomaterials and delay wound healing, while tolerogenic DCs are capable of down-regulating the immune cells and resolve inflammation [11]. Activated immunogenic DCs promote T-cell proliferation and secrete pro-inflammatory cytokines, e.g. IL-1β, IL-6, IL-12, and TNF-α, which further amplify DC maturation by autocrine stimulation. The immature and semi-mature tolerogenic DCs are promoters of tolerance and secrete e.g. IL-10 and TGF-β [45]. Besides PRR engagement, integrin signaling due to binding of DCs to ECM proteins on the biomaterial, may act as an alternative mechanism of DC maturation and activation and should be taken into account in the strategy of modulating immune responses to biomaterials.

3.4.4. Mast cells

Mast cells are a leukocyte subset represented in most tissues and are best known for their role in allergy. However, they play an important protective role as well, being intimately involved in host defense and wound healing. In the innate immune response, they are an important source of pro-inflammatory mediators and cytokines, containing many granules that are rich in histamine, and producing prostaglandins and cytokines that promote inflammation [35]. Together with tissue-resident macrophages and DCs, mast cells are responsible for the recruitment of inflammatory cells in the innate immune response, i.e. chemotaxis of PMNs and monocytes through secretion of e.g. IL-1β, TNF-α, and MCP-1 [11,28,29]. Besides functioning in host defense mechanisms, mast cells participate more generally in the orchestration of inflammatory responses, e.g. through IL-10 secretion, and tissue remodeling, through secretion of proteases and anti-inflammatory cytokines, such as IL-4 [46]. They express a large set of receptors allowing them to respond to a large variety of stimuli, with activation of specific receptors leading to specific actions. Therefore, mast cell functions are highly dependent on the physiological context, as small differences in the mast cell environment may yield variant or even opposite actions [46].

3.5. The chronic inflammatory response

Once neutrophils, monocytes and macrophages have entered the site of injury or infection in the acute phase of the response, they collaborate to remove the foreign entity [39]. The transition of the acute inflammatory response to the chronic inflammatory response is signified by the departure of the PMNs and infiltration of more macrophages and lymphocytes, which give rise to new tissue formation [8,10,31].

3.5.1. Macrophages

Generally, when the acute phase of inflammation has not sufficed to clear the source of infection within the first 2 days after implantation, macrophages become the dominating force in the persisting inflammatory response. Macrophages are recruited by many of the same signals as neutrophils but have a longer life span. Tissue-resident macrophages have a life span up to months [27,28]. The primary role of macrophages is to function as a common guardian cell of which the main function in homeostasis is to clear the interstitial environment of extraneous cellular material through phagocytosis [44]. Macrophages are professional phagocytes with extraordinary synthetic and secretory capacities and exert key controlling influences on wound healing and fibrosis responses [31].

A resting macrophage is activated by microbial products, immune complexes, chemical mediators, certain ECM proteins, and T-cell-derived cytokines. An adherent macrophage on a biomaterial is activated to initiate phagocytosis and cytokine secretion, hereby directing the inflammatory and wound healing response to the biomaterial [10]. Several of the key biomaterial-dependent chemokines and cytokines (e.g. IL-1β, IL-6, IL-8, and TNF-α) have the potential to induce multiple autocrine and paracrine effects in the chronic inflammatory and wound healing phases, as well as a time-dependent switch in cytokine secretion from acute to chronic phase phenotype [31]. Uptake of apoptotic neutrophils can stimulate macrophages to release mediators that suppress the inflammatory response, e.g. TGF-β, IL-10 and prostaglandin E$_2$ (PGE$_2$) [39]. In bridging the innate and adaptive immune response, macrophages can fuse to become multinucleated giant cells and act as APCs to activate leukocytes which are responsible for the adaptive immune response, e.g. through expression of co-stimulatory molecules that are essential for T-cell activation [27,37].

Beside their function as phagocytes and APCs, it is assumed that macrophages play a prominent role in a successful wound healing response through the synthesis of growth factors such as TGF-β, basic fibroblast growth factor (bFGF), platelet-derived growth factor (PDGF), and vascular endothelial growth factor (VEGF), which promote cell proliferation and synthesis of ECM molecules by resident cells [10,35]. TGF-β is a potential stimulator of ECM production, promoting both fibronectin and collagen synthesis in fibroblasts, and decreasing collagen breakdown. With respect to angiogenesis, bFGF is probably one of the major growth factor families involved, being strongly mitogenic for endothelial cells, directing their migration and proliferation. PDGF recruits neutrophils and monocytes, stimulates the activation of macrophages, and induces expression of TGF-β [33]. Production of VEGF by cells present in the damaged microenvironment is induced by both IL-1β and IL-10, stimulating vasculogenesis and angiogenesis [38].

3.5.2. Macrophage phenotypes

Macrophages show remarkable plasticity, which allows them to efficiently respond to environmental signals and change their phenotype concordantly. The different macrophage phenotypes are identified and distinguished according to markers present at the cell surface and profiles of cytokine and gene expression. Both the acute and the chronic inflammatory response can markedly alter the physiology of macrophages [44]. Furthermore, surface topology and molecular organization of biomaterials affects macrophages, and the cell-surface interaction can change quantity and identity of secreted pro-inflammatory cytokines and chemokines, gene expression patterns, and downstream remodeling events [47].

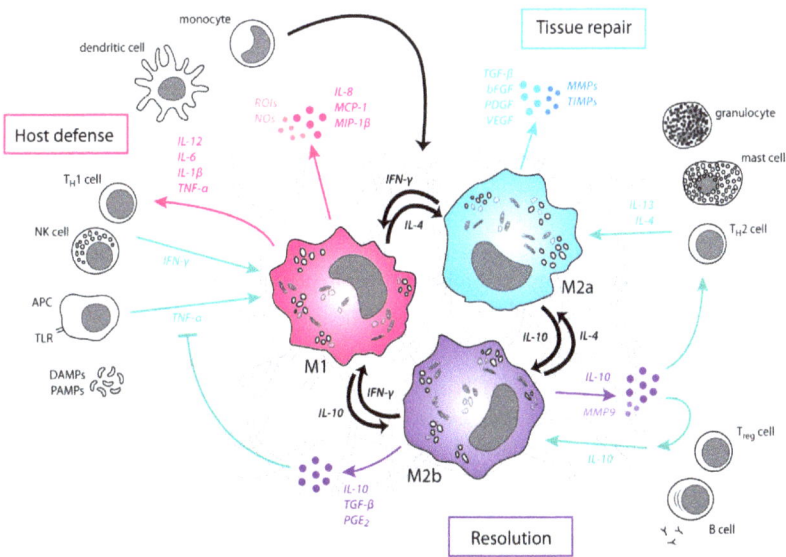

Figure 3. Schematic representation of macrophage plasticity. Macrophages can adapt their phenotype in response to environmental cues provided via paracrine or autocrine signaling. Illustrated are extremities within the continuous spectrum of macrophage polarization states ('M1', 'M2a', 'M2b') (adapted from [11,44]). Illustration by Anthal Smits.

Two main macrophage phenotypes have been suggested, classified as "M1" and "M2", mirroring the T helper 1 (T_H1) and T helper 2 (T_H2) cell polarization [48,49] (figure 3). The pro-inflammatory, cytotoxic macrophage phenotype, signified as M1, is characterized by the promotion of pathogen killing and is associated with classic signs of inflammation. These classically activated macrophages are involved in killing intracellular pathogens, up-regulation of pro-inflammatory cytokines, inhibition of anti-inflammatory cytokines, and synthesis of oxygen and nitrogen radicals, making them a crucial part of host defense [10,11,44,45,47]. Their activation is stimulated by pro-inflammatory cytokines, e.g. IFN-γ (released by T_H1 cells or NK cells), TNF-α (released by APCs), IL-1β, IL-6, and IL-12, but also by PAMPs, DAMPs, hypoxia, and abnormal matrix, such as pathological collagen deposition [11,29]. Activated M1 macrophages also secrete pro-inflammatory cytokines themselves, i.e. TNF-α, IL-1, IL-6, IL-12, and IL-23, inducing T_H1 cell responses [45]. Furthermore, they produce low levels of anti-inflammatory IL-10 [29,48]. Macrophages activated by a biomaterial are typically of the M1 phenotype and can promote the invasion of additional inflammatory cells by secreting chemokines such as IL-8, MCP-1, and MIP-1β. They also secrete degradative enzymes and display high phagocytic activity [11]. Via the production of a variety of enzymes that degrade ECM components, such as matrix metalloproteinases (MMPs), collagenase, and elastase, M1 macrophages are crucial in matrix destruction and tissue reorganization, allowing them to quickly migrate through injured tissues [45]. However, prolonged activation of M1 macrophages can lead to tissue damage.

Immuno-regulation, tissue repair, and constructive tissue regeneration are promoted by the anti-inflammatory macrophage phenotype, signified as M2. These macrophages inhibit pro-inflammatory cytokine secretion, promote anti-inflammatory cytokine secretion, and up-regulate mannose receptors which are necessary for FBGC-formation and play a role in matrix remodeling [10,47]. This alternative macrophage activation is stimulated by the release of IL-4 and IL-13 by T_H2 cells, cytokines (e.g. IL-10, TGF-β), glucocorticoids, and apoptotic cells [29,35,50]. In contrast to M1 macrophages, M2 macrophages typically produce high levels of IL-10 and low levels of IL-12, leading to T_H2 cell responses [45,48]. These macrophages show reparative actions by promoting angiogenesis, production of pro-fibrogenic factors resulting in enhanced fibrinogenic activity of fibroblasts, over-expression of certain ECM proteins, and differential secretion of MMPs and tissue inhibitors of metalloproteinases (TIMPs) [10,49].

The M2 phenotype can be divided into two subsets, i.e. wound healing (M2a) and regulatory (M2b) macrophages (figure 3) [11,44]. Wound healing macrophages are mainly triggered by IL-4, released by mast cells, granulocytes, or T_H2 cells, which down-regulates pro-inflamma-tory cytokine secretion by the macrophage. These macrophages promote wound healing processes by contributing to the production of ECM proteins, such as fibronectin, and by the activation of fibroblasts [11]. Although M2a macrophages exert anti-inflammatory activities, they are not capable of down-regulating immune responses. Regulatory macrophages are triggered by a variety of signals, e.g. IL-10, apoptotic cells, immune complexes, and glucocorticoids. Their main task is to limit inflammation and to dampen the immune response, restoring homeostasis while limiting the development of fibrosis [11,49]. They achieve this by releasing high levels of IL-10, which is a very potent immune-suppressive cytokine acting through inhibition of IL-6 signaling and NF-κB activation [38].

Macrophages seem to retain their plasticity and respond to environmental signals. The activation of stimulus-specific transcription factors is likely to dictate the functionalized polarization of macrophages through effects on inducible gene promoters with specific features, translating signals in the microenvironment of the macrophage into a polarized phenotype [51]. The progression from an inflammatory macrophage phenotype (M1) toward a more regenerative/anti-inflammatory macrophage phenotype (M2a/b) correlates with a change in cytokine secretion profile by T helper cells changing from type 1 (T_H1) to type 2 (T_H2), promoting resolution of the inflammation [8]. The phenotype of a macrophage population can change over time but a single biochemical marker to distinguish between populations has not been identified [44]. It is suggested that macrophages possess a continuum of phenotypes for distinct biological functions, showing overlap of biomarkers and functions for M1 and M2 macrophages [45]. The primary three macrophage phenotypes suggested here, i.e. pro-inflammatory, wound healing, and regulatory, can blend into a continuum of secondary phenotypes that serve a wide variety of functions [44]. It is also unknown whether uncommitted macrophages are recruited to the site of scaffold remodeling and subsequently stimulated to differentiate locally or whether phenotype-committed macrophages are selectively recruited to sites of remodeling, depending on the antigens or substrates that are present [47]. The molecular determinants that precisely control macrophage plasticity, e.g. switching between polarization states, are to a large extend unknown, which makes targeting transcription factors for modulatory aims a challenge [51].

3.5.3. Lymphocytes

In the chronic phase of the inflammatory response, lymphocytes appear at the site of inflammation together with macrophages [31]. Lymphocytes play a role in the adaptive immune response, involving major histocompatibility complex (MHC) class I and class II molecules, expressed on the surface of APCs, and recognized by receptors and co-receptors on T cells. In general, MHC class I molecules present peptide antigens derived from pathogens that replicate intracellularly and whose proteins are present in the cytosol of the cell, to cytotoxic $CD8^+$ T cells. MHC class II molecules present peptides obtained from pathogens and their products that are present in the extracellular milieu and have been taken up into the endocytic vesicles of phagocytic cells, to helper $CD4^+$ T cells. The $CD4^+$ T_H1 cells and cytolytic $CD8^+$ T cells migrate to the infected tissue, where they activate macrophages to kill antigen-bearing pathogens. This response is referred to as the cell-mediated immune response. On the other hand, $CD4^+$ T_H2 cells and B-lymphocytes (B cells) perform their functions in the lymphoid tissues, where T_H2 cells activate B cells to produce antibodies against target antigens, called the humoral immune response [29,30].

Accumulation of T cells is associated with the expression of MCP-1 few days after injury, with production of the chemokines interferon-γ-inducible protein-10 (IP-10), and monokine induced by interferon-γ (MIG), of which macrophages appear to be a major source [35]. T cells become activated via interactions with APCs, i.e. macrophages, DCs, and B cells, which present processed antigens bound to MHC molecules on their cell surfaces. Additional co-stimulatory interactions with specific molecules on APCs are required upon lymphocyte activation, i.e. interaction between CD80 or CD86 on the APC and CD28 on the T-cell surface [30]. Characteristics of activation include expression of specific cell surface markers and production of the classic activation cytokines IL-2 and IFN-γ [31]. T cells will undergo clonal expansion by proliferation and up- or down-regulation of their effector function. When T cells are activated but not co-stimulated, they become anergic, a mechanism for suppression of inappropriate immune reactivity. Via this mechanism, cells that may have been inappropriately activated, undergo apoptosis, and are removed by macrophages. For example, anti-inflammatory IL-10 induces antigen specific anergy of T helper cells, helping in the prevention of excessive inflammation [31].

Macrophages and lymphocytes are capable of activating each other through direct and indirect mechanisms [31]. Activated T cells induce production of pro-inflammatory cytokines IL-1β, TNF-α, and IL-6, and chemokines IL-8, MCP-1, and MIP-1β by macrophages in a contact-dependent manner. T cells promote the adhesion of macrophages to biomaterials and their subsequent fusion, as well as biomaterial-dependent cytokine production, having consequences for the biocompatibility of the biomaterial [31]. NK cells, a lymphocyte subset next to T and B cells, are potential sources of IL-4 and IL-13 and may promote the FBR by inducing macrophage fusion into FBGCs [31].

3.6. Inflammatory resolution and wound healing

After the inflammatory stimulus has been eliminated, the ongoing inflammatory response must be resolved to avoid excessive tissue damage and to initiate the healing process. During the resolution of inflammation, further infiltration of leukocytes is prevented and removal of debris from the inflamed site is promoted, thereby restoring tissue homeostasis [39]. The process of resolution is an active process requiring signals that turn off neutrophil infiltration and, at the same time, promote the uptake and clearance of apoptotic cells and debris. Lipid mediators, e.g. lipoxins and resolvins, seem to have a key role in this process, and the resolution of inflammation is accompanied by an active switch in the types of lipid mediator found at the inflamed site [28,39]. During the inflammatory response, prostaglandins and cytokines that amplify inflammation are generated by various cell types, including neutrophils, monocytes, and macrophages. Following this, PGE_2 and prostaglandin D2 (PGD_2) gradually promote the synthesis of anti-inflammatory and pro-resolving mediators, such as lipoxins. Another mechanism of inflammatory resolution is inactivation of chemokines through cleavage by MMPs, terminating inflammatory cell influx [39].

The initiation of wound healing is generally marked by the arrival of fibroblasts for the production of ECM proteins, and of endothelial cells for angiogenesis. They occur within the 3 to 5 days of monocyte invasion and activation of resident macrophages, resulting in the formation of granulation tissue [27]. Granulation tissue formation is a wound healing response in which fibroblasts and endothelial cells recruited by macrophages, invade and proliferate within the inflamed tissue in an attempt to establish structure and homeostasis at the local inflammation site [11,27]. Granulation tissue consists of a dense population of macrophages, fibroblasts, and neovasculature embedded within a loose matrix of fibronectin, collagen, and hyaluronic acid, serving as an intermediary substrate [31,33]. Fibroblasts are mesenchyme-derived cells with their primary function being to produce and remodel the local ECM, providing scaffolding and framework to repair the wound [3]. The persistent presence of macrophages within the granulation tissue ensures constant remodeling of the tissue matrix and constant recruitment of fibroblasts and endothelial cells [27].

The outcome of tissue regeneration or scar formation, i.e. fibrosis, is dependent on the duration of the chronic response that contributes to cytokine production and formation of granulation tissue [8]. Fibrosis is the excessive deposition of matrix components that results in destruction of normal tissue architecture and compromised tissue function and arises from a continuous injuring stimulus, excessive synthesis or decreased degradation [33]. Synthetic and degradative functions of fibroblasts are controlled and regulated by signals from the matrix, as well as leukocyte cytokines and growth factors, wherein macrophages and their phenotype play an important role [27,52].

4. The foreign body response to biomaterials

The implantation of a biomaterial can intensify the inflammatory response by inducing a foreign body response (FBR). The FBR at the tissue-material interface is composed of macrophages and foreign body giant cells (FBGCs) and forms the end-stage response of the inflammatory and wound healing responses following implantation of a medical device, prosthesis, or biomaterial [10,29]. Typically, within 2-4 weeks the foreign material is encapsulated within an almost avascular, fibrous connective tissue, depending on the porosity of the biomaterial [52]. The FBR is characterized by the presence of macrophages and FBGCs together with the components of granulation tissue. Macrophages and FBGCs are believed to exert critical effects on both tissue and implanted material, e.g. degradation, and chemokine and cytokine production [31].

4.1. Macrophage fusion

Macrophages develop integrins, which play a major role in the adhesion of macrophages to a biomaterial and in the IL-4-induced macrophage fusion to form FBGCs [10]. Macrophage-integrin binding to the protein layer on the biomaterial surface provides intracellular signals that can modulate macrophage behavior, such as cytoskeletal rearrangements and the formation of adhesion structures, called podosomes. There is extensive interplay between intracellular signaling molecules activated by integrin binding and cytoskeletal proteins. Disruption of the adhesion signals promotes anoikis, i.e. apoptosis induced by cell detachment from its supportive matrix. A hypothesis is that macrophage fusion to form FBGCs is an escape mechanism to avoid apoptosis [10].

Macrophages adhere to the surface of an implanted biomaterial when they are unable to phagocytose the material due to a large material-to-cell size ratio. Phagocytosis of large, non-degradable implanted materials usually does not occur due to the size disparity. When the particle size in phagocytosis >5 μm, frustrated phagocytosis may occur instead, a process in which ROIs are secreted aimed to degrade the biomaterial [10,29]. Macrophages fuse with other macrophages to form multinucleated FBGCs, associated with chronic inflammation arising from the persistent presence of a foreign body. These multinucleated cells are characteristic of granulomatous inflammation and show abundant chromatin with scattered nuclei in an irregular pattern [31]. The fusion of macrophages to form FBGCs serves to prolong the life span of these frustrated macrophages, allowing continued release of cytokines and growth factors [27].

Lymphocytes also seem to play a critical role in the FBR. They have been observed to associate with adherent macrophages and FBGCs, and enhance macrophage adhesion and fusion, while the presence of macrophages stimulates lymphocytes to proliferate [31]. Dependent on the biomaterial, next to macrophages, lymphocytes themselves also produce inflammatory mediators [10,31]. Lymphocytes enhance adherent macrophage and FBGC activation in terms of inflammatory cytokine production via paracrine (indirect) and juxtacrine (direct) means [10]. T cells have been demonstrated to promote macrophage adhesion and fusion via paracrine effects, however, close association of lymphocytes and macrophages also suggests direct signaling which has been shown to dominate at later time points of their interaction [11].

4.2. Macrophage phenotype in fusion

The phenotype of the macrophages involved has been shown to play an important role in biomaterial scaffold remodeling [10,11,52]. The fusion of adherent macrophages to FBGCs is typically associated with a phenotype switch of the macrophages over time, going from a more pro-inflammatory activation state (M1) to a more anti-inflammatory activation state (M2). M1 versus M2 macrophage activation has led to morphological variants of multinucleated giant cells *in vitro* [10]. The M2 activation cytokines IL-4 and IL-13 promote macrophage fusion and the formation of large FBGCs with randomly arranged nuclei and high degrees of cytoplasmic spreading, while the M1 activation cytokine IFN-γ induces more limited degrees of macrophage fusion with resultant Langerhans-type giant cells. However, the activation state of fusing macrophages is neither M1-like, nor M2-like but rather an in-between state in the continuous spectrum of macrophage polarization. This suggests that biomaterial activation is unique in the process of inflammation [10,11].

The fusion of M2-activated macrophages into FBGCs is stimulated by IL-4 and IL-13, assumed to be secreted by activated T cells [11]. The precise origins of FBGC-inducing cytokines at the implant site remain unclear, with T_H2 cells, NK cells, eosinophils, basophils, and mast cells as possible candidates [31]. Both IL-4 and IL-13 were found to up-regulate mannose receptors on fusing macrophages, which mediate endo- and phagocytosis, with localization of the receptor at the fusion interface [10]. MCP-1 is also involved in FBGC formation though not by recruiting cells but rather by guiding macrophage chemotaxis toward each other [10,11].

Biomaterial-adherent macrophages and FBGCs seem to show combined action of biomaterial degradation and down-modulation of pro-inflammatory mediators. Perhaps the presence of macrophage fusion and FBGC formation on biomaterial surfaces represents host down-modulation of pro-inflammatory cytokine production, possibly via phagocytic removal of macrophages actively releasing these cytokines [31]. Next to promoting M2 phenotype and macrophage fusion, IL-4 prevents apoptosis of biomaterial-adherent macrophages by inducing shedding of TNF-α receptor I, preventing this TNF-α-mediated process [11].

4.3. Biomaterial degradation and fibrosis

Macrophages and FBGCs mediate biomaterial degradation by concentrating phagocytic and oxidative activities at the interface between the cell and the biomaterial. During frustrated phagocytosis, macrophages and FBGCs release degradative mediators such as ROIs, degradative enzymes, and acid into the privileged zone between the cell membrane and the biomaterial surface such that immediate buffering or inhibition of these mediators is delayed or reduced [10]. In this process the phagocytic activity of macrophages decreases, while their degradative capacity increases [11].

FBGCs have the potential to be responsive to cellular signals via cell surface receptor expression as well as actively participate in the inflammatory response through the production of cytokines [10]. They produce anti-inflammatory cytokines, e.g. IL-10, which may be counter-regulated by the proteolytic and pro-oxidant microenvironment. Additionally, FBGCs are thought to release pro-fibrotic factors, e.g. TGF-β and PDGF, which trigger the action of fibroblasts and endothelial cells. Continuous action of FBGCs is assumed to result in prolonged fibroblast activation and excessive biomaterial-associated matrix deposition, leading to impaired wound healing and excessive fibrosis [11]. Therefore, FBGC formation has appeared to be an undesirable phenomenon with a negative impact on biocompatibility, producing cytokines that bias wound healing cells toward a fibrogenic phenotype [31]. Efforts in the design of the biomaterial for *in situ* tissue engineering of heart valves should enhance the biocompatibility, limiting macrophage fusion into FBGCs. Surface chemistry-dependent modulation of the protein layer may enable different receptor binding and signaling in the immune cells leading to altered cellular responses, promoting wound healing while sustaining implant function [11].

5. Modulating the immune response

The implantation of any biomaterial initiates an immune response. However, the extent and severity of this response can be modulated by adapting scaffold properties. As described in the previous sections, the immune response is a multi-phased cascade involving many different components. The combined effect of these components will determine the end-stage outcome of the immune response, ranging from pathological fibrotic repair to fully functional regeneration of the original tissue. By interfering with specific elements within this inflammatory cascade, the downstream outcome can be drastically affected, for better or for worse. In this plane of intersection, immuno-modulating scaffolds for *in situ* tissue engineered heart valves are being developed. The development of such a 'smart' scaffold bridges multiple length-scales and is dependent on a multitude of scaffold features. Biological scaffolds inherently come with a natural architecture and a cocktail of signaling components, which would be difficult to replicate with a synthetic counterpart. Synthetic scaffolds, on the other hand, offer a more dedicated control of individual elements in comparison to biological scaffolds. Either scaffold type can be modified within its own framework. There is a legion of possibilities to modify scaffolds over various interdependent scales, ranging from tuning biomaterial surface chemistry, scaffold architecture and mechanical properties, to the incorporation of bioactives and targeting of specific cell types. Apart from the scaffold itself, the implantation procedure contributes to the immune response. The method of implantation affects the degree of inflammation [27], and as such should be taken into account in scaffold design.

5.1. Biomaterial surface engineering

Biocompatibility and thrombogeneity are particularly important during the onset of the immune response. Immediately after implantation, blood proteins precipitate onto the biomaterial surface, creating an inflammatory milieu that determines the activation of the complement and coagulation cascades. Biomaterial surface chemistry influences the proteins that adsorb, which mediates subsequent interactions with immune cells and may lead to their activation [8]. Factors that affect the amount, composition, and conformation of proteins within the initial layer include the hydrophobicity/hydrophilicity of a surface, as well as its charge and the distribution of charged groups [32]. Incorporation of anti-fouling properties into the biomaterial surface has proven an efficient method to block non-specific protein binding and promote specific biomolecule-binding. This is typically achieved by modifications with hydrophilic polymers, such as poly(ethylene glycol) (PEG), that act as molecular spacers and create a hydrophilic microenvironment that can resist non-specific protein adsorption and cell binding [53].

Biomaterial surface topography and micron-scale architecture can modulate the cell-scaffold interactions that influence immune cell activation, alignment, infiltration, and fusion. Variations in surface roughness and topography affect cell adhesion, morphology, and cytokine secretion. The cell-surface interaction can change quantity and identity of secreted pro-inflammatory cytokines and chemokines, the gene expression pattern, and downstream remodeling events [11,47]. For example, one of the key cellular immune response mechanisms which can be targeted for control of biocompatibility is the mechanism for macrophage adhesion [31,54]. Macrophage fusion on biomaterial surfaces is material dependent, indicating that the surface must have an appropriate array of adsorbed proteins in order for adherent cells to adopt the necessary phenotype to fuse into FBGCs [10]. Furthermore, surface roughness of electrospun fibers has been shown to affect blood activation [55], illustrating the importance of appropriate surface engineering, in particular in the early phases of inflammation.

5.2. Scaffold architecture

Cell infiltration into the scaffold is one of the prerequisites for succesful tissue regeneration. It was shown that early infiltration of immune cells determines the degree of downstream ECM production and remodeling [56]. Cell infiltration is primarily determined by the scaffold architecture, or microstructure. Decellularized homograft/xenograft valves have shown limited cell infiltration, resulting in poor tissue remodeling and even degeneration. In contrast, decellularized *in vitro* tissue-engineered valves have shown fast repopulation with host cells and tissue remodeling following a distinct demarcation line. It has been suggested that this critical difference in cell infiltration is due to a lack of the dense, native-like microstructural arrangement in tissue-engineered valves, as opposed to native valves [57].

For synthetic scaffolds, the importance of scaffold architecture is even more evident. In contrast to natural ECM, cells are typically unable to rapidly break down synthetic biomaterials in order to migrate. Therefore, cell infiltration into a synthetic scaffold is generally dependent on the available pore size, or void space [58,59]. Apart from overall cell infiltration, the pore size can also affect cell phenotype. For example, pore size has shown to be an important factor in the degree of macrophage fusion and material encapsulation. Porous implants with uniform spherical pores of 30-40 μm were shown to elicit healing with minimal fibrosis, high vascularity, and a higher M2/M1 macrophage ratio [52]. It has to be noted however, that the optimal pore size is not generic and has to be tailored to the application.

Synthetic scaffolds for heart valve tissue engineering typically consist of nano- or microfibers, with a high surface area-to-volume ratio. This fibrous architecture dictates the behavior of infiltrating cells. In addition to the void space, the fiber diameter and inter-fiber distance determine cell adhesion, spreading and proliferation [60,61]. Fiber diameter has also shown to affect platelet adhesion and coagulation activation [55]. Fiber alignment guides cell orientation and migration via contact guidance. Furthermore, it was shown that fiber alignment enhanced cell infiltration into a nanofibrous PLLA scaffold [62]. Novel processing techniques to produce fibrous 3D scaffolds with adjustable void space and/or aligned fibers (e.g. low-temperature electrospinning [63]), enhance the degrees of freedom in scaffold modification via 3D architecture (figure 4). For complex structures, such as the aortic valve, multi-layered scaffolds might be required to achieve suitable local cues [59,64].

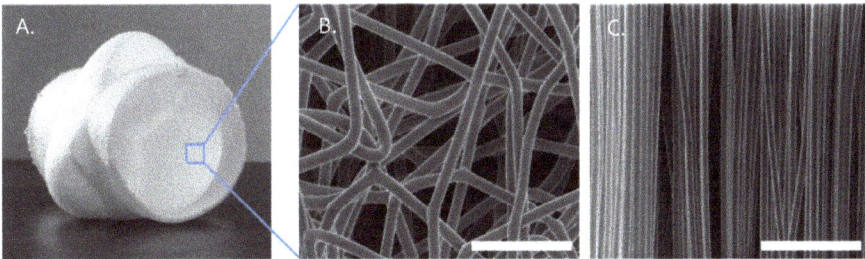

Figure 4. (A) Photograph of an electrospun poly(ε-caprolactone) heart valve demonstrating 3D valve architecture, and scanning electron micrographs of its microstructure showing either random (B) or aligned microfibers (C) (scalebar = 100 μm; images courtesy of M. Simonet and G. Argento).

5.3. Mechanical properties and degradation rate

Heart valve scaffolds require appropriate mechanical properties to endure the cyclic stresses and strains exerted by the hemodynamic environment. However, next to proper functioning in the hemodynamic environment, scaffold mechanical properties play an important role on the cellular level. The macromechanical properties are determined by the intrinsic material properties, the scaffold architecture and the degradation rate. The intrinsic material properties (e.g. stiffness) and the scaffold architecture (e.g. anisotropy) determine the local stresses and strains experienced by the cell. It is well recognized that mechanical conditioning is an important stimulus for ECM production and remodeling. It has been hypothesized that polymeric scaffolds can divert loads from the cells, so-called 'cell shielding', resulting in hampered ECM production. Furthermore, the scaffold or matrix stiffness can modulate the differentiation of cells into pathological phenotypes, e.g. osteoblastic or myofibroblastic, in response to mechanical and biochemical cues [5]. Therefore, efficient transduction of loads from the biomaterial to the cells is crucial. Elastomers typically exhibit adequate mechano-transduction properties, making them a favorable class of materials for application as synthetic scaffolds [25].

Mechanical integrity of the scaffold is dependent on the degradation rate of the material, or rather on the balance between material degradation and ECM production. Accelerated material degradation can result in mechanical instability and valve failure. On the other hand, long-term presence of the biomaterial results in prolonged macrophage activity. Macrophages typically persist at the implantation site until the biomaterial is completely resorbed. When uncontrolled, this may lead to excessive chronic inflammation resulting in fibrosis, calcification, and/or degeneration. Mineralization of synthetic or biologic scaffolds is end-stage pathology, generally irreversible and untreatable. This underlines the importance of timely degradation of the biomaterial. Apart from proper material selection, degradation rate of polymers is tunable by varying copolymer ratios [3]. Variations in degradation kinetics of materials are also employed for controlled delivery of bioactives, for example by introducing fast-degrading fibrin gel [65] or synthetic or biological microspheres [23,66] into the scaffold.

5.4. Incorporation of bioactives

Throughout the course of the immune response, signaling factors orchestrate the actions of the immune cells. By incorporating bioactive factors into the biomaterial scaffold, the cellular niche can be modulated locally. These biochemical factors can direct local cellular function, or promote recruitment of specific cell types via chemotaxis. Additionally, the crosstalk between immune cells and tissue cells can be enhanced, regulating the healing process [11]. Since these signaling factors play a role in a specific phase of the immune response, spatio-temporal control of growth factor or cytokine release has been the aim for many tissue engineering scaffolds. For example, long-term release of stromal cell-derived factor 1α (SDF-1α) from porous PLGA scaffolds has demonstrated to result in reduced numbers and degranulation of mast cells at the scaffold in a subcutaneous mouse model. This led to downstream alterations in the inflammatory cascade, jumpstarting regeneration with enhanced participation of progenitor cells, increased angiogenesis and decreased fibrosis [67]. De Visscher et al. developed heart valves constructed from photo-oxidized bovine pericardium, which were impregnated with SDF-1α in combination with fibronectin to improve the SDF-1α presentation to the cells. Implanted in the pulmonary position in sheep, these valves demonstrated improved homing of primitive cells and normal functioning at 5 months follow-up [68]. Other pro-angiogenic factors, such as VEGF, have shown to play a similar role in vascularization and endothelialization via recruitment of bone marrow-derived circulating cells, with an essential paracrine role for myeloid cells [69]. Injectable hydrogels featuring a sustained release of VEGF, either or not combined with PDGF, have shown to enhance angiogenesis [70,71]. Dual delivery of MCP-1 and VEGF was applied to promote early monocyte invasion as well as angiogenesis. This was shown to increase mature vessel formation via enhanced endothelial and smooth muscle cell recruitment and displayed a trend of macrophage polarization to the M2 type in a time- and dose-dependent manner [66]. MCP-1 has demonstrated to be a potent immune-modulatory factor, leading to successful remodeling and regeneration of a PCL/PLLA blood vessel graft in mice [23]. Decellularized porcine aortic valves coated with a fusion protein of fibronectin and hepatocyte growth factor (HGF) demonstrated modest acceleration of infiltration of tissue cells, particularly in the valve leaflet, after implantation in a dog model [72].

Single extracellular molecules can impact both pro-inflammatory and anti-inflammatory pathways in different cell types participating in the repair response [35]. The shift from pro-inflammatory to anti-inflammatory response is generally mediated by lipoxins, protectins, and resolvins, actively promoting resolution of infection and tissue repair. Lipoxins are arachidonic acid (AA) derivatives generated by lipoxygenases, and stop the influx of neutrophils, promote the uptake of apoptotic neutrophils by macrophages and recruit additional monocytes to help clear away dead cells and tissue debris [28,39]. Incorporation of such bioactive components may enhance the resolution of the inflammatory response, avoiding uncontrolled chronic inflammation. Resolution of inflammation is also mediated by glucocorticoids, which inhibit inflammatory cell activation by withdrawing the synthesis of inflammatory mediators, and promote resolution of inflammation by enhancing anti-inflammatory cytokine release [29,54]. Glucocorticoids have been shown to modulate the phenotype of infiltrating macrophages and lymphocytes and could thus be used locally to regulate the cellular response [54].

An alternative to incorporating specific signaling moieties into a scaffold is to preseed the scaffold with cells that act as natural signaling factories. Cells, typically bone marrow-derived mononuclear cells, harvested from the host are directly seeded into a scaffold, which is subsequently implanted in a single operation. Although the preseeded cells are cleared from the scaffold within several days after implantation, they mediate the immune response via paracrine signaling by secreting a natural cocktail of growth factors and cytokines. This approach has shown prosperous results in clinical trials using synthetic blood vessel grafts [24]. Furthermore, a similar approach using decellularized tissue-engineered heart valves has shown promising short-term results after 4 week implantation in the pulmonary position in non-human primates [73].

Apart from boosting selected signaling molecules, biomaterials can be designed to tether endogenously released factors to promote a regenerative microenvironment. Natural occurring GAGs have been identified to bind and modify inflammatory factors like interleukins and chemokines, e.g. IL-10 [11]. Subtle differences in GAG structure and/or sequence might be sensed by signaling molecules, guiding their interaction with the ECM and mediating their presentation to leukocytes [11]. In this way, physiological cytokine concentrations are ensured, reducing the risk of adverse side-effects. Heparan sulfate is well-recognized as a natural binding site for many growth factors and cytokines, a feature which has been exploited by developing heparin-mimetic peptide nanofibers that are capable of binding growth factors such as VEGF and HGF [74].

Clearly, the use of bioactives or on-the-fly harvestable cells is a powerful tool to create immune-modulating scaffolds. Methods using covalent immobilization of factors [65], microspheres with controlled degradation profiles [66] or hollow-fiber electrospinning techniques [59] enable optimized spatio-temporal control of one or multiple factors. Furthermore, advanced hydrogels have been developed to offer on-demand, remote-controlled release using a magnetic field [75]. With state-of-the-art supramolecular polymers it is possible to engineer cell-responsive substrates [76], offering truly 'smart' scaffolds that can interact with their environment to mediate the host response to the biomaterial.

5.5. Cell recruitment and differentiation

The inflammatory response is mainly driven by colonization of the scaffold by blood-derived cells. The nature of the infiltrating cells and their differentiation were demonstrated of pivotal importance to control the delicate balance between fibrotic or functional regenerated ECM production. Of all the cells involved in the immune response, several cell populations can be identified as target cells for *in situ* heart valve tissue engineering.

Macrophages are the predominant mediators throughout the entire immune response, making them an attractive therapeutic target [77]. Although, the precise nature of macrophage plasticity and polarization has yet to be illuminated, it has been shown that early macrophage phenotype determines the end-stage outcome in various biological matrices. In particular, an increased ratio of M2/M1 macrophages correlates to enhanced remodeling, which is likely mediated by differential attraction of secondary cells [78]. By promoting the M2 phenotype, either via specific recruitment or local polarization, the inflammatory response may instantly be directed towards healing instead of inflammation [48,52]. With the identification of multiple subtypes, it is likely that the various macrophage phenotypes play a critical role throughout the various stages of acute inflammation, the healing phase and the resolution of inflammation (figure 5).

ECM production and remodeling is governed by the attraction of secondary cells to the scaffold, consisting of mature (myo-)fibroblasts and endothelial cells, as well as various stem/progenitor cells, released into the circulation by the bone marrow. Furthermore, it has been suggested that adult valve interstitial cells are continuously replenished via circulating endothelial or mesenchymal cell precursors derived from the bone marrow and subsequently undergo endothelial-to-mesenchymal-transition (EndoMT) [5]. Circulating progenitors, such as endothelial progenitor cells (EPC), can have a significant influence on the inflammatory response [4,12,79]. EPC are hypothesized to be an important target cell for endothelialization. Rapid formation of an endothelium over a scaffold is desirable as it acts as a dynamic and selective barrier by maintaining a nonthrombogenic surface, controlling the transfer of molecules across the layer, and regulating immune and inflammatory reactions. The endothelial layer also interacts with underlying cells to regulate their growth and proliferation [12].

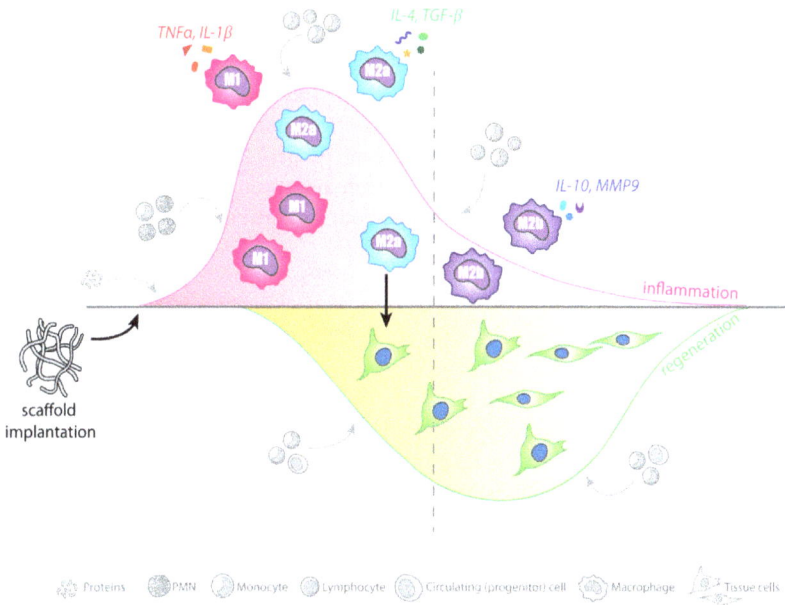

Figure 5. Hypothesized role of the various macrophage polarization states throughout the process of inflammation and tissue regeneration in response to scaffold implantation. Illustration by Anthal Smits.

Mesenchymal stem cells (MSCs) proliferate during the healing phase, directed by cytokines secreted by nearby cells, e.g. activated platelets and macrophages, and by ECM components such as collagen peptides and fibronectin [29]. MSCs produce an immunoprivileged environment by preventing the activation and proliferation of DCs, T cells, macrophages, and PMNs through direct cell-cell interactions and paracrine signaling [8]. Cells derived from immunoprivileged regions have been delivered to promote cell engraftment and protect grafts against autoimmune and allogeneic rejection. These cells secrete a range of factors, eg. TGF-β and IL-10, inducing regulatory T-cell differentiation/expansion, which enhances immuno-protection [8].

Recruitment and adhesion of target cell types can be achieved by offering binding domains on the scaffold, for example using supramolecular building blocks with cell-specific peptide sequences [76,79]. When combined with anti-fouling materials, such as PEG, this results in highly selective substrates.

5.6. Minimally invasive implantation methods

Independent of the biomaterial, the injury incurred during the implantation process will trigger an immune response, due to the disruption of host tissue and induction of cell damage. Besides substantial mortality and morbidity risks, invasive open heart surgery for heart valve replacement causes extensive tissue damage, giving rise to DAMPs, which prime the system for an enhanced immune response [29]. As an alternative, various transvascular, catheter-based techniques, as well as alternative minimally invasive surgical techniques, such as the transapical approach, have been developed [4,80,81]. This has implication for the scaffold design as the scaffold must be crimped and incorporated into a stent. Upon delivery at the valve annulus, the scaffold must also be able to expand properly, be held in place and instantly function within the hemodynamic environment. Transapical valve implantation of preseeded decellularized tissue engineered heart valves into both the aortic and pulmonary position has already proven feasible in pre-clinical models [82,83].

6. Challenges and pitfalls

In situ tissue engineering of heart valves represents a quick, cheap, and on-demand approach. Immunomodulatory scaffolds hold great promise for future application and commercialization. However, some priority challenges remain to be addressed in the translation from bench to bed.

6.1. ECM formation versus fibrosis

One of the main challenges for *in situ* tissue engineering is to stimulate functional ECM formation without inducing fibrosis. To maintain functionality of the valve, rapid ECM formation is required in order to overtake the load-bearing role of the degrading scaffold. However, cells and molecules that are stimulatory for ECM production have been designated as pro-fibrotic mediators. This poses a paradoxal challenge. Macrophage plasticity is a striking example. M2 macrophages have been identified as pro-wound healing cells, promoting ECM production by secretion of IL-4 and TGF-β. On the other hand, both IL-4 and TGF-β are strong inducers of fibrosis if not tightly regulated. Chemokines, such as MCP-1, have been identified as pro-fibrotic mediators by attracting fibrocytes and stimulation of M2 polarization [84,85]. On the other hand, MCP-1 inhibition leads to delayed or inhibited wound healing [86]. Fibrocytes are blood-borne mesenchymal stem cell progenitors with a fibroblast/myofibroblast-like phenotype (CD34$^+$/CD45$^+$/collagen type I$^+$) that similarly have been related to both ECM formation and fibrosis. The same holds for EndoMT-derived (myo-)fibroblasts. However, the local activation state of recruited myofibroblasts, rather than the source, determines their ECM remodeling activity. For example, TLR-signaling promotes fibroblasts to differentiate into collagen-producing myofibroblasts [84]. Valvular interstitial cells (VICs) in the adult valve have a quiescent myofibroblast-like phenotype. Regulating the activation state of colonizing myofibroblasts in the scaffold is pivotal in the prevention of fibrosis and obtaining a VIC-like population. The TGF-β pathway is one of the main players in this process. Furthermore, IL-10 has been shown to inhibit fibrosis in numerous animal models [84], underlining that timely resolution of inflammation is one of the main challenges for *in situ* tissue engineering.

6.2. Hemodynamic environment

In cardiovascular *in situ* tissue regeneration, the hemodynamic environment plays a key role by directing cell recruitment and cell differentiation. The mechanical load applied to the heart valves is a powerful regulator of cell phenotype, influencing many cell functions such as orientation, replication, growth factor production, and collagen synthesis [33]. In cardiovascular devices, apoptosis is often induced by shear stress arising from the blood flow [10]. Shear stress also has a significant effect on adhesion of circulating cells to the valve scaffold. Direct intimal binding of cells to the ventricular side of the leaflet is unlikely due to high shear forces during systole. In contrast, end-systolic and diastolic turbulations on the aortic side of the leaflet typically result in low shear stresses that allow for cell adhesion to the scaffold [4].

So far, the exact mechanism behind cell population of heart valve replacements with host cells remains elusive. For blood vessels, animal studies have identified trans-anastomotic ingrowth as the main source of host tissue cells in the scaffold [87]. However, this is most likely an animal model-dependent phenomenon, as it is known that trans-anastomotic ingrowth is very limited in humans [88]. Therefore, the use of humanized animal models or *in vitro* model systems [89] is indispensible in evaluating scaffold performance for future clinical applications.

6.3. Comorbidity and impaired wound healing

Little is known about the effect of the pathological status of a tissue, organ, or patient on the fate of a tissue engineered heart valve. It is reasonable to believe that the pre-existing pathology or existing risk factors would influence wound healing and long-term outcomes of valve implantation. One of the most complicated aspects of designing a replacement scaffold for diseased tissue would be the incorporation of measures which prevent the device from succumbing to the same fate as the diseased tissue it is replacing [12].

Impaired wound healing conditions include advanced age, diabetes mellitus (insulin resistance), vascular diseases (e.g. atherosclerosis), and obesity, in which adipose tissue functions as initiator of the chronic inflammatory response. Diabetic patients have significantly impaired wound healing as they are relatively immunocompromised and have higher blood glucose levels affecting leukocyte function [90]. Diabetes and advanced age are associated with delayed or impaired wound healing through a reduced ability to transition from an M1 to an M2 macrophage phenotype [52]. Malnutrition adversely affects wound healing by prolonging inflammation, inhibiting fibroblast function, and reducing angiogenesis and collagen deposition. For example, carbohydrates are needed for collagen synthesis, and ω-3-fatty acids are needed for modulation of the arachidonic acid pathway, resolving inflammation [90].

The patient's regenerative potential is dependent on age. The concentration of progenitor cells in human blood decreases with age [4]. Furthermore, aging typically leads to impaired angiogenesis and local immunity is altered due to lack of growth factors, increased neutrophil invasion and higher number of mature macrophages. Levels of TGF-β in wounds of elderly are, like fetal, markedly reduced, which is possibly related to reduced scarring with age [35]. Next to regeneration potential, the rate at which the scaffold degrades may also be age-specific due to variations in cell availability.

Any chronic disease which affects the cardio-respiratory system may adversely affect the supply of oxygen and other nutrients required for wound healing. Although hypoxia is one of the chemoattractants for neutrophils and macrophages, oxygen is needed for their optimal function and to allow phagocytosis. Oxygen is also essential for collagen deposition as it acts as a substrate in the hydroxylation of proline and lysine residues. Smoking affects oxygen partial pressures and causes more wound healing complications and it is likely that smoking may also affect immune function and collagen deposition [90].

The use of diseased cells or tissues in humanized animal models or *in vitro* model systems [89] may aid in gaining insight in the effects of comorbidities on valve regeneration.

6.4. Patient heterogeneity

In vivo remodeling of tissue engineered heart valves displays considerable variability among patients, owing to biological heterogeneity among individuals in physiological tissue remodeling potential [5]. This heterogeneity could be a result of mutations or polymorphisms in key proteins central to ECM synthesis and remodeling [2]. The goal is to understand and potentially control human variation in different facets of biomaterial-tissue interaction and the healing process by developing robust or even patient-tailored scaffolds.

To cope with patient-to-patient heterogeneity, an important issue in tissue engineering of aortic heart valves will be the real-time noninvasive and non-destructive assessment of mechanical properties both *in vitro* and *in vivo* to ensure tissue quality and function [5]. The challenge here is to find appropriate methodologies to evaluate the evolving structural remodeling and functionality, especially in a noninvasive manner so that the valve can be followed over time [5]. One way of approaching this issue is developing imaging modalities and discovering new biomarkers of inflammation which would help further understanding of inflammatory diseases and discerning events related to inflammation in heart valve tissue-engineered implants [12]. When applied to engineered heart valves, developed biomarkers should correlate directly with success and failure in order to generate outcome measurements, such as laboratory assays or imaging results that substitute for and reflect the mechanism of a significant clinical event or characteristic, e.g. stenosis, calcification, or infection [5]. An important consideration is whether calcification, the major pathologic process in valve degeneration, will be problematic. Evidence suggests that calcification may not be a major problem as long as the scaffold is ultimately resorbed and/or not intrinsically mineralizable, the interstitial cells are viable, and the ECM is capable of remodeling [5].

For the translation from bench to bed, there must be understanding of the mechanisms involved and development of biomarkers, assays and tools for the assessment of valve regeneration. Surrogate and true endpoints must be defined to characterize and assure the quality of the tissue constructs, and predict outcomes as early as possible [5]. Key targets for characterizing tissue-engineered constructs include tissue composition, cellular gene expression and phenotype, ECM, and other key effectors of tissue remodeling and tissue quality [5].

7. Conclusion

The complexity of the immune response poses a challenging environment for *in situ* tissue engineering of heart valves [46]. Clearly, a better understanding of the underlying pathways appears crucial for controlling the fate of implanted biomaterial scaffolds and modulating inflammatory reactions in such a way as to induce tissue regeneration and remodeling and prevent fibrosis and/or degeneration [12]. Remaining largely unknown are the specifications of the optimal components (i.e. cells, scaffold and potentially biological modulators) and process conditions (mechanical and metabolic) that will facilitate the formation of optimal substitute heart valve tissues, whose function best emulates the structure, function, and extended durability of a natural valve in vivo [5]. However, the prosperous results of synthetic and biological scaffolds so far demonstrate the ground-breaking potential of *in situ* tissue engineering for heart valves.

Acknowledgements

This work was supported by a grant from the Dutch government to the Netherlands Institute for Regenerative Medicine (NIRM, grant No. FES0908). This research forms part of the Project P1.01 iValve of the research program of the BioMedical Materials institute, co-funded by the Dutch Ministry of Economic Affairs, Agriculture and Innovation. The financial contribution of the Nederlandse Hartstichting is gratefully acknowledged.

Author details

S. L. M. van Loon, A. I. P. M. Smits, A. Driessen-Mol, F. P. T. Baaijens and C. V. C. Bouten*

*Address all correspondence to: C.V.C.Bouten@tue.nl

Department of Biomedical Engineering, Eindhoven University of Technology, MB, Eindhoven, The Netherlands

References

[1] El-Hamamsy I, Eryigit Z, Stevens LM, Sarang Z, George R, Clark L, et al. Long-term outcomes after autograft versus homograft aortic root replacement in adults with aortic valve disease: a randomised controlled trial. Lancet 2010 Aug 14;376(9740):524-31.

[2] Mendelson K, Schoen FJ. Heart valve tissue engineering: concepts, approaches, progress, and challenges. Ann Biomed Eng 2006 Dec;34(12):1799-819.

[3] Bouten CV, Dankers PY, Driessen-Mol A, Pedron S, Brizard AM, Baaijens FP. Substrates for cardiovascular tissue engineering. Adv Drug Deliv Rev 2011 Apr 30;63(4-5):221-41.

[4] Mol A, Smits AI, Bouten CV, Baaijens FP. Tissue engineering of heart valves: advances and current challenges. Expert Rev Med Devices 2009 May;6(3):259-75.

[5] Schoen FJ. Heart valve tissue engineering: quo vadis? Curr Opin Biotechnol 2011 Oct; 22(5):698-705.

[6] Sacks MS, Schoen FJ, Mayer JE. Bioengineering challenges for heart valve tissue engineering. Annu Rev Biomed Eng 2009;11:289-313.

[7] Breuer CK, Mettler BA, Anthony T, Sales VL, Schoen FJ, Mayer JE. Application of tissue-engineering principles toward the development of a semilunar heart valve substitute. Tissue Eng 2004 Nov;10(11-12):1725-36.

[8] Boehler RM, Graham JG, Shea LD. Tissue engineering tools for modulation of the immune response. Biotechniques 2011 Oct;51(4):239-40, 242, 244.

[9] Mol A, Driessen NJ, Rutten MC, Hoerstrup SP, Bouten CV, Baaijens FP. Tissue engineering of human heart valve leaflets: a novel bioreactor for a strain-based conditioning approach. Ann Biomed Eng 2005 Dec;33(12):1778-88.

[10] Anderson JM, Rodriguez A, Chang DT. Foreign body reaction to biomaterials. Semin Immunol 2008 Apr;20(2):86-100.

[11] Franz S, Rammelt S, Scharnweber D, Simon JC. Immune responses to implants - a review of the implications for the design of immunomodulatory biomaterials. Biomaterials 2011 Oct;32(28):6692-709.

[12] Simionescu A, Schulte JB, Fercana G, Simionescu DT. Inflammation in cardiovascular tissue engineering: the challenge to a promise: a minireview. Int J Inflam 2011;2011:958247.

[13] Badylak SF. The extracellular matrix as a biologic scaffold material. Biomaterials 2007 Sep;28(25):3587-93.

[14] Weber B, Emmert MY, Schoenauer R, Brokopp C, Baumgartner L, Hoerstrup SP. Tissue engineering on matrix: future of autologous tissue replacement. Semin Immunopathol 2011 May;33(3):307-15.

[15] Keane TJ, Londono R, Turner NJ, Badylak SF. Consequences of ineffective decellularization of biologic scaffolds on the host response. Biomaterials 2012 Feb;33(6):1771-81.

[16] Klopsch C, Steinhoff G. Tissue-engineered devices in cardiovascular surgery. Eur Surg Res 2012;49(1):44-52.

[17] Schoen FJ, Levy RJ. Calcification of tissue heart valve substitutes: progress toward understanding and prevention. Ann Thorac Surg 2005 Mar;79(3):1072-80.

[18] Dijkman PE, Driessen-Mol A, Frese L, Hoerstrup SP, Baaijens FP. Decellularized homologous tissue-engineered heart valves as off-the-shelf alternatives to xeno- and homografts. Biomaterials 2012 Jun;33(18):4545-54.

[19] White JK, Agnihotri AK, Titus JS, Torchiana DF. A stentless trileaflet valve from a sheet of decellularized porcine small intestinal submucosa. Ann Thorac Surg 2005 Aug;80(2): 704-7.

[20] Hoerstrup SP, Sodian R, Daebritz S, Wang J, Bacha EA, Martin DP, et al. Functional living trileaflet heart valves grown in vitro. Circulation 2000 Nov 7;102(19 Suppl 3):III44-III49.

[21] Schmidt D, Dijkman PE, Driessen-Mol A, Stenger R, Mariani C, Puolakka A, et al. Minimally-invasive implantation of living tissue engineered heart valves: a comprehensive approach from autologous vascular cells to stem cells. J Am Coll Cardiol 2010 Aug 3;56(6):510-20.

[22] Pektok E, Nottelet B, Tille JC, Gurny R, Kalangos A, Moeller M, et al. Degradation and healing characteristics of small-diameter poly(epsilon-caprolactone) vascular grafts in the rat systemic arterial circulation. Circulation 2008 Dec 9;118(24):2563-70.

[23] Roh JD, Sawh-Martinez R, Brennan MP, Jay SM, Devine L, Rao DA, et al. Tissue-engineered vascular grafts transform into mature blood vessels via an inflammation-mediated process of vascular remodeling. Proc Natl Acad Sci U S A 2010 Mar 9;107(10): 4669-74.

[24] Hibino N, McGillicuddy E, Matsumura G, Ichihara Y, Naito Y, Breuer C, et al. Late-term results of tissue-engineered vascular grafts in humans. J Thorac Cardiovasc Surg 2010 Feb;139(2):431-6, 436.

[25] Wu W, Allen RA, Wang Y. Fast-degrading elastomer enables rapid remodeling of a cell-free synthetic graft into a neoartery. Nat Med 2012 Jul;18(7):1148-53.

[26] Yokota T, Ichikawa H, Matsumiya G, Kuratani T, Sakaguchi T, Iwai S, et al. In situ tissue regeneration using a novel tissue-engineered, small-caliber vascular graft without cell seeding. J Thorac Cardiovasc Surg 2008 Oct;136(4):900-7.

[27] Gonzales-Simon A, Eniola-Adefeso O. Host Response to Biomaterials. In: Bhatia S, editor. Engineering Biomaterials for Regenerative Medicine. 1 ed. Cambridge: Springer New York; 2012. p. 143-59.

[28] Barton GM. A calculated response: control of inflammation by the innate immune system. J Clin Invest 2008 Feb;118(2):413-20.

[29] Norton LW, Babensee JE. Innate and Adaptive Immune Responses in Tissue Engineering. In: Meyer U, Handschel J, Wiesmann HP, Meyer T, editors. Fundamentals of Tissue Engineering and Regenerative Medicine. Springer Berlin Heidelberg; 2009. p. 721-47.

[30] Parham P. The Immune System. 2 ed. Garland Science; 2005.

[31] Anderson JM, McNally AK. Biocompatibility of implants: lymphocyte/macrophage interactions. Semin Immunopathol 2011 May;33(3):221-33.

[32] Ekdahl KN, Lambris JD, Elwing H, Ricklin D, Nilsson PH, Teramura Y, et al. Innate immunity activation on biomaterial surfaces: a mechanistic model and coping strategies. Adv Drug Deliv Rev 2011 Sep 16;63(12):1042-50.

[33] Mutsaers SE, Bishop JE, McGrouther G, Laurent GJ. Mechanisms of tissue repair: from wound healing to fibrosis. Int J Biochem Cell Biol 1997 Jan;29(1):5-17.

[34] Nilsson B, Ekdahl KN, Mollnes TE, Lambris JD. The role of complement in biomaterial-induced inflammation. Mol Immunol 2007 Jan;44(1-3):82-94.

[35] Eming SA, Hammerschmidt M, Krieg T, Roers A. Interrelation of immunity and tissue repair or regeneration. Semin Cell Dev Biol 2009 Jul;20(5):517-27.

[36] von Hundelshausen P, Weber C. Platelets as immune cells: bridging inflammation and cardiovascular disease. Circ Res 2007 Jan 5;100(1):27-40.

[37] Tsirogianni AK, Moutsopoulos NM, Moutsopoulos HM. Wound healing: immunological aspects. Injury 2006 Apr;37 Suppl 1:S5-12.

[38] Grimstad O, Sandanger O, Ryan L, Otterdal K, Damaas JK, Pukstad B, et al. Cellular sources and inducers of cytokines present in acute wound fluid. Wound Repair Regen 2011 May;19(3):337-47.

[39] Soehnlein O, Lindbom L. Phagocyte partnership during the onset and resolution of inflammation. Nat Rev Immunol 2010 Jun;10(6):427-39.

[40] Harris HE, Raucci A. Alarmin(g) news about danger: workshop on innate danger signals and HMGB1. EMBO Rep 2006 Aug;7(8):774-8.

[41] Ziegler-Heitbrock L, Ancuta P, Crowe S, Dalod M, Grau V, Hart DN, et al. Nomenclature of monocytes and dendritic cells in blood. Blood 2010 Oct 21;116(16):e74-e80.

[42] Shi C, Pamer EG. Monocyte recruitment during infection and inflammation. Nat Rev Immunol 2011 Nov;11(11):762-74.

[43] Shantsila E, Wrigley B, Tapp L, Apostolakis S, Montoro-Garcia S, Drayson MT, et al. Immunophenotypic characterization of human monocyte subsets: possible implications for cardiovascular disease pathophysiology. J Thromb Haemost 2011 May;9(5): 1056-66.

[44] Mosser DM, Edwards JP. Exploring the full spectrum of macrophage activation. Nat Rev Immunol 2008 Dec;8(12):958-69.

[45] Kou PM, Babensee JE. Macrophage and dendritic cell phenotypic diversity in the context of biomaterials. J Biomed Mater Res A 2011 Jan;96(1):239-60.

[46] Beghdadi W, Madjene LC, Benhamou M, Charles N, Gautier G, Launay P, et al. Mast cells as cellular sensors in inflammation and immunity. Front Immunol 2011;2:37.

[47] Badylak SF, Valentin JE, Ravindra AK, McCabe GP, Stewart-Akers AM. Macrophage phenotype as a determinant of biologic scaffold remodeling. Tissue Eng Part A 2008 Nov;14(11):1835-42.

[48] Biswas SK, Chittezhath M, Shalova IN, Lim JY. Macrophage polarization and plasticity in health and disease. Immunol Res 2012 Sep;53(1-3):11-24.

[49] Murray PJ, Wynn TA. Protective and pathogenic functions of macrophage subsets. Nat Rev Immunol 2011 Nov;11(11):723-37.

[50] Gordon S, Martinez FO. Alternative activation of macrophages: mechanism and functions. Immunity 2010 May 28;32(5):593-604.

[51] Lawrence T, Natoli G. Transcriptional regulation of macrophage polarization: enabling diversity with identity. Nat Rev Immunol 2011 Nov;11(11):750-61.

[52] Brown BN, Ratner BD, Goodman SB, Amar S, Badylak SF. Macrophage polarization: an opportunity for improved outcomes in biomaterials and regenerative medicine. Biomaterials 2012 May;33(15):3792-802.

[53] Yu Q, Zhang Y, Wang H, Brash J, Chen H. Anti-fouling bioactive surfaces. Acta Biomater 2011 Apr;7(4):1550-7.

[54] Rolfe B, Mooney J, Zhang B, Jahnke S, Le S, Chau Y, et al. The Fibrotic Response to Implanted Biomaterials: Implications for Tissue Engineering. In: Eberli D, editor. Regenerative Medicine and Tissue Engineering - Cells and Biomaterials. InTech; 2011. p. 551-68.

[55] Milleret V, Hefti T, Hall H, Vogel V, Eberli D. Influence of the fiber diameter and surface roughness of electrospun vascular grafts on blood activation. Acta Biomater 2012 Jul 27.

[56] Hibino N, Yi T, Duncan DR, Rathore A, Dean E, Naito Y, et al. A critical role for macrophages in neovessel formation and the development of stenosis in tissue-engineered vascular grafts. FASEB J 2011 Dec;25(12):4253-63.

[57] Dijkman PE. Tissue-engineered heart valves for minimally invasive surgery. PhD thesis. Eindhoven University of Technology, The Netherlands; 2012.

[58] Balguid A, Mol A, van Marion MH, Bank RA, Bouten CV, Baaijens FP. Tailoring fiber diameter in electrospun poly(epsilon-caprolactone) scaffolds for optimal cellular infiltration in cardiovascular tissue engineering. Tissue Eng Part A 2009 Feb;15(2): 437-44.

[59] Szentivanyi A, Chakradeo T, Zernetsch H, Glasmacher B. Electrospun cellular microenvironments: Understanding controlled release and scaffold structure. Adv Drug Deliv Rev 2011 Apr 30;63(4-5):209-20.

[60] Li WJ, Cooper JA, Jr., Mauck RL, Tuan RS. Fabrication and characterization of six electrospun poly(alpha-hydroxy ester)-based fibrous scaffolds for tissue engineering applications. Acta Biomater 2006 Jul;2(4):377-85.

[61] Lowery JL, Datta N, Rutledge GC. Effect of fiber diameter, pore size and seeding method on growth of human dermal fibroblasts in electrospun poly(epsilon-caprolactone) fibrous mats. Biomaterials 2010 Jan;31(3):491-504.

[62] Kurpinski KT, Stephenson JT, Janairo RR, Lee H, Li S. The effect of fiber alignment and heparin coating on cell infiltration into nanofibrous PLLA scaffolds. Biomaterials 2010 May;31(13):3536-42.

[63] Simonet M, Driessen-Mol A, Baaijens FP, Bouten CV. Heart valve tissue regeneration. In: Bosworth L, Downes S, editors. Electrospinning for tissue regeneration.Cambridge: Woodhead Publishing Limited; 2011. p. 202-24.

[64] Pham QP, Sharma U, Mikos AG. Electrospun poly(epsilon-caprolactone) microfiber and multilayer nanofiber/microfiber scaffolds: characterization of scaffolds and measurement of cellular infiltration. Biomacromolecules 2006 Oct;7(10):2796-805.

[65] Chiu LL, Radisic M. Scaffolds with covalently immobilized VEGF and Angiopoietin-1 for vascularization of engineered tissues. Biomaterials 2010 Jan;31(2):226-41.

[66] Jay SM, Shepherd BR, Andrejecsk JW, Kyriakides TR, Pober JS, Saltzman WM. Dual delivery of VEGF and MCP-1 to support endothelial cell transplantation for therapeutic vascularization. Biomaterials 2010 Apr;31(11):3054-62.

[67] Thevenot PT, Nair AM, Shen J, Lotfi P, Ko CY, Tang L. The effect of incorporation of SDF-1alpha into PLGA scaffolds on stem cell recruitment and the inflammatory response. Biomaterials 2010 May;31(14):3997-4008.

[68] De Visscher G, Lebacq A, Mesure L, Blockx H, Vranken I, Plusquin R, et al. The remodeling of cardiovascular bioprostheses under influence of stem cell homing signal pathways. Biomaterials 2010 Jan;31(1):20-8.

[69] Grunewald M, Avraham I, Dor Y, Bachar-Lustig E, Itin A, Jung S, et al. VEGF-induced adult neovascularization: recruitment, retention, and role of accessory cells. Cell 2006 Jan 13;124(1):175-89.

[70] Silva EA, Mooney DJ. Spatiotemporal control of vascular endothelial growth factor delivery from injectable hydrogels enhances angiogenesis. J Thromb Haemost 2007 Mar;5(3):590-8.

[71] Sun Q, Silva EA, Wang A, Fritton JC, Mooney DJ, Schaffler MB, et al. Sustained release of multiple growth factors from injectable polymeric system as a novel therapeutic approach towards angiogenesis. Pharm Res 2010 Feb;27(2):264-71.

[72] Ota T, Sawa Y, Iwai S, Kitajima T, Ueda Y, Coppin C, et al. Fibronectin-hepatocyte growth factor enhances reendothelialization in tissue-engineered heart valve. Ann Thorac Surg 2005 Nov;80(5):1794-801.

[73] Weber B, Scherman J, Emmert MY, Gruenenfelder J, Verbeek R, Bracher M, et al. Injectable living marrow stromal cell-based autologous tissue engineered heart valves:

first experiences with a one-step intervention in primates. Eur Heart J 2011 Nov;32(22): 2830-40.

[74] Mammadov R, Mammadov B, Guler MO, Tekinay AB. Growth factor binding on heparin mimetic peptide nanofibers. Biomacromolecules 2012 Sep 10.

[75] Zhao X, Kim J, Cezar CA, Huebsch N, Lee K, Bouhadir K, et al. Active scaffolds for on-demand drug and cell delivery. Proc Natl Acad Sci U S A 2011 Jan 4;108(1):67-72.

[76] Dankers PY, Harmsen MC, Brouwer LA, van Luyn MJ, Meijer EW. A modular and supramolecular approach to bioactive scaffolds for tissue engineering. Nat Mater 2005 Jul;4(7):568-74.

[77] Koh TJ, DiPietro LA. Inflammation and wound healing: the role of the macrophage. Expert Rev Mol Med 2011;13:e23.

[78] Brown BN, Londono R, Tottey S, Zhang L, Kukla KA, Wolf MT, et al. Macrophage phenotype as a predictor of constructive remodeling following the implantation of biologically derived surgical mesh materials. Acta Biomater 2012 Mar;8(3):978-87.

[79] Fioretta ES, Fledderus JO, Burakowska-Meise EA, Baaijens FP, Verhaar MC, Bouten CV. Polymer-based scaffold designs for in situ vascular tissue engineering: controlling recruitment and differentiation behavior of endothelial colony forming cells. Macromol Biosci 2012 May;12(5):577-90.

[80] Lutter G, Ardehali R, Cremer J, Bonhoeffer P. Percutaneous valve replacement: current state and future prospects. Ann Thorac Surg 2004 Dec;78(6):2199-206.

[81] Walther T, Dewey T, Borger MA, Kempfert J, Linke A, Becht R, et al. Transapical aortic valve implantation: step by step. Ann Thorac Surg 2009 Jan;87(1):276-83.

[82] Emmert MY, Weber B, Behr L, Frauenfelder T, Brokopp CE, Grunenfelder J, et al. Transapical aortic implantation of autologous marrow stromal cell-based tissue-engineered heart valves: first experiences in the systemic circulation. JACC Cardiovasc Interv 2011 Jul;4(7):822-3.

[83] Emmert MY, Weber B, Wolint P, Behr L, Sammut S, Frauenfelder T, et al. Stem cell-based transcatheter aortic valve implantation: first experiences in a pre-clinical model. JACC Cardiovasc Interv 2012 Aug;5(8):874-83.

[84] Wynn TA. Cellular and molecular mechanisms of fibrosis. J Pathol 2008 Jan;214(2): 199-210.

[85] Sun L, Louie MC, Vannella KM, Wilke CA, LeVine AM, Moore BB, et al. New concepts of IL-10-induced lung fibrosis: fibrocyte recruitment and M2 activation in a CCL2/ CCR2 axis. Am J Physiol Lung Cell Mol Physiol 2011 Mar;300(3):L341-L353.

[86] Low QE, Drugea IA, Duffner LA, Quinn DG, Cook DN, Rollins BJ, et al. Wound healing in MIP-1alpha(-/-) and MCP-1(-/-) mice. Am J Pathol 2001 Aug;159(2):457-63.

[87] Hibino N, Villalona G, Pietris N, Duncan DR, Schoffner A, Roh JD, et al. Tissue-engineered vascular grafts form neovessels that arise from regeneration of the adjacent blood vessel. FASEB J 2011 Aug;25(8):2731-9.

[88] Zilla P, Bezuidenhout D, Human P. Prosthetic vascular grafts: wrong models, wrong questions and no healing. Biomaterials 2007 Dec;28(34):5009-27.

[89] Smits AI, Driessen-Mol A, Bouten CV, Baaijens FP. A mesofluidics-based test platform for systematic development of scaffolds for in situ cardiovascular tissue engineering. Tissue Eng Part C Methods 2012 Jun;18(6):475-85.

[90] Young A, McNaught CE. The physiology of wound healing. Surgery (Oxford) 2011 Oct; 29(10):475-9.

Permissions

The contributors of this book come from diverse backgrounds, making this book a truly international effort. This book will bring forth new frontiers with its revolutionizing research information and detailed analysis of the nascent developments around the world.

We would like to thank Elena Aikawa, MD, PhD, for lending her expertise to make the book truly unique. She has played a crucial role in the development of this book. Without her invaluable contribution this book wouldn't have been possible. She has made vital efforts to compile up to date information on the varied aspects of this subject to make this book a valuable addition to the collection of many professionals and students.

This book was conceptualized with the vision of imparting up-to-date information and advanced data in this field. To ensure the same, a matchless editorial board was set up. Every individual on the board went through rigorous rounds of assessment to prove their worth. After which they invested a large part of their time researching and compiling the most relevant data for our readers. Conferences and sessions were held from time to time between the editorial board and the contributing authors to present the data in the most comprehensible form. The editorial team has worked tirelessly to provide valuable and valid information to help people across the globe.

Every chapter published in this book has been scrutinized by our experts. Their significance has been extensively debated. The topics covered herein carry significant findings which will fuel the growth of the discipline. They may even be implemented as practical applications or may be referred to as a beginning point for another development. Chapters in this book were first published by InTech; hereby published with permission under the Creative Commons Attribution License or equivalent.

The editorial board has been involved in producing this book since its inception. They have spent rigorous hours researching and exploring the diverse topics which have resulted in the successful publishing of this book. They have passed on their knowledge of decades through this book. To expedite this challenging task, the publisher supported the team at every step. A small team of assistant editors was also appointed to further simplify the editing procedure and attain best results for the readers.

Our editorial team has been hand-picked from every corner of the world. Their multi-ethnicity adds dynamic inputs to the discussions which result in innovative outcomes. These outcomes are then further discussed with the researchers and contributors who give their valuable feedback and opinion regarding the same. The feedback is then collaborated with the researches and they are edited in a comprehensive manner to aid the understanding of the subject.

Apart from the editorial board, the designing team has also invested a significant amount of their time in understanding the subject and creating the most relevant covers. They scrutinized every image to scout for the most suitable representation of the subject and create an appropriate cover for the book.

The publishing team has been involved in this book since its early stages. They were actively engaged in every process, be it collecting the data, connecting with the contributors or procuring relevant information. The team has been an ardent support to the editorial, designing and production team. Their endless efforts to recruit the best for this project, has resulted in the accomplishment of this book. They are a veteran in the field of academics and their pool of knowledge is as vast as their experience in printing. Their expertise and guidance has proved useful at every step. Their uncompromising quality standards have made this book an exceptional effort. Their encouragement from time to time has been an inspiration for everyone.

The publisher and the editorial board hope that this book will prove to be a valuable piece of knowledge for researchers, students, practitioners and scholars across the globe.

List of Contributors

Ioan Tilea and Cristina Maria Tatar
Internal Medicine Clinic, Division of Cardiology, University of Medicine and Pharmacy Tirgu Mures, Romania

Brindusa Tilea
Infectious Disease Clinic, University of Medicine and Pharmacy Tirgu Mures, Romania

Horatiu Suciu, Mihaela Ispas and Razvan Constantin Serban
Cardiology Clinic, Emergency Clinical County Hospital Tirgu Mures, Romania

Dena Wiltz, C. Alexander Arevalos, Liezl R. Balaoing, Alicia A. Blancas, Matthew C. Sapp, Xing Zhang and K. Jane Grande-Allen
Department of Bioengineering, Rice University, Houston, TX, USA

Elaine E. Wirrig and Katherine E. Yutzey
The Heart Institute, Cincinnati Children's Hospital Medical Center, Cincinnati, Ohio, USA

Erik Fung
Section of Cardiology, Heart & Vascular Center, Dartmouth-Hitchcock Medical Center, Lebanon, New Hampshire, USA
Geisel School of Medicine at Dartmouth, Dartmouth College, Hanover, New Hampshire, USA

Masanori Aikawa
Center for Excellence in Vascular Biology, Cardiovascular Division, Brigham and Women's Hospital and Harvard Medical School, Boston, Massachusetts, USA

Claudia Goettsch
Center for Interdisciplinary Cardiovascular Sciences, Cardiovascular Medicine, Brigham and Women's Hospital, Harvard Medical School, Boston, MA, USA

Elena Aikawa
Center for Excellence in Vascular Biology, Cardiovascular Medicine, Brigham and Women's
Hospital, Harvard Medical School, Boston, MA, USA

Robert B. Hinton
The Heart Institute, Division of Cardiology, Cincinnati Children's Hospital Medical Center, USA

L. Mourino-Alvarez
Department of Vascular Physiopathology, Hospital Nacional de Paraplejicos, SESCAM,Toledo, Spain

C.M. Laborde
Laboratory of Biochemistry, Hospital Nacional de Paraplejicos, SESCAM, Toledo, Spain

M.G. Barderas
Proteomic Unit, Hospital Nacional de Paraplejicos, SESCAM, Toledo, Spain

Laura Iop and Gino Gerosa
Department of Cardiac, Thoracic and Vascular Sciences School of Medicine, University of Padua, Padua, Italy

S. L. M. van Loon, A. I. P. M. Smits, A. Driessen-Mol, F. P. T. Baaijens and C. V. C. Bouten
Department of Biomedical Engineering, Eindhoven University of Technology, MB, Eindhoven, The Netherlands

www.ingramcontent.com/pod-product-compliance
Lightning Source LLC
Chambersburg PA
CBHW070735190326
41458CB00004B/1178